Molecular Approach to Cancer Management

Molecular Approach to Cancer Management

Gajanan V. Sherbet

Newcastle University, Newcastle upon Tyne, United Kingdom

The Institute for Molecular Medicine, Huntington Beach, CA, United States

ELSEVIER

ACADEMIC PRESS

An imprint of Elsevier

Academic Press is an imprint of Elsevier
125 London Wall, London EC2Y 5AS, United Kingdom
525 B Street, Suite 1800, San Diego, CA 92101-4495, United States
50 Hampshire Street, 5th Floor, Cambridge, MA 02139, United States
The Boulevard, Langford Lane, Kidlington, Oxford OX5 1GB, United Kingdom

Notices

Knowledge and best practice in this field are constantly changing. As new research and experience broaden our understanding, changes in research methods, professional practices, or medical treatment may become necessary.

Practitioners and researchers must always rely on their own experience and knowledge in evaluating and using any information, methods, compounds, or experiments described herein. In using such information or methods they should be mindful of their own safety and the safety of others, including parties for whom they have a professional responsibility.

To the fullest extent of the law, neither the Publisher nor the authors, contributors, or editors, assume any liability for any injury and/or damage to persons or property as a matter of products liability, negligence or otherwise, or from any use or operation of any methods, products, instructions, or ideas contained in the material herein.

British Library Cataloguing-in-Publication Data
A catalogue record for this book is available from the British Library

Library of Congress Cataloging-in-Publication Data
A catalog record for this book is available from the Library of Congress

ISBN: 978-0-12-812896-1

For Information on all Academic Press publications
visit our website at https://www.elsevier.com/books-and-journals

Publisher: Mica Haley
Acquisition Editor: Rafael Teixeira
Editorial Project Manager: Tracy Tufaga
Production Project Manager: Julia Haynes
Cover Designer: Christian Bilbow

Typeset by MPS Limited, Chennai, India

Dedication

To Sai Baba

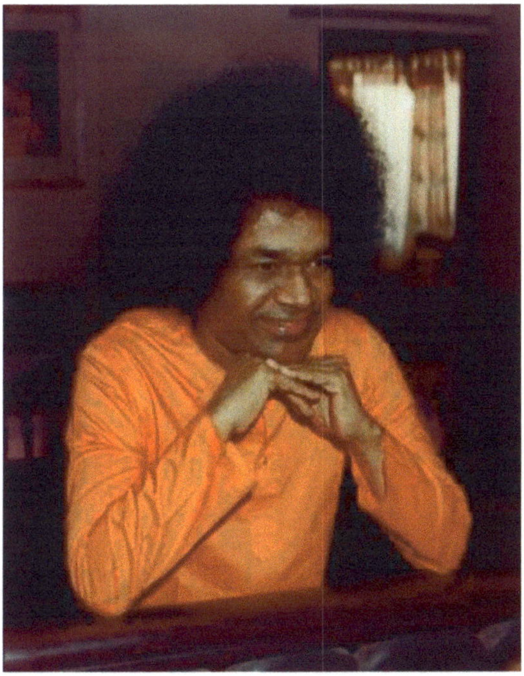

Contents

Preface

ஒல்லும்வா யெல்லாம் வினைநன்றே ஒல்லாக்கால்
செல்லும்வாய் நோக்கிச் செயல்

(Thirukkural chapter 68, verse 673)
When a natural course is clear, take prompt action.
When it is not, seek a novel path of function.

Thiru Valluvar
(Tamil Poet Second Century AD, India)

The development of novel modes of treatment of disease is fraught with problems of drug tolerance, toxicity and side effects notwithstanding stringent evaluation at the pre-clinical and clinical levels. This applies most crucially to cytotoxic therapy, but probably nearly equally in many forms of therapy. Molecular modes of approach based on genomic organisation, metabolic pathways and the operation of signalling systems have been the focus of research for some time not because they might obviate any drug-related effects altogether but because they carry the potential of providing targeted treatment. One should hasten to say that molecular approach is not a novel approach. What is novel is that several ways of identifying suitable targets have come to light in recent days. Many targets for molecular intervention have been recognised and have been or may be beneficially exploited. Diseases not infrequently are caused by abnormal activation of enzymes and their substrates. A multiplicity of factors triggers immune dysfunction and leads to the pathogenesis of autoimmune diseases. Aberrant genetic factors determine and modulate cellular processes, behaviour, and cancer invasion and metastasis. Enzymes, which can degrade and restructure the extracellular matrix, have been associated with cardiovascular and cerebral vascular diseases, arthritis, multiple sclerosis, obesity, cancer invasion and metastasis.

I have previously enlarged upon the intensive effort directed towards the identification of molecular targets amenable to elaboration and development into novel therapeutic strategies for cancer management. Many genetic determinants are identifiable that possess the ability to regulate cell cycle progression and cell proliferation, and promote tumour growth and metastasis or suppress metastatic spread. They induce cellular features and behavioural changes distinguished in the epithelial mesenchymal transition, the emergence of the cancer stem cell phenotype and the invasive faculty exhibited by cancer cells. Importantly, it is notable that these genetic determinants may offer themselves as molecular targets at the genetic level itself or in their downstream signalling and potentially accessible to be targeted for therapy (Sherbet, 2011a, 2013). Here I have attempted to provide a more focused but fathomable and comprehensible view of neoplastic conditions.

I acknowledge with thanks the help and support I have received from Professors Satnam Dlay and Barrie Mecrow. I thank Dr M.S. Lakshmi for reading the manuscript and making helpful suggestions and also for providing the translation of the verse from Thirukkural. I thank without reservation the Elsevier editorial team for their assistance and advice.

Gajanan V. Sherbet
Newcastle University of Newcastle upon Tyne, United Kingdom
The Institute for Molecular Medicine, Huntington Beach, CA, United States

Abbreviations

ABC ATP-binding cassette transporters
ADAMTS a disintegrin and metalloproteinase with thrombospondin motifs
ALK anaplastic lymphoma kinase
ALK1 activin-like receptor kinase 1 (type 1 receptor for TGF-β). These kinases referred to with epithets 1, 2, 5, etc., to distinguish them from the anaplastic lymphoma kinase ALK
AMOT angiomotin
AMPK AMP-activated protein kinase
Ang-1 angiopoietin-1
Ang-2 angiopoietin-2
ANGPL angiopoietin-like protein
AREG amphiregulin
ASK1 apoptosis signal regulating kinase 1
ATF-2 activated transcription factor
BBB blood–brain barrier
BCC basal cell carcinoma
bHLH basic helix loop helix (transcription factors)
BMP bone morphogenetic protein
BTLA B and T lymphocyte attenuator, CD272
CAM chorioallantoic membrane
CDH11 cadherin 11
c-di-GMP cyclic di-GMP
cIAP cellular inhibitor of apoptosis proteins, a member of the IAP family
CIN cervical intraepithelial neoplasm
c-met tyrosine kinase receptor of HGF
CMG2 capillary morphogenesis gene 2
CNS central nervous system
COX cyclooxygenase
CpG-ODN CpG oligodeoxynucleotide
CREB cAMP response element binding protein
CRISPR clustered regularly interspaced short palindromic repeats
CRM1 chromosome region maintenance 1; exportin1

CSC cancer stem cell
CSF cerebrospinal fluid
CSL CBF1/RBP-Jk, suppresser of hairless, Lag-1 acronym
CTGF connective tissue growth factor
CTLA4 cytotoxic T-lymphocyte antigen-4, CD152
CXCR CXC motif chemokine receptor
d-1MT 1-methyl-d-tryptophan
DAG diacylgycerol
DCIS ductal carcinoma in situ
DDR discoidin domain receptor
Dhh Desert Hedgehog
DLL Delta-like ligand of Notch
DMSO dimethyl sulphoxide
DR death receptors of TRAIL signalling
DSB double strand DNA break
EAE experimental autoimmune encephalomyelitis
ECM extracellular matrix
EF oedema factor component of LeTX
EGFR epidermal growth factor receptor
EMT epithelial mesenchymal transition
eNOS endothelial nitric oxide synthase
EPCAM epithelial cell adhesion molecule
ER oestrogen receptor
ERE oestrogen response element
ERK extracellular signal-regulated kinase (of MAPK family)
ES embryonic stem cell
FAK focal adhesion kinase
FGF fibroblast growth factor
FGFR FGF receptor
FOX forkhead-box
GCT ovarian granulosa cell tumours
GGPP geranylgeranyl pyrophosphate
GPCR G-protein coupled receptor
GPx glutathione peroxidase
HAT histone acetyl transferase
HCC hepatocellular carcinoma
HDAC histone deacetylase
HER2 human epidermal growth factor receptor-2
HGF hepatocyte growth factor
Hh Hedgehog
HHT hereditary haemorrhagic telangiectasia
HIF hypoxia-inducible factor
HMG high mobility group proteins

HMG-CoA 3-hydroxy-3-methylglutaryl-coenzyme A
HMGCR HMG-CoA reductase
HNSCC head and neck squamous cell carcinoma
HSC hematopoietic stem cells
HUVEC human umbilical vein endothelial cells
HVEM herpes virus early mediator
IAP inhibitor of apoptosis protein
ICAM intercellular adhesion molecule
ICD intracellular domain
ICOS inducible T-cell co-stimulator CD278
ID inhibitor of (differentiation) DNA binding protein
IDO indoleamine -2, 3-dioxygenase
IGF insulin-like growth factor
IGFBP IGF-binding proteins
IGFR IGF receptor
Ihh Indian Hedgehog
IKK IκB kinase
IL interleukin
iNOS inducible nitric oxide synthase
IPP isopentenyl pyrophosphate
IRF interferon regulatory factors
IRS insulin receptor substrate proteins
Lats large tumour suppressor;
LBD laminin-binding domain
LeTx anthrax lethal toxin
LF lethal factor of anthrax lethal toxin
LOH loss of heterozygosity
LPS lipopolysaccharide
MAPK mitogen-activated protein kinase
MET mesenchymal epithelial transition
MFAP5 microfibrillar-associated protein 5
miRNA microRNA
MKK1 mitogen-activated proteins kinase kinase 1 (MAP2K1/MEK1)
MMP matrix metalloproteinase
MMTV murine mammary tumour virus
MS multiple sclerosis
MSA methylseleninic acid
MSC mesenchymal stem cells
MST mammalian Sterile20-like kinase
MTA metastasis associated gene family of tumour promoters
mTOR mammalian target of rapamycin
mTORC mTOR complex
N-CAM neural cell adhesion molecule

NDR nuclear Dbf2-related family
NDRG1 N-myc downstream-regulated gene-1
NF-κB nuclear factor kappa-B transcription factor
NGN neurogenins
NIK NF-κB inducing kinase
NO nitric oxide
NOS nitric oxide synthase
NRG neuregulin
NSC neural stem cells
NSCLC non-small cell lung cancer
NuRD nucleosome remodelling and histone deacetylase complex
PA protective antigen component of anthrax lethal toxin
PAR protease activated receptor-2
PD1 programmed cell death protein 1, CD279, encoded by the PDCD1 gene
PDCD4 programmed cell death protein 4 encoded by the PDCD4 gene
PDGF platelet-derived growth factor
PDGFR PDGF receptor
PDK1 phosphoinositide-dependent kinase 1
PDL1 PD1 ligand
PFS progression free survival
PGE2 prostaglandin E2
PI3K phosphoinositide 3-kinase
PKA protein kinase A
PKC protein kinase C
PLC phospholipase C
Poly (A:U) poly (adenylic–uridylic acid)
Poly (I:C) poly (inosine-cytidylic acid)
PR progesterone receptor
PRCP prolylcarboxypeptidase
PREP prolylendopeptidase
PTCH PATCHED, an element in Hedgehog signalling
RAGE receptor for advanced glycation end products
RANK receptor activator of nuclear factor kappa-B ligand
RANKL receptor activator of nuclear factor kappa-B ligand
RASSF RAS-association domain family protein
RGD arginine-glycine-aspartic acid sequence
RKIP Raf kinase inhibitor protein
ROS reactive oxygen species
RTK receptor tyrosine kinases
SARAH Salvador 1/RASSF1A/Hippo domain
SAV1 Salvador
SBP1 selenium-binding protein 1

Shh Sonic Hedgehog
SIRP signal regulatory protein
SMO smoothened, an element in Hedgehog signalling
SPARC secreted protein acidic and rich in cysteine (osteonectin)
SUFU suppressor of Fused, an element in Hedgehog signalling
TAB TAK-binding protein
TAK TGF-β activated kinase
TALEs transcription activator-like effectors
TAT transactivator of transcription domain
TAZ transcriptional co-activator with a PDZ-binding motif
TCR T-cell receptor
TDG thymine/DNA/glycosylate demethylase
TEAD TEA domain transcription factors
TEM8 tumour endothelial marker 8
TET ten–eleven translocation family enzymes
TF tissue factor cell surface receptor (thromboplastin)
TFP trifluoperazine
TGF transforming growth factor
TIMP tissue inhibitor of metalloproteinase
TIRAP toll-interleukin 1 receptor domain-containing adaptor protein
TLR Toll-like receptor
TNBC triple negative breast cancer
TNF tumour necrosis factor
TNM tumour node metastasis staging
tPA tissue plasminogen activator
TRAIL tumour necrosis factor-related apoptosis-inducing ligand
TRIF TIR domain-containing adaptor protein-inducing IFN-β
TRX thioredoxin
TRXR thioredoxin reductase
TSA trichostatin A
TSP thrombospondin
TSR TSP repeat motif
TXNIP thioredoxin interacting protein
uPA urokinase type plasminogen activator
uPAI uPA inhibitor
uPAR uPA receptor
VEGF vascular endothelial growth factor
VISTA V domain-containing Ig suppressor of T-cell activation
WISP Wnt inducible signalling pathway protein
YAP Yes-associated protein
ZFP zinc-finger proteins
ZOL zoledronate (zoledronic acid)

Introduction

Genetic and epigenetic modes of approach to molecular-targeted therapy have been intensely explored over several years with laudable and fruitful efforts directed towards cancer management. It has often been argued that therapeutic targets can be identified on the basis of certain basic criteria such as signalling pathways that can be influenced by the modulation of many elements such as hormonal and growth factor responses and motility factors. The remodelled cell membrane and the ECM (extracellular matrix) and cyto-skeletal components can be valuable as targets. Many molecular targets can be closely identified with tumour growth, cell proliferation and apoptosis. Also some foci of interest may be differentially expressed in situ and invasive and metastatic disease, such as for instance the metastasis promoter and suppresser genes (Sherbet, 2008, 2011a, 2011b, 2013).

Here my effort is directed to dissecting the practicability of targeted molecular therapy that has gained currency with the rapid advances in our understanding of the molecular bases of the crucial biological traits of cancer cells such as modes of regulation cell proliferation and apoptosis and the signalling systems linked with invasion and metastasis. The components of these molecular modes of function and of associated cascades of signal transduction have been viewed as potential molecular targets for controlling the growth and secondary spread of cancer.

CHAPTER 1

Modulation of Growth Factor Signalling in Targeted Therapy: Role of the Epidermal Growth Factor Family and Their Receptors

A major family of biological response modifiers are growth factors of the epidermal growth factor (EGF) family and their receptors the EGFRs. These subserve prominent functions in cell differentiation and morphogenesis, cell proliferation and apoptosis and also in tumorigenesis. Mutations or overexpression of growth factor receptors have been linked with aggressive behaviour of tumours and poor prognosis. Several growth factor ligands have been identified; they are synthesised as transmembrane proteins with an extracellular amino N-terminal region possessing the EGF module, a transmembrane domain and a C-terminal intracellular cytoplasmic region.

The extracellular region with the EGF module is released by proteolytic cleavage at a position in the vicinity of the cell membrane as the growth factor that can function in autocrine, paracrine or endocrine modes, and amid these modes activates EGFR (erbB1/HER1), human epidermal growth factor receptor 2 HER2 (erbB2), erbB3 (HER3) and erbB4 (HER4). The EGFR family receptors are one-pass transmembrane proteins and share many structural features, including a shared pattern of ligand–receptor interaction of specificity and transactivation. This course of transactivation might be useful in practical terms in devising strategies of combination therapy to overcome potential resistance to inhibitory monoclonal antibodies or receptor tyrosine kinase (RTK) inhibitors.

RECEPTOR TYROSINE KINASES AS MOLECULAR TARGETS

An obvious approach to controlling tumour growth would be by targeting RTKs. Of note are EGFR, FGFRs (fibroblast growth factors) and the growth factors themselves. The monoclonal humanised antibodies such as

Molecular Approach to Cancer Management. DOI: http://dx.doi.org/10.1016/B978-0-12-812896-1.00001-5

trastuzumab and pertuzumab against HER2 extracellular domain are used as first-line monotherapy or in combination with conventional therapy in stage 3 (locally advanced) and stage 4 metastatic breast cancer. Trastuzumab possibly has a dual role in that besides inhibiting the RTK there are indication that it can suppress neovascularisation. Not only can it inhibit tumour growth, but it is known to be able to reduce vascular endothelial growth factor (VEGF) expression, thus effectively inhibit microvascular density and vascular permeability (Le XF et al., 2008). In experimental animals, it has inhibited corneal neovascularisation and in parallel reduced VEGF expression in the epithelial and endothelial layers of the cornea (Guler et al., 2009).

HER2 in Cancer

Trastuzumab has provided a successful way of treating breast cancers with high HER2 expression and gene amplification (Cobleigh et al., 1999; Shepard et al., 2008; Vogel et al., 2002). Of particular interest is that some patients with low grade and node-negative HER2+ breast cancer seem to run a higher risk of recurrence and therefore potentially could benefit greatly from the trastuzumab treatment (Gonzalez-Angulo et al., 2014; Tovey et al. 2009).

These findings underscore the importance of the EGFR family to cancer progression and prognosis and as a most valuable route for targeted treatment and management of patients. Targeting growth factor function especially the sharp focus on HER2 receptors has been amply justified, for around a quarter of breast cancers express HER2 and this markedly correlates with aggressive behaviour and poor prognosis. The phenotypic outcome of HER2 signalling includes not only enhanced cell proliferation but also suppression of apoptosis, promotion of invasion and angiogenesis. Specific targeting of cytotoxic drugs to HER2 would provide dual benefits of growth control and suppression of invasion. Besides, trastuzumab can compound its biological effects arising from HER2 inhibition by inhibiting angiogenesis and in this way prevent metastatic spread.

HER2 and Suppression of Its Signalling Pathway

With this background, one can suggest that much additional benefits can be derived from looking at the components of the pathways such Akt and ERK/mitogen activated protein kinase (MAPK) of growth factor/receptor signalling. EGFR family members are established activators of PI3K/Akt (see Sherbet, 2003). The Akt pathway is said to be constitutively active when EGFR, HER2 and ErbB3 are overexpressed (Longva et al., 2005). With the acceptance that ErbB3 can dimerise with HER2, it seems possible that these two receptors might collaborate in proliferative signalling. Normanno et al.

(2002) showed that inhibition of EGFR kinase by ZD1839 (geftinib) produced a synergistic inhibition of breast cancer cells when combined with trastuzumab. ZD1839 inhibited phosphorylation of both MAPK and Akt. Trastuzumab on its own seemed to inhibit Akt but not MAPK. Compatible findings have been described. The anti-EGFR cetuximab, not trastuzumab, inhibited the phosphorylation of MAPK and Akt. Not unexpectedly, cetuximab downregulated EGFR, but not HER2 (Yamazaki et al., 2012). Basically combining EGFR inhibition with trastuzumab is synergistic in effect with inhibition of both Akt and MAPK signalling and suppression of cell cycle progression as shown some time ago (D'Alessio et al., 2010). The PI3K inhibitor GDC-0941 suppressed Akt/MAPK/ERK signalling and inhibited cell proliferation in HER2+ cells (Yao et al., 2009).

Combination of the PI3K inhibitor buparlisib with trastuzumab seems to be well tolerated. Administered at 100 mg/day dose level (the single-agent maximum tolerated dose), the combination resulted in partial response in two breast cancer patients (17%) and stable disease (≥6 weeks) in seven breast cancer patients (58%) with HER2+ advanced/metastatic disease resistant to trastuzumab (Saura et al., 2014). Yao E et al. (2009) found that HER2 inhibition is an essential component of the effects of GDC-0941, but participation of HER3 was ruled out. Recently Park et al. (2014) have shown that HER3 negativity and loss of PTEN are clear risk factors for progression-free survival.

The suppressor gene PTEN obviously would come into the reckoning here by its ability to regulate Akt function. Loss of PTEN or activating mutations of PI3K has strong links to trastuzumab resistance (Dave et al., 2011; Chandarlapaty et al., 2012) in breast cancer as well as other forms of cancer. Indeed, trastuzumab can activate PTEN and inhibit PI3K/Akt signalling and this may be the mainstay of tumour inhibition by trastuzumab. Also in the background of PTEN deficiency, Akt inhibition has been able to counteract trastuzumab resistance (Wang Q et al., 2014). Eto et al. (2014) found that microRNA (miRNA)-21 suppressed PTEN expression and upregulated Akt signalling. When overexpressed, this miRNA enhanced trastuzumab resistance and its suppression appeared to restore the sensitivity of gastric cancer cells. miRNA-21 is often upregulated in cancers and promotes activation of epithelial mesenchymal transition (EMT); it is anti-apoptotic and also able to induce cell proliferation. But miRNA-21 can exert its effects also by other means such as inhibition of expression of certain tumour suppressor genes (see Sherbet, 2011a).

Trastuzumab-mediated inhibition of cell proliferation might involve NF-κB. The latter is activated in many forms of human cancer and associated with the overexpression of several growth factors and their receptors, e.g., EGFR

(Biswas et al., 2000), HER2 (Pianetti et al., 2001) and hepatocyte growth factor (HGF) (Fan S et al., 2005). HER2 has been found to activate NF-κB together with the regulator IκB kinase α (IKKα). IKKα negatively regulates NF-κB on the one hand and on the other also suppresses PTEN. In this way it might be balancing the opposing effects of NF-κB and PTEN on cell survival. Furthermore, NF-κB itself can downregulate PTEN. Thus one can enlist several possible means by which to potentiate the inhibition of cell proliferation by trastuzumab as well as counteract the resistance to the drug encountered frequently.

The EMT is a developmental programme manifesting phenotypic changes in cell morphology, reduced intercellular adhesion and enhanced cell migration. EMT is a major event in tumour progression and has been regarded as a target for preventing tumour progression. EMT is activated in the presence of EGFR and HER2. This provides heightened impetus to the deployment of trastuzumab and EGFR inhibitors in the treatment of epithelial neoplasms. Growth factor induced EMT involves STAT3 functioning via Snail and Twist mediation (Yamashita et al., 2002, 2004; Lo HW et al., 2007; Cheng GZ et al., 2008). Chung SS et al. (2014) noticed that STAT3 occurs in a phosphorylated state in breast tumours overexpressing HER2 and this was associated with the expression of the EMT phenotype together with stem cell markers. They demonstrated that inhibition of STAT3 reversed this phenotypic alteration and have gone on to suggest that combining STAT3 inhibitors might overcome trastuzumab resistance.

E-cadherin is prominently associated with suppression of invasion and its loss leads to the acquisition of cell motility. The transcription factors Snail, ZEB1 and ZEB2 repress E-cadherin transcription and this induces EMT. TWIST is a basic helix loop helix (bHLH) transcription factor. On the other hand, NF-κB could be involved, for it is believed to induce Snail expression. TNF-α is known to induce EMT in a Snail or ZEB1/ZEB2-dependent fashion (Chua HL et al., 2007; Chuang MJ et al., 2008). Indeed NF-κB binds to the Snail promoter and induces its transcription (Barbera et al., 2004).

Trastuzumab and Drug Conjugates in Cancer Management

Targeting and delivery of cytotoxic drugs to cancer cells overexpressing HER2 have had considerable success. Trastuzumab and drug conjugates achieve specificity of delivery and cytotoxicity arising from action of the drug plus the inhibitory effects of trastuzumab itself; this lends to an overall high degree of efficacy. The trastuzumab emtansine (T-DM1) conjugate of the antibody with the anti-mitotic microtubule binding and disrupting drug DM1 (emtansine) has been found to be highly efficient in clinical trials (see Niculescu-Duvaz, 2010; Barok et al., 2014). The antibody-drug conjugate is targeted to HER2-expressing tumour cells, internalised and the cytotoxic drug is released leading to the destruction of the tumour cell. Niculescu-Duvaz (2010) has emphasised the efficacy of the treatment in preventing further progression after chemotherapy or even trastuzumab therapy itself. However, it was recognised subsequently that a majority of HER2+ patients treated with the conjugate did show disease progression. Also patients can be intrinsically resistant to T-DM1 and hence unresponsive or minimally responsive to the conjugate (Barok et al., 2014). Therefore the options of enhancing the efficacy and the benefits of combining the T-DM1 conjugate with other cytotoxic drugs as well as inhibitors of HER2 signal transduction such as RTK and PI3K inhibitors are being evaluated in preclinical studies. T-DM1 was quite effective in trastuzumab refractory metastatic breast cancer and it increased survival without progression. Progression-free survival (PFS) was found also in patients who had been treated with trastuzumab and taxane, when T-DM1 was administered with capecitabine and the RTK inhibitor lapatinib (Tykerb, GW572016) (Krop and Winer, 2014). Intriguing is the improvement in PFS seen in patients given T-DM1 as compared with trastuzumab plus docetaxel (Hurvitz et al., 2013b). The conjugate could be more effective than antibody and drug combination therapy on account of efficient targeting of the drug. Of considerable interest is the report that conjugation of trastuzumab with cytotoxic drugs might be effective in tackling metastases. Garcia et al. (2013) chemically conjugated trastuzumab to Doxorubicin or Taxol. The conjugates were selectively toxic to HER2+ cells. Trastuzumab/Taxol conjugate reduced lung metastases in experimental tumour model. Garcia et al. (2013) suggest that the conjugate targeted the metastatic deposits effectively. Whether the conjugate destroyed metastatic deposits expressing HER2 or prevented the primary tumour from metastasising is a moot point for no evidence of physical targeting of metastases was provided. Nonetheless, this is indeed a significant finding.

Conjugates in which drugs are linked with the antibody through cysteine or lysine residues have a high drug/antibody ratio. Lowering this ratio by site-specific conjugation appears to improve in vivo stability whilst maintaining efficacy (Jackson et al., 2014). Among other factors that would affect, the efficiency of antibody-drug conjugates is the receptor-mediated internalisation and cellular distribution of the conjugate. Internalisation of the monoclonal antibody/receptor complex into the lysosomes is an important event in generating an effective phenotypic outcome. Owen et al. (2013) showed that this is dependent on the molecular nature of the conjugate. It is needless to reiterate that antibody/drug conjugates not only aid the efficacy and specificity of delivery but also help to reduce systemic toxicity of the drug.

Trastuzumab and Angiogenesis

Tumours induce neovascularisation which then provides them access to the vascular system for dissemination to form distant metastases. Logically suppression of neovascularisation has provided an effective means of controlling tumour growth and metastatic spread. VEGF induces tumour vascularisation by binding to its receptor VEGFR. The humanised monoclonal antibody bevacizumab targets VEGFR and inhibits VEGF signalling. Using a murine model of tumour xenografted into the brain, Kodack et al. (2012) showed that combination of HER2 inhibition with VGFR inhibition reduced tumour growth and promoted survival of host animals. They also noted that the benefits might have accrued from the inhibition of angiogenesis as indicated by reduced microvascular density associated with the xenografts. These results are interesting per se. On the negative side, however, one cannot rule out the operation of factors that could have impinged upon the findings such as the iatrogenic interference from the traumatic experimental procedures. Earlier, Lange et al. (2011) reported findings based on an experimental spontaneous metastasis model. They subcutaneouly xenografted the HER2 overexpressing oesophageal adenocarcinoma cell line PT1590 and demonstrated that trastuzumab inhibited tumour growth, microvessel density and spontaneous lung metastases. Many clinical trials currently being carried out have been designed to look at the effectiveness of combining bevacizumab with cytotoxic drugs.

A new approach has been suggested by He J et al. (2013) who have reported that miRNA-199a and miRNA-125b are downregulated in ovarian cancer tissues and cell lines. Their overexpression seems to inhibit tumour-associated angiogenesis. HER2 and HER3 overcome the inhibitory effect of the miRNAs on angiogenesis. Besides HER2, miRNA-125b has other targets; among them are erythropoietin and its receptor (Ferracin et al., 2013).

The Influence of miRNAs on HER2 Function

Given the involvement of miRNAs in many aspects of cell function and behaviour in normal as well as aberrant cell physiology (see Sherbet, 2013), it is inevitable that miRNA might be expected to significantly influence HER2 signalling.

Two important components in the biogenesis and function of siRNAs and miRNAs are Drosha and Dicer. The primary miRNA transcripts are processed by the so-called microprocessor complex formed of the nuclear RNase III Drosha (the catalytic subunit) and the protein DGCR8 (DiGeorge syndrome critical region 8) (the Pasha protein of Drosophila, the subunit that recognises the substrate) into pre-miRNAs. The latter are translocated to the cytoplasm and are further processed by Dicer (see Sherbet, 2013 for references).

Both Drosha and Dicer have been found to be downregulated in breast cancers. Drosha downregulation is seen in HER2 overexpressing high-grade tumours and Dicer in triple negative (ER−/PR−/HER2−) tumours. There seemed to be no obvious relationship to outcome of anthracycline therapy. Both Drosha and Dicer were simultaneously downregulated in a proportion of HER+ tumours (Dedes et al., 2011). However, we have no information about the response to trastuzumab. Recent work has strongly implicated miRNAs in HER2 signalling with the demonstration that some actively regulated HER2 expression by binding to its 3′ UTR (untranslated region). The miRNAs-342-5p and 744* were found to be downregulated in HER2+ breast tumours and in fact the former specifically inhibited the growth of HER2+ cells (Leivonen et al., 2014). Others such as miRNA-19a might be associated with better prognosis in HER+ breast cancer patients (Anfossi et al., 2014). It is needless to add the caveat here that miRNAs might operate through other growth factor signalling systems and alter the expression of receptors by similar binding to 3′ UTR. Given the numerical multiplicity of miRNA species, targeting 3′ UTR in specified genes would be an arduous undertaking. The identification of genes with targetable 3′ UTRs using 3′ UTR constructs is an unenviable task.

Whilst much emphasis is placed on HER2+ breast cancer, the decidedly aggressive triple negative (ER−/PR−/HER2−) breast cancers provide a prime example where the identification of new therapeutic targets would be highly beneficial. Jonsdottir et al. (2012) reported that elevated expression of miRNA-106b could identify patients with high risk of developing metastatic disease within a group of HER2-negative patients. It might be recalled here that the triple negative cancers have a greater propensity to form brain metastases, albeit not always greater than HER2+ tumours.

It is generally accepted that trastuzumab suppresses HER2-mediated growth factor signalling. Possibly this effect might be compounded by inhibition of cell motility/invasion. We know that like EGFR and other growth factor receptors, HER2 also participates in cell migration via the adhesion receptors cadherin or integrin and the cytoskeletal components catenin and talin. HER2-induced cell migration is said to require catenin δ1 (p120 catenin) and this occurs in a Rac1 and CDC-42 GTPase-dependent manner (Johnson et al., 2010). This indeed might be indicative of possible influence of Wnt signalling, which is known to be modulated by some miRNAs by targeting 3′ UTR (Liu Y et al., 2011) and is said to upregulate HMGA2 and promote cell proliferation. The HER2-associated cell migration has included a role for miRNAs. In HER2+ overexpressing breast cancer cells, trastuzumab apparently is able to upregulate miRNA-194 expression and this is believed to suppress cell migration by altering the cytoskeletal machinery (Le XF et al., 2012). Another dimension that may be added to the role of miRNAs in breast cancer is the possible association of miRNAs with mutated breast cancer susceptibility genes. The miRNA-4417 and miRNA-423-3p has been identified with the ability to distinguish between hereditary and non-inherited breast cancers (Estal et al., 2013). However, with molecular genetics being able to detect BRCA mutations with ease, the contribution of these miRNAs in practice might be limited.

The Mammalian Target of Rapamycin Signalling Pathway

The mammalian target of rapamycin (mTOR) pathway involves two mTOR complexes, namely mTORC1 and mTORC2. The mTORC1 complex consists of raptor (the regulatory-associated protein of TOR), G protein β-subunit-*like* protein (GβL) and Pras40. The mTORC1 activates its effectors S6K and 4EBP1 (eukaryotic initiation factor 4E-binding protein 1) and in this way regulates phenotypic changes and enhances ribosomal biosynthesis and cell cycle regulatory proteins for G1–S transition and cell proliferation. The complex mTORC2 has the rictor (rapamycin-insensitive companion of TOR), GβL, mSin1 and Protor which can phosphorylate Akt and might be involved in cytoskeletal reorganisation (Sarbassov et al., 2004, 2005). The relevance of mTOR is underscored by the overexpression of S6K1 in breast cancer and apparent link with poor prognosis. S6K1 functions downstream of Akt and mediates cell proliferation and so mTOR would mediate cell proliferation and cell survival. There is a complex circuitry of feedback regulation between mTORC1 and mTORC2 and DEPTOR. Loss of DEPTOR activates the mTOR complexes and S6K, SGK1 and Akt which lead to cell proliferation and survival. However, when overexpressed, DEPTOR suppresses the feedback inhibition of Akt by mTORC1. The removal of the inhibitory constraint promotes Akt-mediated cell proliferation (Fig. 1.1).

Modulation of Growth Factor Receptor Function by mTOR Signalling

The mTOR signalling cascade is deregulated in many tumours. This signalling system is prominently active in the regulation of autophagy, cell proliferation and survival as well as in angiogenesis. So it emerges as an essential component of tumour inception, growth and progression. The preeminence of this signalling system may be attributed to the perceived integration of EGFR, VEGF, IGFR (insulin-like growth factor receptor), TNFR (tumour necrosis factor receptor) and ER (oestrogen receptor) signalling. On account of its being able to influence manifold signalling systems, mTOR inhibitors are seen as viable therapeutic tools on its own or in combination therapy. It is noteworthy that mTOR inhibitors appear to wield marked effects on cells refractory to EGFR inhibitors. Inhibitors of mTOR seem to be able to restore

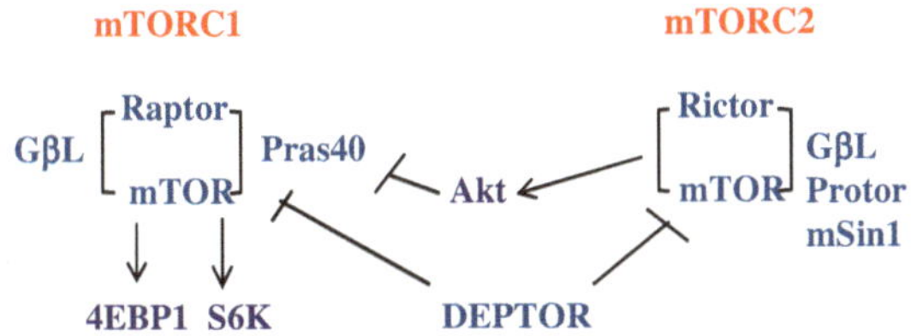

FIGURE 1.1

Depicts the mTOR signalling complexes and their regulation of Akt, 4EBP1 and S6K in the control of cell proliferation. GβL stimulates the kinase activity of mTOR leading to 4EBP1 and S6K function. PRAS40 (proline-rich Akt substrate 40 kDa) is a component of mTORC1 mediates Akt signalling to mTOR. Binding of PRAS40 inhibits mTOR. Both mTORC1 and mTORC2 are inhibited by DEPTOR. There is a complex circuitry of feedback regulation between mTORC1 and mTORC2 and DEPTOR. Loss of DEPTOR activates the mTOR complexes and S6K, SGK1 and Akt, which lead to cell proliferation and survival. However, when overexpressed, DEPTOR suppresses the feedback inhibition of Akt by mTORC1. The removal of the inhibitory constraint promotes Akt-mediated cell proliferation (Peterson et al., 2010). This figure is partly based on Efeyan and Sabatini (2010). The operation of mTOR pathway in cell survival involving PI3K/Akt and MAPK crosstalk, which might be potentially useful in devising combination inhibition of mTOR signalling, is shown in Fig. 1.4. These two figures should be read together.

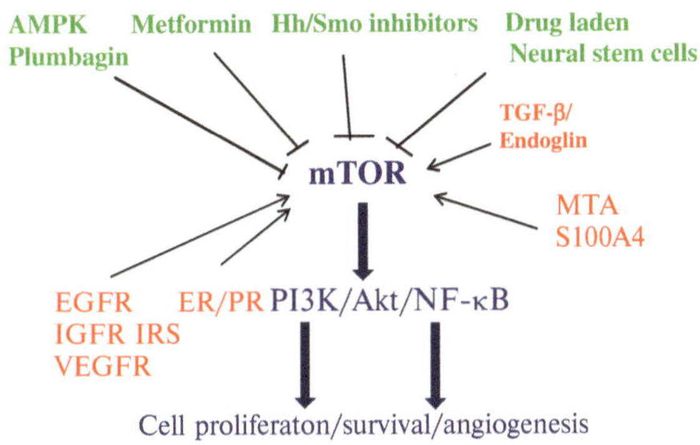

FIGURE 1.2

Portrays the extensive compass of signalling co-ordinated and apparently regulated by mTOR and therefore possibly amenable to modulation using appropriate inhibitors. Inhibition of mTOR brings about corresponding suppression of cell proliferation, survival and angiogenesis. Many allosteric inhibitors of mTOR and RTKs and dual mTOR/PI3K inhibitors have been evaluated. These are not shown here. TGF-β promotes EMT and this possibly occurs via Smad.

the inhibitory effects of EGFR inhibitors of control of growth and VEGF production (Fig. 1.2).

One might interpose here that DEPTOR is an mTOR inhibitor and its overexpression in cancers leads to cell proliferation and survival. This is said to be due to the feedback regulation occurring between mTORC1 and mTORC2 and DEPTOR. When overexpressed, DEPTOR suppresses the feedback inhibition of Akt by mTORC1. The removal of the inhibitory constraint promotes Akt-mediated cell proliferation (Peterson et al., 2009). The downregulation of DEPTOR suppresses cell proliferation together with inhibition of PI3K/Akt in RPMI-8226 multiple myeloma cells and is said to sensitise the cells to melphalan (Zhang HR et al., 2013). This is compatible with the attribution of resistance to melphalan to the inhibition of apoptosis (Chauhan et al., 1997).

Everolimus (mTOR inhibitor) and the EGFR inhibitor gefitinib can suppress EGFR-related signalling of growth and VEGF production (Bianco et al., 2008). The angiogenic and lymphangiogenic effects exerted by FGF-2 have been attributed to mTOR activation (Matsuo et al., 2007). These events correlated with the inactivation of mTOR signalling (Garcia-Maceira and Mateo, 2009).

Of special significance is potential use of mTOR inhibitors in the management of triple negative breast cancer (TNBC), which is said to be resistant to rapamycin. But it has been described as effective in supressing tumour growth in combination cytotoxic agents in animal tumour models and in vitro. Lee C et al. (2008) reported that YB-1, a transcription factor, which is highly expressed in breast cancer, induced signal transduction by promoting dimerisation of HER2 and EGFR. Interestingly, YB-1 promoted cell survival by activating the mTOR/Akt pathway. Suppression of YB-1 can block cell proliferation in HER2 overexpressing cells as well as TNBC cell lines. The EGFR/mTOR pathway could also operate and enhance cell invasion (Zhang H et al., 2014). Combination of everolimus plus trastuzumab and paclitaxel has had much effect in trastuzumab-resistant HER2+ overexpressing breast cancers (Hurvitz et al., 2013a).

Of some interest in this context is the report that metformin inhibits cancer stem cells (CSCs) in a murine tumour model of MMTV-HER2. In this model, metformin downregulated HER2 and EGFR, and, among other things, also mTOR signalling (Zhu P et al., 2014). Whilst these findings are relevant with regard to potential benefits of metformin in the management of TNBCs, it ought to be recognised the effects might have occurred by a totally different mode of action. Metformin inhibits cell proliferation and exerts marked anti-inflammatory effects, arrests cell cycle progression and induces apoptosis and is seen as an effective anti-cancer agent. A major effector metformin is AMPK, but possibly it can act independently of AMPK and there is some agreement that AMPK might function by inhibiting mTOR. Metformin activates AMPK and inhibits mTOR signalling but it can also directly target mTOR quite independently of AMPK (Dowling et al., 2011, see also Sherbet, 2013 for further discussion). It ought to be pointed out also that the suggestion that metformin might inhibit CSC is not a new thought. It was shown previously to be able to inhibit CSCs identifiable with high CD44 and low CD24 expression and to suppress mTOR signalling. The recent findings of Lionello et al. (2014) have suggested the potential value of mTOR signalling in the induction of angiogenesis. They found that the expression of mTOR and EGFR was closely linked and also with enhanced microvascular density.

Molecular Therapeutics of HER2-Positive Tumours Metastatic to the Brain

Many tumour types are known to metastasise to the brain, e.g., breast cancer, small cell lung carcinoma, melanomas, colon cancers and kidney tumours. The incidence of central nervous system (CNS) metastasis varies from 20% in lung cancer, followed by melanoma (7%) and breast cancers (5%) to as low as 2% in colorectal cancer (Barnholz-Sloan et al., 2004). Indeed, lung and breast carcinomas and melanomas metastatic to the brain form around 2/3 of all cancers (Nayak et al. 2012). Progression to CNS metastasis is rare in the cases of tumours such as hepatocellular carcinoma (HCC) where the incidence of brain metastasis might be encountered in well below 1% of cases (Kim M et al., 1998; Han MS et al., 2013). HCCs do metastasise to other sites such as the lung, which is a prominent metastatic site (Uchino et al., 2011).

One can quite legitimately enquire into the causes of this apparent propensity to form brain metastases displayed by some tumours in order to develop strategies to contain this brain seeking proclivity and to improve therapeutic management of patients with brain metastases. Recent years have seen a marked increase in the incidence of brain metastases in patients with HCC and this has been attributed prolonged survival resulting from therapy (Shao YY et al., 2011). Indubitably improvements in the modes of patient management in terms of diagnosis and treatment would lead to the progression of the primary tumour to the CNS (Nayak et al., 2012). But looking specifically at the incidence of CNS metastasis of breast cancer, there must exist intrinsic tumour features that facilitate the formation of CNS metastases. For it is notable that whilst overall incidence of breast cancer metastasis to the brain only 5%, HER2+ tumours show a markedly greater propensity at around 25%. High-grade ER negative, EGFR+ and HER2 overexpressing breast cancers possess a greater propensity to metastasise to the brain (Hicks et al., 2006; Miller et al., 2003).

Several factors might contribute to the dissemination of tumours to the brain (Fig. 1.3) and these can markedly influence the development of new strategies of treatment of brain metastases. An important concept has been formulated that therapy with trastuzumab might create a "sanctuary-site" for tumour in the brain. It has been argued that trastuzumab is unable to

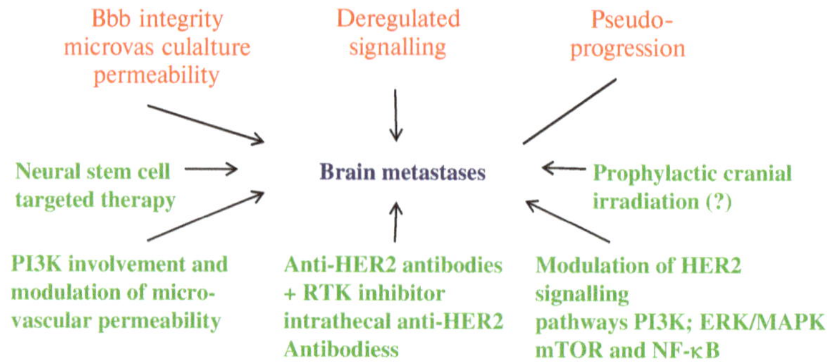

FIGURE 1.3

Factors relevant to the dissemination of HER2+ breast tumours to the brain. Detection of pseudo-progression is an important consideration in the management of patients. *From Patil, A., and Sherbet, G.V, 2015. Therapeutic approach to the management of HER2-positive breast cancer metastatic to the brain. Cancer Lett. 358, 93–99.*

penetrate the blood brain barrier (BBB). The levels of trastuzumab in the CSF are low in comparison with that in the serum but it has been found to increase following radiotherapy, which possibly compromises BBB integrity (Stemmler et al., 2007). This lends weight to the argument that the CNS is a sanctuary-site in patients on trastuzumab (Lin NU and Winer, 2007).

We have recently reviewed much evidence of the EGF family growth factors and their receptors on cell proliferation, apoptosis, and differentiation and tumorigenesis. Mutations or overexpression EGFR family receptors have been associated with aggressive tumours and poor prognosis for patients. That HER2+ breast cancers might display preferential metastasis to the brain has been broadly accepted, although a clonal link between HER2+ component of the primary neoplasm and the formation of HER2+ brain metastases is yet to be firmly established. A further interesting facet of the story is that HER3 overexpressing tumours can also metastasise specifically to the brain and often HER3 is expressed concomitantly with HER2 (Berghoff et al., 2014), but in this scenario HER3 makes a negative contribution to the overall survival of HER2+ patients post-metastasis.

Many new avenues of therapeutic approach based on the manipulation of the signal transduction systems associated with HER2 function have been envisaged (Fig. 1.4), notably Akt and ERK/MAPK of growth factor/receptor signalling. Genetic alterations involving EGFR, HER2 and PTEN have been encountered more frequently in brain metastases than in primary breast cancers (Hohensee et al., 2013). Recently Bachmann et al. (2013) found a high degree of correspondence in HER2 status of matched brain metastases and primary breast cancers, unlike with ER/PR (progesterone receptor) status. Also

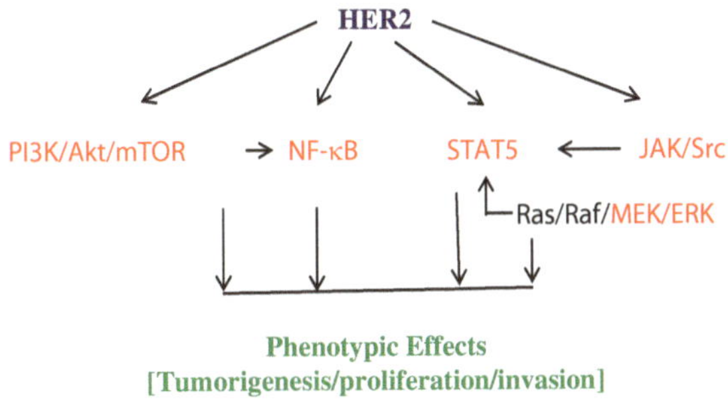

FIGURE 1.4

The major pathways of HER2 signalling in cell proliferation, tumorigenesis, invasion and eventual metastatic deposition are shown here. HER2 can signal directly via the PI3K/Akt/mTOR and NF-κb or JAK/STAT or indirectly through the JAK/Src pathway. Ras/Raf/MEK/ERK function via STAT or other transcription factors, e.g., CREB. *From Patil, A., and Sherbet, G.V, 2015. Therapeutic approach to the management of HER2-positive breast cancer metastatic to the brain. Cancer Lett. 358, 93–99.*

HER2+ patients showed a shorter interval, though not statistically sustained, to the manifestation of brain metastasis than did HER2-negative patients. Yap YS et al. (2012) found that anti-HER2 treatment greatly prolonged the time to the formation of brain metastasis. Renfrow and Lesser (2013) have reviewed evidence indicating that targeting HER2 with the RTK inhibitor lapatinib and capecitabine can prevent or increase the time to CNS progression and also reduce metastatic lesions in the CNS. One can see an additional advantage in the finding that in primary tumours and in brain metastases PI3K is frequently constitutively active. Inflammatory cytokines are associated with vascular dysfunction from vascular dilation and enhanced permeability. Often these cytokines signal via the STAT pathways, which can be phosphorylated by PI3K and MAPK. Thus PI3K activation could result in significant compromise of the integrity of the BBB enabling the entry of disseminated cancer cells into the brain. In other words, counteracting the deregulated PI3K might serve dual function of preventing the loss of BBB integrity as well as inhibiting growth factor signalling.

Growth factor function involves another signalling system viz. mTOR signalling pathway, which is active in cell proliferation and survival signalling. It is deregulated in many forms of tumour. The transcription factor NF-κB is the final effector of many signalling systems. The mTOR and NF-κB pathways interact and mutually regulate each other's signalling. In fact, mTOR is said to control NF-κB downstream of Akt in the background of PTEN deficiency (see Sherbet, 2011a, 2013). Trastuzumab-mediated inhibition of cell proliferation might involve NF-κB. The latter is activated in many forms of human cancer and associated with the overexpression of many growth factors and their receptors, e.g., EGFR, HER2, HGF (Biswas et al., 2000; Pianetti et al., 2001; Fan S et al., 2005).

The mTOR inhibitor everolimus and the EGFR inhibitor ZD1839 (gefitinib) can suppress EGFR-related signalling of growth and VEGF production (Bianco et al., 2008). The efficacy of combining mTOR inhibitors with trastuzumab in advanced breast cancer has been looked at quite seriously. Much research is also being carried out to exploit the HER2/mTOR route to managing breast cancer metastases to the brain. The inhibition of EGFR kinase by ZD1839 produces a synergistic inhibition of breast cancer cells when combined with trastuzumab. ZD1839 inhibits phosphorylation of both MAPK and Akt (Normanno et al., 2002). Geftinib is in clinical trials to evaluate its effects on metastasis to the brain of NSCLC (NCT00614809, NCT01951469, NCT00238251).

Neural Stem Cells in Targeted Treatment of Brain Metastases

Stem cell transplantation therapy has gained much credence in the past few years. The bone marrow contains two stem cell populations, viz. mesenchymal stem cells (MSCs) and haematopoietic stem cells (HSC). MSCs promote the proliferation and differentiation of HSC. MSCs are pluripotent cells capable of self-renewal, which can be induced to differentiate into several cell lineages. MSCs can effectively modulate the immune system.

An exciting new approach is the employment of neural stem cells, which show marked tropism to brain lesions. Neural stem cells have been genetically engineered to express therapeutic anti-cancer gene products and can effectively target brain metastases and suppress growth of the lesions (Menon et al., 2009). Targeted delivery and activation of prodrugs using neural stem cells have been tested successfully. Most of these studies are to be deemed to be at the experimental stage but nonetheless needs to be highlighted on account of their high clinical potential.

Wang C et al. (2012) transduced the cytosine deaminase gene (CDA) and the thymidine kinase (TK) gene into neural stem cells. Cytosine deaminase converts 5-fluorocytosine (5-FC) to 5-fluorouracil (5-FU) and TK converts ganciclovir (an acyclic nucleoside analogue of 2′-deoxyguanosine inhibitor of DNA synthesis) into its toxic active form. In an experimental metastasis system, the neural stem cells targeted brain metastases arising from lung cancer cells injected into the host animals and effectively reduced the size of the metastases besides prolonging survival. Targeted delivery of carboxylesterase that enabled the conversion of camptothecin-11 to an inhibitor of topoisomerase SN-38 has also been reported. Unhappily but inevitably the experimental procedures involved are too invasive.

In the context of deploying this technology to inhibit HER2 signalling, one should cite the work of Frank et al. (2009). They transiently co-transfected neural stem cells with plasmids carrying the heavy and light chains of an anti-HER2 antibody identical in sequence to trastuzumab. Upon intravenous introduction, these genetically modified stem cells targeted breast cancer xenografts in host animals. The stem cells were found in the tumour and inhibited the growth of the xenografts. The diapedesis of cancer cells across the vascular endothelium occurs at sites where the structural integrity of the endothelium is compromised. One has to ask if the BBB impedes the entry of neural stem cells into the brain and more specifically if endothelial permeability is a determining factor in the localisation of neural stem cells in the target. MSCs have the ability to migrate across the BBB (Liu L et al., 2013). So one would expect that when the stem cells have migrated across the brain endothelium, a proportion of them would home into the metastatic lesion and restrain its growth by secreting anti-HER2 antibodies. The molecular environment of the metastases, such as the production of proangiogenic growth factors, which can promote neural stem cell migration into the metastases (Díaz-Coránguez, 2013), would inevitably come into the reckoning (see Patil and Sherbet, 2015 for a detailed discussion).

CLINICAL EVALUATION OF mTOR INHIBITORS

Several clinical evaluations of everolimus in combination with other mTOR inhibitors, e.g., rapamycin and temsirolimus, and RTK inhibitors as well as established chemotherapeutic agents are currently being carried out in many forms of early and advanced disease. Studies are also being designed to look at the efficacy of combining mTOR inhibitors with trastuzumab in advanced breast cancer. Perhaps it might be a little premature to over emphasise the potential role of mTOR signalling in TNBC and take an over optimistic view of the latent benefits. A recent study by Nakajima et al. (2014) of a significant number of TNBCs came up with no correlation of EGFR expression with p-Akt or p-mTOR expression or with any clinical features. There were no activating mutations or amplification of EGFR gene in the TNBC samples they investigated.

The breast cancer oral everolimus-2 (BOLERO-2) trial has focused on hormone receptor-positive and HER2-negative advanced breast cancer. Hormone receptor-positive tumours form a large subtype, which responds to treatment with non-steroidal aromatase inhibitors. However, disease progression does take place with the development of resistance believed to result from the deregulation of PI3K/Akt/mTOR pathway. Of note in the context of management of patients with this tumour subtype is the combination of aromatase inhibitors with mTOR inhibition. The combination does improve PFS irrespective of age. Both elderly and younger patients show similar and comparable levels of side effects although more deaths might occur of patients on treatment. These aspects need careful consideration in patient management (Pritchard et al., 2013).

Combination of everolimus with the aromatase inhibitor exemestane has been approved recently by the US Food and Drug Administration and the European Medicines Agency (EMA/CHMP/402772/2012) for the treatment of hormone receptor-positive, HER2-negative advanced breast cancer. Several clinical trials are underway (see ClinicalTrials.gov NIH). The BOLERO-2 study has shown that this combination markedly improves PFS as compared with exemestane alone (Yardley et al., 2013; NCT00863655). Diaby et al. (2014a) have confirmed the benefits of BOLERO-2 using HUI (Health Utilities Index) to assess health status HRQL (health-related quality of life), but they do question the cost effectiveness of the treatment (Diaby et al., 2014b). Nonetheless, patient welfare cannot remain a matter of erudite analyses, and with patient welfare in mind it would be imprudent to throw away the benefits. Cost considerations cannot at any time assume priority over benefits to the patients. The everolimus and exemestane combination is reportedly more efficacious than everolimus with the anti-oestrogen Fulvestrant (Bachelot et al., 2014), but the latter combination has shown benefit in some patients (see Massarweh et al., 2014).

Overall, it might be reasonable to conclude that everolimus might lend itself to producing a twofold reduction in tumour burden as indicated by the analysis of responses in patients with solid tumours (Ravaud et al., 2014). However, as a note of caution, one should add that this study as well as others (see Sivendran et al., 2014) have emphasised the accompaniment of marked metabolic side effects with everolimus administration.

The HER2/mTOR Route to Patient Management

HER2+ breast cancers have shown a marked propensity to metastasise to the brain. This general premise has been broadly accepted. But this has not been tested with paired primary tumours and corresponding metastases. Genetic alterations involving EGFR, HER2 and PTEN have been encountered more frequently in brain metastases than in primary breast cancers (Hohensee et al., 2013). Intratumoral heterogeneity of HER2 expression cannot be ruled out and hence a clonal relationship between metastases and HER2+ component of the primary tumour cannot be established. Nonetheless, it is noteworthy that HER2 status has shown a remarkably high levels of correspondence between matched brain metastases and primary breast cancer (Bachmann et al., 2013). Notwithstanding the caveats, the relationship is indeed valuable for patient management.

It may be argued that brain metastases are an outcome of enhanced patient survival derived from HER2+ inhibition and the inability of monoclonal antibodies to cross the BBB (Singh et al., 2014). Molecular subtype luminal A (ER+ or PR+ or ER+/PR+, HER2−) and B (ER+ or PR+ or ER+/PR+, HER2+) (see Komen, 2014) form the majority of tumours and TNBC (with low level of the tetraspan tight junction protein claudin) around a fifth of breast cancers. The molecular subtype HER2+ luminal tumours show higher frequency of brain metastases as compared with TNBCs. HER2+ tumours carry a greater risk of metastasis to the brain, but so also do around a fifth of TNBCs (Minisini et al., 2013; Aversa et al., 2014). According to Berghoff et al. (2014), HER3 overexpression was associated with more frequent brain only metastasis. They found that HER3 overexpression was associated with HER2 overexpression. HER3 overexpression does appear to make a negative contribution to overall survival of HER2+ patients post-metastasis. So the occurrence of brain only metastasis of HER3+ tumours is somewhat intriguing when viewed in the light of the ability of growth factor ligands to activate both HER2 and HER3. If further studies confirm this scenario, HER3 could turn out to be a useful feature for patient management. Of interest in this context is the possibility that management of HER2+ tumour metastatic to the brain has been attempted with a combination of PI3K/Akt and mTOR inhibitors together with HER2 inhibition with trastuzumab. Also worthy of note is the report by Swain et al. (2014) that treatment with anti-HER2 monoclonal antibodies and the anti-mitotic docetaxel can delay tumour progression to brain metastases. These studies underscore the potential of active adjuvant therapy to manage the progression of HER2+ tumours to the CNS. Yap YS et al. (2012) reviewed a large series of breast cancer patients and concluded that anti-HER2 treatment prolonged (virtually doubled) the time to the formation of brain metastasis. The targeting HER2 with the RTK inhibitor lapatinib and capecitabine can prevent or increase the time to CNS progression and also reduce metastatic lesions in the CNS (Renfrow and Lesser, 2013).

Combinations of everolimus with EGFR and HER2 inhibitors have been investigated in advanced disease. The combination of everolimus and lapatinib has been described as being well tolerated and may have stabilised the disease in a proportion of patients (Gadgeel et al., 2013). Andre et al. (2014) conducted a placebo-controlled double blind trial with trastuzumab-resistant, HER2-positive, advanced breast cancer. They reported that the median PFS was 7.00 months with everolimus and 5.78 months with placebo. Adverse events were encountered in the everolimus group. A significant increase in PFS was seem upon addition of everolimus to trastuzumab and the anti-mitotic vinorelbine (nor-5′-anhydrovinblastine), but as the authors themselves have stated, this has to be viewed in the light of the adverse effects noted. Some histologic phenotypes of metastatic renal cell carcinoma have shown limited response to temsirolimus or everolimus; 7% partial responses, and 49% had stable disease but disease progression was noted in 44% of patients. Tumour shrinkage was seen in a third of the patients (Voss et al., 2014).

Resistance to mTOR Inhibition

Preclinical evaluations have encountered resistance to mTOR inhibitors and this is a valid rationale for exploring combining mTOR inhibitors with inhibitors other signalling pathways that can interact with and influence mTOR signalling. Much emphasis has been placed on mTORC2/Akt and Ras/MAPK/Akt pathway. Sarbassov et al. (2005, 2006) stated that Rictor/mTORC2 regulates Akt signalling. Given that PI3K/Akt/mTOR pathway is activated in many tumours and given its activation in patients in HER2+ breast cancers, earnest efforts have been underway for some time to tackle intrinsic and acquired resistance also to trastuzumab therapy. Combinations of PI3K inhibitors and mTOR inhibitors alongside HER2 inhibition have provided valuable data that support the clinical evaluations of these inhibitors.

O'Brien et al. (2014) have described the in vitro and in vivo effects of PI3K inhibitors an mTORC1-specific inhibitor and a PI3K/mTOR dual inhibitor. All the inhibitors tested inhibited cell proliferation and in vivo induced the regression of trastuzumab-resistant xenografts. The authors make an additional point that when the dual inhibitor was employed they found no feedback activation of PI3K and this is an important finding that supports the value of combination of PI3K and mTOR signal inhibition, notwithstanding the fact that individually both PI3K and mTOR inhibitors were equally effective.

Brouxhon et al. (2014) have reported that soluble E-cadherin is able to activate both MAPK and PI3K/Akt pathway mediating mTOR signalling and promote tumour growth and invasion in an experimental tumour model. Of much interest is that suppression of soluble cadherin led to the inhibition of tumour growth and invasion. Insulin-like growth factor (IGF)/insulin receptor substrate 1 (IRS1) can also activate PI3K/Akt signalling. There is a view that negation of RTK signalling using phosphatases can supplement the effects of mTOR inhibitors.

PTEN mutations not only enhance Akt but also promote mTOR signalling. Dual inhibition of PI3K and mTOR with PF-05212384 accentuates the induction of apoptosis by the RTK inhibitor PF-00299804 (Zhu Y and Shah, 2014). Similar are the findings that geftinib synergises with another PI3K/ mTOR dual inhibitor (see Katanasaka et al., 2014). Whilst in the background of the presence of PTEN dual inhibitors might be able to induce apoptosis by colluding with PTEN, some inhibitors can and do induce autophagy. Such an alternative phenotypic route has been suggested for the dual inhibitor NVP-BEZ235 (Hong SW et al., 2014). Although this work was carried out in tumour cell cultures, it would be helpful to note that the PTEN background might be not critical in determining the application of dual inhibitors in disease control.

There is much evidence that RTK inhibitors can function synergistically with mTOR. The IGF type 1 receptor plays an important part in cell growth and survival. It also increases cell motility, transformation and protect cells from apoptosis. Upon ligand binding, IGF1R undergoes autophosphorylation and this leads to the engagement and phosphorylation of the substrates IRS1 and IRS2. Some of these phenotypic changes occur through the modulation of E-cadherin expression. As shown in Fig. 1.5, Akt can inhibit mTORC1/S6K and the latter is able to inhibit IRS1. So there are further opportunities to compound the inhibition by influencing mTORC1. Humanised anti-IGF-IR monoclonal antibodies effectively inhibit cell proliferation. A demonstrably significant synergy has been found in the function of anti-IGF-IR antibodies

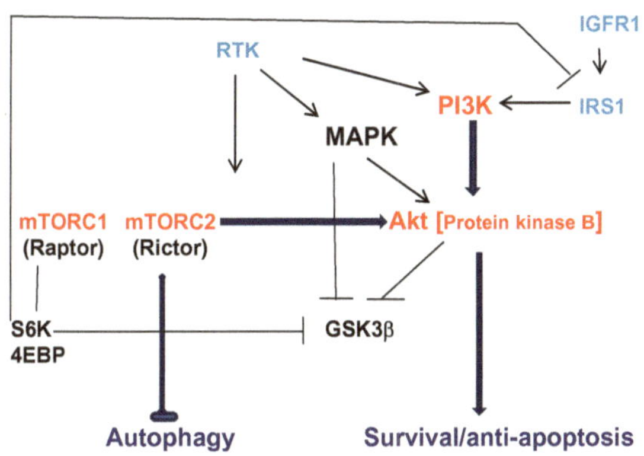

FIGURE 1.5

Summarises the role of mTOR pathway in cell survival involving PI3K/Akt and MAPK signalling crosstalk potentially useful in devising combined inhibition of mTOR signalling. The PI3k/Akt system activates mTORC1, which suppresses autophagy. However, mTORC2 can activate Akt, so it has been suggested that mTORC2 could indirectly negatively regulator autophagy. IGFR, insulin-like growth factor receptor; IRS, insulin receptor substrate.

with temsirolimus on renal carcinoma cells in vitro (Cardillo et al., 2013). A phase I clinical trial employing the monoclonal antibody CP-751871 with everolimus in patients with advanced sarcomas and other solid tumours was carried out some time ago but results are not available (NCT00927966; Quek et al., 2010).

Anaplastic Lymphoma Kinase-Positive NSCLC and Crizotinib and Second/Third Generation RTK Inhibitors

Crizotinib, an aminopyridine-based RTK inhibitor, has come to the fore on account of its success in the treatment of advanced NSCLC carrying the ROS1 rearrangement. The ROS1 kinase is related by significant sequence homology to the anaplastic lymphoma kinase (ALK). The rearranged ROS1 forms fusion proteins with several partners. In the fusion proteins the kinase domain of ROS1 is constitutively active and promotes cell proliferation. The ROS fusion kinase is encountered in many tumours, including approximately 1% of NSCLC patients. The constitutively active fusion kinase is an important target for therapy using the crizotinib.

Crizotinib was reported previously to produce significant responses in phases I and II clinical trials with possible improvements in patient survival (Hung JJ et al., 2013; Shaw et al., 2014; Russell et al., 2011). It has been described as more efficient as a first-line treatment as compared with pemetrexed (an anti-folate)-plus-platinum chemotherapy as first-line agents (Solomon et al., 2014). More recent studies have confirmed that crizotinib improves PFS and that it could be regarded as a first-line treatment option for ALK+ NSCLC patients (Blackhall and Cappuzzo, 2016). Crizotinib has had FDA approval as a first-line treatment option, but in Europe that option is available for ALK+ patients who have had no pretreatment. In Italy patients with previous chemotherapy may be eligible (Cortinovis et al., 2016). A powerful case has been made for administering the second generation of ALK inhibitor ceritinib as first-line therapy. However, in the event that resistance to the drug develops, the second line option is chemotherapy. According to results of a phase III study presented at the ESMO (2016), ceritinib was superior to chemotherapy, in respect of median PFS and increased overall response rate. Alectinib and ceritinib have been suggested as second line options in crizotinib failure. Overall, expert opinion seems to favour the protocol of administering a second generation ALK inhibitor in the event of crizotinib failure as the standard treatment ALK+ positive lung cancer (ESMO, 2016). Crizotinib, ceritinib and alectinib have all been attributed with clear CNS responses with regard to metastases. But crizotinib shows poor CNS penetration and justifiably a case can be made for agents that have more efficient access to the CNS to obtain CNS responses. The effects of alectinib on CNS metastases are striking in respect of the overall response rate of CNS lesions and complete CNS response (Gadgeel et al., 2014; Ou SH et al., 2016). Lorlatinib and brigatinib, the newer inhibitors, have produced marked CNS responses.

Combination of crizotinib with other RTK inhibitors has been tested in pleural mesothelioma. Inhibitors of PI3K, a downstream target of ALK kinase and the PI3K/mTOR dual inhibitor GDC-0980 have effectively suppressed cell proliferation and cell migration in vitro. Suppression of growth was also noticed of xenografts of mesothelioma cells in murine hosts (Kanteti et al., 2016). In fact, the resistance to crizotinib might be a result of the activation of interacting proliferation pathways such as EGFR and c-met/PI3K. The EGFR family signalling system is active in NSCLC in common with many other neoplasms. Mutations in EGFR and amplification of c-met have been found to be important factors in the development of resistance to crizotinib (Chen JH et al., 2008). This would be likely outcome, for crizotinib would be expected to inhibit both ALK and c-met (Nwizu et al., 2011). ALK+ cells may be sensitive in terms of growth inhibition to simultaneous use of ALK, c-met and EGFR (Li C et al., 2015). Therefore combining ALK inhibitors with anti-EGFR monoclonal antibodies or the HER2-neutralising trastuzumab, which can also inhibit EGFR, is worthy of investigative effort. Janne et al. (2016) employed the pan-EGFR antibody dacomitinib, with crizotinib, following failure of first-line chemotherapy. The combination was not beneficial and was associated with unacceptable toxicity. However, this should not dissuade attempts to use inhibitors of EGFR/HER2 with ALK inhibitors. This group had earlier reported good clinical activity with dacomitinib as first-line treatment in NSCLC patients (Janne et al., 2014). Needless to say that the prevailing genetic environment is an important consideration in that they found the responses were superior among patients who carried activating mutations of EGFR. It would be worthwhile bearing in mind in this context that EGFR RTK inhibitors have a good record of generating 60%–80% response of CNS metastases in patients carrying EGFR mutations (Dempke et al., 2015).

Inhibition PI3K together with ALK inhibitors, which also inhibit c-met, might be viable options. Engelman et al. (2008) have supported the use of PI3K/mTOR inhibitors. It may be noted here that inhibitors of the PI3K/mTOR pathway are effective against tumours carrying PIK3CA mutations. They have also suggested that MEK inhibitors would be potentially useful against tumours with KRAS mutations. The latter have been linked with resistance to crizotinib. Resistance to alectinib also develops over time and this is associated with the activation of growth factor signalling pathways such as IGFR, HER3 and c-met pathways (Isozaki et al., 2016). Tackling the activated alternative signalling pathways would again be an obvious means to overcome the acquired resistance.

It would be reasonable to suggest that ALK+ NSCLC patients with advanced could derive significant benefits from crizotinib and the later generation inhibitors. Indeed, much progress is afoot in the development of new ALK inhibitors that can overcome drug resistance and also effectively generate CNS responses. Entrectinib is a new inhibitor on the horizon, which is said to be a powerful inhibitor of ALK, ROS1 and RTKs. It is being evaluated in vitro and in xenograft studies. Entrectinib has induced regression of human tumour xenografts. Early clinical evaluation seems promising with discernible objective response in patients with colon cancer and NSCLC (Ardini et al., 2016). Alectinib has been tested on an NSCLC cell line, which is crizotinib-resistant and carries ALK mutations. Xenografted tumours have also displayed regression (Yoshimura et al., 2016). It has also produced marked CNS responses. Lorlatinib is a new inhibitor, which possesses better CNS penetration, and it is being evaluated in phase I/II clinical trials. Preclinical studies have shown that it is effective in vitro and in xenografts models against crizotinib-resistant NSCLC. When combined with PI3K and PI3K/mTOR inhibitors, lorlatinib has proved to be able to overcome ALK inhibitor resistance. Brigatinib is a dual inhibitor of ALK and EGFR, effective against crizotinib-resistance and also effective against CNS metastases (see Wu et al., 2016).

CHAPTER 2

The TGF-β Family Accessory Type III Receptor Function in Cancer Progression

TGF-β performs diverse and pleiotropic physiological functions participating in cell adhesion, migration and proliferation, as a part of normal growth and differentiation. The signalling cascade is distinguishable into the canonical and non-canonical pathways. The ligands transduce their effects through a relatively uncomplicated system of two types of receptor, the type I and type II (RI and RII) receptors and type III accessory receptors together with the activation of the downstream Smad proteins in the canonical pathway. The cascade of activation involves binding of the ligand to type II receptor, recruits the type I receptor and phosphorylates it. This in turn phosphorylates and activates the R-Smads. The ligand induces the phosphorylation of Smad2 and Smad3 in the activin and Smads1, 5 and 9 in the bone morphogenetic protein (BMP) pathways. The activation of these Smads in turn activates R-Smad, which forms a complex with Smad4 to activate the transcription of responsive genes. Smad6 and Smad7 are inhibitory Smads that inhibit R-Smad activation. The inhibitory Smads can be activated by both TGF-β/activin and TGF-β/BMP pathways. The activation of Smads2 and Smad3 would be expected to promote cell proliferation, but ligands that activate the antagonistic Smads6 and Smad7 would inhibit cell proliferation. TGF-β is itself able to induce the expression of the inhibitory Smads, which could be a part of the self-regulatory mechanisms. To expand on the role of Smad7 aside from TGF-β, other growth factors such as EGF can activate Smad3. Again, EGF can be negatively regulated Smad7. However, inflammatory cytokines like IFN-γ induce the expression of Smad7. Smad7 may have ambivalent, indeed a dual, role in cancer and has been associated with either suppression or the promotion of tumour growth. This could relate to the prevailing intracellular microenvironment. An important provision would be that the type III accessory receptors exert differential effects on cell proliferation.

The Smad proteins are not activated in the non-canonical signalling system. The non-canonical signalling pathways include the PTEN, PI3K/Akt,

Molecular Approach to Cancer Management. DOI: http://dx.doi.org/10.1016/B978-0-12-812896-1.00002-7

Ras/Raf/ERK1-2 (extracellular signal-regulated kinase)/MAPK (mitogen activated protein kinase) and integrin signalling systems. Thus TGF-β is able to exert a wide spectrum of phenotypic by this dual signal transduction system (see Sherbet, 2011a). It is essential to appreciate that contrast and dichotomy of function in any effort to use the components of the TGF-β signal transduction for developing drug-related strategies.

THE FUNCTIONAL CONSIDERATIONS OF ENDOGLIN AND BETAGLYCAN

The canonical Smad signalling system involves regulatory components; among them are endoglin (CD105), a 180-kDa homodimeric transmembrane protein and the 250–350 kDa proteoglycan betaglycan. Betaglycan is also transmembrane protein. Endoglin and betaglycan belong to the family of glycoproteins, which possess the characteristic zona pellucida (ZP) module of approximately 260 aminoacid residues in the extracellular domain. The ZP module is involved in the oligomerisation of glycoproteins and also in protein–protein interactions. The ectodomains undergo proteolytic cleavage at a site close to the membrane to secrete a soluble fragment. Both soluble forms of the auxiliary receptors appear to take part in TGF-β signalling. Endoglin and betaglycan carry significant sequence homology in their transmembrane and cytoplasmic domains. The cytoplasmic domain is highly conserved in the proteins belonging to this class. The transmembrane and cytoplasmic fragment of betaglycan may be a substrate of γ-secretase. Inhibitors of the latter suppress TGF-β signalling implicating the transmembrane and cytoplasmic segment in the signalling process.

Endoglin and betaglycan are often described as accessory type III receptors. Essentially they facilitate the binding of the TGF-β family ligands to types I and II receptors. Type III receptor might indeed function in both ligand-dependent and -independent signalling. Endoglin acts upstream of the activin receptor-like kinase 1 (ALK1)/Smads1, 2 and 3 cascade. It binds TGF-β receptors to recruit TGF-β family ligands to form active complexes. TGF-β binds to endoglin in the presence of RII, but endoglin can bind RII even when the ligand is absent. In endothelial cells, ALK5 and the endothelial cell-specific ALK1 promote endoglin activity in the presence of RII. The TGF-β family ligands activin-A and BMPs can bind endoglin in consort with other receptors (see Sherbet, 2011a for references).

Betaglycan was identified some time ago to function as a co-receptor for TGF-β. It has several binding sites and high affinity for TGF-β and accentuates signalling by TGF-β and TGF-β family ligands. The ectodomain (external domain) of betaglycan has two ligand binding regions, one in the distal and a second one in proximal half in relation to the membrane. The ectodomain displays a bi-lobular structure, with each lobule folding and binding TGF-β independently of the other (Mendoza et al., 2009). Functionally, betaglycan leads to the suppression of cell proliferation and invasion. The soluble form of betaglycan is expressed at reduced levels in many forms of cancer suggesting that it might in fact inhibit TGF-β signalling. Betaglycan can mediate TGF-β ligand-dependent or -independent signalling through the canonical Smad system and the non-Smad pathways.

THE PARADOXICAL FUNCTIONS OF ENDOGLIN IN ANGIOGENESIS AND TUMOUR PROGRESSION

Endoglin was identified some time ago as the candidate HHT (hereditary haemorrhagic telangiectasia type 1 associated with blood vessel abnormalities) gene (McAllister et al., 1994). It shares some sequence homology in the transmembrane and intracellular domain with betaglycan. The extracellular domain of endoglin contains an RGD (Arg-Gly-Asp) sequence and so potentially could be participating in cell adhesion phenomena. This sequence does not occur in the extracellular domain of betaglycan. This might account for possible differences in the mechanisms of regulation of cell adhesion by the endoglin and betaglycan, viz. RGD-mediated regulation in the former and Cdc42-dependent alterations of the actin cytoskeletal dynamics in the latter (Oh SY et al., 2013). Filopodia, which may have a bearing on the migratory behaviour cells, are formed in MCF10A and HMEC mammary epithelial cells by the mediation of betaglycan and CDC42 and take place in a β-arrestin-dependent fashion. More significant is that TGF-β signalling is regulated in a collaborative fashion by endoglin and betaglycan. Betaglycan forms a complex with endoglin. Since endoglin can interact with TGF-β receptors type II and type I (Wong SH et al., 2000), it could be that betaglycan recruits endoglin to form the receptor complexes.

Endoglin subserves a dual role in endothelial function, angiogenesis and tumour progression. It is highly expressed in vascular endothelial cells in embryogenesis and also in some disease states. It participates in many normal and abnormal physiological processes of angiogenesis. It has been associated with tumour development and dissemination, both dependent upon adequate vascularisation. Endoglin shows some specificity of expression in endothelia and has been linked with endothelial proliferation and cell migration. These are markedly inhibited together with inhibition of capillary formation, diminished eNOS (endothelial nitric oxide synthase) activity and reduced vascular endothelial growth factor (VEGF) secretion in murine endothelial cells that were endoglin (+/−) in comparison with endoglin (+/+) cells (Jerkic et al., 2006). A subsequent confirmed finding is the eNOS reduction but not the reduction in VEGF in haploinsufficient cells (Duwel et al., 2007). So overall these findings are consistent with reduction of angiogenesis with reduced endoglin production. Whether endoglin influences the barrier function of endothelia and potentially influence the diapedesis of tumour cells into the vasculature is unresolved at present, with markedly opposite views being expressed in this regard.

It has been noted that endoglin expression positively relates to tumour progression. With the perceived overexpression in tumour vasculature, the specificity of expression in endothelial cells, tissue regeneration and inflammatory phenomena, and with the recognition of its potential ability to modulate angiogenesis, endoglin has been regarded as a viable target for inhibition of tumour-associated angiogenesis and inhibition of tumour growth and metastasis. Its expression is upregulated in some tumour types such as ovarian and breast cancers and can also promote metastatic spread. Pancreatic cancer cells have been reported to display higher levels of endoglin as compared with normal epithelium accompanied by higher cell invasion and higher expression of markers associated with the induction of epithelial mesenchymal transition (EMT), but there was no correlation with survival (Fujiwara et al., 2013). Others have found that endoglin expression is associated with poor disease prognosis. It would be necessary to establish whether endoglin per se is associated with metastatic ability. In head and neck squamous cell carcinoma, endoglin expression has paralleled that of the tumour/metastasis promoter gene S100A4 (Oliveira et al., 2014; see also Sherbet, 2008, 2011, 2014 for S100A4), but intriguingly, the methylation status of S100A4 showed no relationship to metastasis.

Some growth factors can switch endoglin signalling from canonical to non-canonical pathways. These considerations are of utmost importance in deploying anti-endoglin antibodies as a treatment modality. PTEN, PI3K/Akt, Ras/Raf/ERK1-2/MAPK and integrin signalling could be involved in endoglin participation in cell proliferation, apoptosis, cell adhesion and migration. Equally valid is the postulate that reduction of endoglin in the vascular endothelium enhances invasion and in this way promotes tumour progression. This occurs in prostate carcinoma cell lines where downregulated expression of endoglin has correlated with progression (see Lopez-Novoa and Bernabeu, 2012; updated 2016).

Several reasons can be adduced for the generation of these opposing biological effects in tumour development. This could be a reflection of the well-established TGF-β function as a tumour suppressor in the early stages but a promoter of progression in later stages of tumour development. Other possible reasons include the ability to promote endothelial integrity, potential differential affinity and specificity in ligand-receptor binding, different modes of targeting of receptors by the ligands and the recruitment of different Smads in downstream signalling. Indeed, endoglin can function via the canonical as well as the non-canonical pathways.

Although the modes of action of endoglin are not fully understood, antibodies raised against endoglin have been used in experimental and clinical investigations with a view to regulating the growth and spread of tumours. TRC105 is a humanised anti-endoglin monoclonal antibody that has been studied in recent years. Administration of TRC105 has been found to markedly reduce angiogenic markers in the circulation (Liu Y et al., 2014). In the treated subjects there was an increase in soluble endoglin. Release of endoglin from the cell membrane has been suggested to be a result of coupling of endoglin with matrix metalloproteinase (MMP) at the cell surface (Kumar et al., 2014). Shedding of endoglin in the soluble form is said to occur late in the normal course of tumour progression. Therefore antibody-mediated induction of shedding of endoglin might retard progression of the disease. There is no definitive evidence at present relating to the significance of soluble endoglin to clinical stage of the disease. There is also the possibility, discussed in a section below, that the appearance of the soluble receptor in the circulation might upregulate immunological response. Given that TGF-β signalling can activate EMT and induce invasion and metastasis, suppression of this signalling pathway by manipulating the function of the auxiliary receptors has been viewed as a viable option. On account of its association as a key element determining invasion, tumour-associated angiogenesis and in tissue regeneration and inflammatory phenomena, endoglin has naturally been focused on as a potential therapeutic target.

THERAPEUTIC TARGETING OF ENDOGLIN

TEW-7197 is a serine/threonine kinase inhibitor of ALK5. ALK5 is highly expressed in many tumours and is involved in promotion of tumour growth and migration and possibly also in the suppression of anti-tumour immune responses. ALK5 promotes endoglin activity in the presence of TGF-β/RII and indeed endoglin and ALK5 are closely involved in the regulation of EMT activation. These consequential outcomes of the TGF-β/ALK5 signalling are crucial in tumour progression. TEW-7187 inhibits the phosphorylation of ALK5 and blocks the TGF-β/ALK5 pathway leading to the suppression of tumour growth. The safety and tolerability of this drug is being addressed in a clinical trial with advanced stage solid tumours (NCT02160106).

Rosen et al. (2012) reported a multicentre phase I (NCT00582985) clinical study of the effects of the anti-endoglin monoclonal antibody TRC105 in advanced or metastatic solid cancers of various types. There was moderate progression free disease in evaluable patients over 2–4 months, often supported by assessment of the expression of appropriate markers. This early study has been followed up with more clinical trials of combination of TRC105 with the angiogenesis inhibitor bevacizumab in glioblastoma, colorectal cancer and adrenal cell carcinoma, and with Pazopanib, a receptor tyrosine kinase inhibitor, which suppresses angiogenesis, in soft tissue sarcoma. Inhibitors of the activin-like kinase class of receptors by pyridinylimidazoles (patent WO 2001062756 A1) and SD-208 (Zaiman et al., 2008) have been described. The latter has shown to be inhibitory of invasion in vitro. It also reduced tumour growth and the number and size of metastases in syngeneic hosts but not athymic nude mice (Ge R et al., 2006). The perceived inhibitory effects on angiogenesis are of much practical significance in combating metastatic spread and SD-208 does warrant further study of this aspect of its action.

Other inhibitors of ALK5 and related kinases are the analogous compound A-77-01 and A-83-01. These exhibit similar biological properties. The TGF-βRI/ALK5 kinase inhibitor LY 2157299 is being evaluated in pre-clinical and clinical studies (Bueno et al., 2008; Liu Z et al., 2009; Li W et al., 2009; Tojo et al., 2005; Workman, 2005; Gras, 2014). These have been shown to suppress tumour growth or inhibit induction by TGF-β of EMT transition. The problem nonetheless is the solubility of the compounds. These studies are generally carried out in vitro or using animal tumour models and the drugs are carried in dimethyl sulfoxide. On the horizon as some of them have been labelled, they have yet to see much basic elucidation of biological properties. However, the ability to inhibit EMT is per se a highly significant attribute of these compounds so much so that in spite of the lack of focus on them it would not be appropriate to rule them out of or indeed rule them in into consideration in the clinical setting. In fact, the inhibitor LY 2157299 is being assessed in clinical trials involving hepatocellular carcinoma, recurrent glioblastoma and metastatic pancreatic cancer. It is needless to reiterate that it has been effective in suppressing Smad phosphorylation in many tumour cell lines including triple negative breast cancer (TNBC) cells (see Gras, 2014).

The ALK1 antibody PF-03446962 is being evaluated in the clinical trials. This monoclonal antibody has shown some benefits in patients with advanced solid tumours together with indication of inhibition of the angiogenic prolife. At the minimum tolerated dose, there were adverse effects which have been described as manageable (Goff et al., 2016). A study of hepatocellular carcinomas suggests that the antibody could be exerting an anti-angiogenic effect. Simonelli et al. (2016) found lower levels of VEGFR3 in patients with stable disease as compared with those who had progressive disease. The outcome was not encouraging in urothelial cancers. No anti-tumour activity was noticed in refractory disease. In fact, VEGF and IL-8 levels had increased (Necchi et al., 2014). Further ambiguity concerning the possible effects on angiogenesis arises when one considers an earlier report. Van Meeteren et al. (2012) had argued that the antibody does not affect the VEGF signalling axis and had no effect on the proliferation and migration of endothelial cells. But, it did inhibit BMP/endoglin signalling and inhibit endothelial sprouting. This runs counter to the conventional view that VEGF stimulates endothelial cell sprouting and migration. It may be mentioned in this context that telangiectasia has been reported as a side effect, which does indicate that the vascular system is targeted by the administration of the antibody.

BETAGLYCAN IN CANCER INVASION AND METASTASIS

Betaglycan has been shown to inhibit the metastasis of in vivo xenografts of human GCTs (ovarian granulosa cell tumours) and human GCT cells. Bilandzic et al. (2014) reported that in their experimental model TGF-β induced the metastatic process by activating the NF-κB/MMP2 pathway and that betaglycan suppressed this pathway and reduced MMP2 levels and in this way inhibited metastasis. However, their data show a considerable range of MMP levels in the control and betaglycan-treated cells and so making a distinction not fully justifiable. The suppression of peritoneal metastasis was quite marked. It ought to be remarked however that the formation of peritoneal metastases is more a reflection of adhesive interaction between the cancer cell and the peritoneum and that ovarian cancer cells are only minimally invasive. But betaglycan can and does suppress angiogenesis, invasion and metastasis. The mode of action by which this is brought about is still uncertain. The suppression of metastasis can result from reduced angiogenesis resulting from the repression of MMPs, but one has to have proper assessment of intra- and tumour-associated microvascular density to be certain that that is the case.

There is a thought that soluble betaglycan, i.e., the ectodomain of betaglycan released from the cells is a determinant of metastasis suppression. The soluble betaglycan would sequester TGF-β and prevent its function. Experimentally generating soluble betaglycan markedly inhibits TGF-β-mediated cell invasion. Elderbroom et al. (2014) looked at the effects of soluble betaglycan using the experimental model in which breast cancer cells were injected into athymic mice via the tail vein. Unfortunately this latter test does not simulate the metastatic process but simply shows that the adhesion of cells in the lungs was indeed influenced by soluble betaglycan. Hanks et al. (2013) have suggested that the loss of betaglycan from the tumour cells might suppress TGF-β signalling by upregulating immunological response to the tumour. In both these cases it is difficult to visualise how the ectodomain in situ or cleaved from the cell could differ in altering the cell adhesive functions or the generation of immunological responses. Nevertheless, it is recognised that proteoglycans in situ do markedly affect adhesive interactions between cells and the substratum. Syndecans would have such effects on adhesive interactions that would affect the migratory behaviour of cells. It is unclear at present how the shedding of the betaglycan ectodomain affects the signalling properties of the transmembrane and cytoplasmic domain. It may be recalled here that the cytoplasmic domain of syndecan-2 is essential for TGF-β signalling. In fact it is involved with interactions with the cytoskeleton and PDZ domain proteins that function to scaffold the membrane receptors to the cytoskeleton (also see discussion below).

THE BETAGLYCAN-INHIBIN PATHWAY

The obvious routes of suppressing TGF-β signalling are by recourse to the inhibition of the kinases involved, as noted before, and by the inhibition of the downstream Smad signalling. Therefore, an important consideration in the present context is the interaction with other members of the TGF-β family of which activins and inhibins have acquired some significance since the demonstration by Lewis et al. (2000) that betaglycan binds inhibin with high specificity. This is quite likely to sequester ALK2 and prevent endoglin-mediated suppression of cell invasion via ALK2 and downstream Smad1 activation. The BMPRII might also function via the Smad pathway and interact with ALK2 signalling with both contributing individually to generate the phenotypic effect (Breen et al., 2013). Again these effects of BMP are liable to be abrogated by betaglycan-mediated sequestration of ALK2 for BMP requires ALK2 for its biological effect (Vale et al., 2004). Thioredoxin has been suggested as a possible inhibitor of Smad signalling. But then it can inhibit caspase-mediated apoptosis via TGF-β1/ASK1 participation (Saitoh et al., 1998; Sanchez-Capelo, 2005). However, Zhao and Hoffmann (2006) engineered thioredoxin with a Smad-binding motif from the co-factor peptide SARA (Smad anchor for receptor activation). This thioredoxin-SARA peptide reduced the levels of Smad2 and Smad3 and inhibited TGF-β-induced activation of EMT.

THERAPEUTIC POTENTIAL OF BETAGLYCAN

As discussed earlier, betaglycan can suppress angiogenesis, invasion and metastasis. The soluble form of betaglycan can suppress metastatic progression by sequestering and subverting TGF-β function. Even in the face of much evidence of its ability to suppress tumour progression, there seems to be very little activity in testing inhibition of TGF-β signalling by taking advantage of the suppressor function of betaglycan. A linear peptide derived from ectodomain of betaglycan, viz. Peptide 144 (P144) inhibits TGF-β1-dependent signalling pathway (Heminda et al., 2009). Both P144 and a second peptide P17 inhibit the development of laser-induced choroidal neovascularisation. The inhibitory effects are accompanied by parallel reduction in the expression of VEGF and reduced MMP activity (Zarranz-Ventura et al., 2013). However, the precise mechanisms of its action are unclear. One encounters a generalised statement that P144 interacts with and inhibits TGF-β binding to betaglycan. Since TGF-β is itself inhibited by betaglycan, one has to have more information on the molecular orientations of P144, TGF-β and betaglycan in the inhibitory process. Zubeldia et al. (2013) pretreated colon adenocarcimoma cells with TGF-β and introduced them into murine hosts and found that the treatment had increased the growth of primary tumours and liver metastases. But upon systemic introduction of P144 or P17, there was a reduction in primary tumour burden and only half the number of hosts were found with metastases as compared with hosts bearing TGF-β-treated cancer cells. The metastatic lesions showed reduced proliferation and enhanced apoptosis and a downregulation of EMT markers and angiogenesis. However, there is no evidence that vascular density associated with the primary tumour was diminished as a consequence of P114/P17 administration. An interesting finding in terms of mechanisms is that the therapeutic function of P144-mediated suppression of TGF-β occurs by the agency of CD4 + CD25 + Foxp3 (forkhead/winged-helix transcription factor) + regulatory T cells and not directly attributable to tumour cells themselves (Llopiz et al., 2009). The latter are indicative of immune responses elicited upon challenge with extraneous antigens or tumour antigens.

The relevance of soluble betaglycan to cancer invasion and metastasis needs to be addressed in more detail. Indeed, there is a need to elucidate how P144 stands in relation to the soluble betaglycan. Also there is paucity of information about how P144 or other peptides derived from the ectodomain of betaglycan affect the biological behaviour of cells. With the suggested relationship between soluble betaglycan and metastatic spread, it might be worthwhile probing the possibility of engaging soluble betaglycan with P144. A clinical trial aimed at determining the effects, efficacy and safety of topical application of P144 in skin fibrosis in systemic sclerosis has been carried out (NCT00574613).

THE ROLE OF ARRESTINS IN TGF-β SIGNALLING

Arrestins are a family of four proteins that regulate the transduction of signals initiated by GPCRs (G-protein coupled receptors). Arrestins can promote signal transduction by engaging tyrosine kinases of PKA/PKC, PI3K, Src and GPCR/MAPK systems. They can promote signal routing linked with the transcription factors NF-κB and mdm2 pathways. So essentially they can influence a wide spectrum of phenotypic effects including cell proliferation and apoptosis. Interestingly, arrestins have come into the picture of TGF-β signalling too. They have been implicated to interact with many signalling pathways, including TGF-β, with a scaffolding task to signalling proteins of several transduction cascades (see Fang Y et al., 2003; Sherbet, 2011a).

You HJ et al. (2009) showed some time ago that betaglycan interacts with β-arrestin 2 and suppresses NF-κB pathway, an important pathway in cancer invasion and metastasis. β-Arrestin 2 has also been linked with betaglycan mediated effects on cell motility (Oh SY et al., 2013). The β-arrestin 2/endoglin complex apparently downregulates c-myc and cyclin D1 leading to inhibition of cell proliferation and this does not occur when the complex is disrupted (Pan CC et al., 2012). Qin R et al. (2014) have studied the β-arrestin pathway in the perceived correlation of enhanced β-arrestin 1 expression with clinical stage of CML (chronic myeloid leukemia) patients. In a murine model β-arrestin 1 depletion has led to enhanced survival. They envisage the binding of β-arrestin 1 to EZH2 of the Polycomb family and the promotion of CML progression by regulating the BCR/ABL fusion gene H4 acetylation. The demonstration here is unequivocal that β-arrestin 1 seems to enhance histone H4 acetylation to further affect gene expression. Histone acetyl transferases acetylate histones and lead to increased transcription of genes. However, EZH2 proteins are involved in maintaining several genes in transcriptional repression. So possibly, β-arrestin 1/EZH2 complex might suppress transcription inhibition by EZH2. The potential modes of functioning of the pathway have not been unravelled by Qin et al. (2014). Equally, suppressor genes such as Kisseptin might be involved in arrestin/GPRS/MAPK pathway. The KiSS-1 gene was identified as a suppressor of invasion and metastasis (see Sherbet, 2013). Kisseptin can activate GPR54 and MAPK signalling. β-arrestin 1 has been shown to inhibit GPR54-mediated signalling to ERK/MAPK (see Szereszewski, 2010). Therefore the promotion of progression might have occurred by the participation of more than one signalling system.

SYNDECANS IN TGF-β SIGNALLING AND TUMOUR PROGRESSION

Syndecans are another class of proteoglycans the loss of which promotes tumour progression. Syndecans are transmembrane proteins with an N-terminal signal sequence and an ectodomain-containing consensus sequences for heparin-binding extracellular ligands including growth factors, extracellular matrix proteins, cell adhesion molecules, among others. Syndecans function as co-receptors for these ligands and facilitate their recruitment to specific receptors and enable transduction of the ligand signal (see Carey, 1997). In this way the syndecans can influence apoptosis and cell proliferation as well as invasion and metastasis. Syndecans have also been attributed with the ability to suppress endothelial cell migration and inhibit angiogenesis. These validate the importance attributed to syndecans in signal transduction. However, their involvement in anti-angiogenesis as demonstrated by De Rossi and Whiteford (2013) is to be regarded as putative since most of their evidence is derived from in vitro assays. Although syndecan-1 is downregulated in many tumour types, in some tumours it is not downregulated or the levels of expression do not relate to disease state, as in germ cell tumours. Syndecan-4 was highly expressed in the tumour cells in seminomas. The expression in the stromal component correlated with disease stage, vascular/lymphatic invasion and nodal metastasis. In non-seminomas, there was a loss of syndecan-4 expression in both tumour and stromal compartments. The loss of the syndecan in the tumour cells correlated with disease spread, but unlike the seminomas, the stromal levels did not correlate with disease state (Labropoulou et al., 2013). This is somewhat paradoxical, since non-seminomas grow and spread more rapidly than do the seminomas.

An important caveat is the variability of the effect of syndecans. They can exert contradictory effects, often dependent upon the tumour type and the localisation of the proteoglycan. The loss of their ectodomain or deletions in the cytoplasmic tail can generate different biological effects on adhesion and cell migration with consequence for cancer invasion and metastasis. Indeed, in the context of angiogenesis, one should recognise that syndecans have also been attributed with the ability to suppress endothelial cell migration and inhibit angiogenesis. Nonetheless, the suppressor gene RKIP (raf kinase inhibitor protein) inhibits HMGA2 (high mobility group protein A2), an established EMT activator, and suppresses the expression of syndecan-2 giving the beneficial outcome of suppressing EMT and tumour progression (see Fig. 23.1).

In breast cancer high expression of syndecan has been reported to be associated with higher histological grades and inversely related to hormonal receptor status. High expression was related to poor overall and disease-related survival. The HER2+ subtype (ER−, PR−, HER2+) and TNBCs have been found to express syndecan-1 at higher levels than luminal tumours and the latter at levels higher than non-metastasising control tumours (Nguyen et al., 2013). In the light of these findings, the possibility has to be considered that in the ER−/PR− environment a switching of signalling to syndecans might be taking place. Consistent with higher expression with progressive disease a recombinant antibody OC-46F2 which specifically recognises the extracellular domain of syndecan-1 has been found to inhibit tumour growth and angiogenesis in experimental human melanoma models. When this antibody was administered to animals bearing tumours that were formed from the implantation of melanoma cells, a significant (approximating 75%) reduction in tumour volume occurred and there was also a marked suppression of VEGFR2 expression in the tumours obtained from the antibody-treated animals (Orecchia et al., 2013). Syndecans, not unlike other proteoglycans such as endoglin and betaglycan discussed earlier, are shed from the cell surface in a soluble form. Heparanases and MMPs initiate proteolytic cleavage of the extracellular domain of syndecan leading to the shedding of the soluble syndecan. Soluble syndecan-1 has been suggested as a potential marker to distinguish between benign and malignant disease and even to predict survival (Mundt et al., 2014). But overall, syndecans have received scant attention in clinical studies barring attempts to see whether serum levels of syndecan-1 might predict inflammatory bowel disease and malignant mesothelioma.

CHAPTER 3

Insulin-Like Growth Factor Signalling as a Target to Control Tumour Progression

Insulin and insulin-like growth factors (IGFs) transduce their signals by binding to specific receptors IGFR1 and IGFR2 with the agency of intermediate components called the insulin receptor substrate (IRS) proteins. The IRS proteins are famously associated with cell proliferation, migration and survival signals generated by growths factors. Another important component of IGF function is the IGF-binding proteins (IGFBPs), which regulate the biological activity of IGFs by interfering with their interaction with IGFRs. IGFs signal prominently via PI3K/Akt and the mitogen activated protein kinase (MAPK) systems. They regulate the apoptosis family genes. The mTOR pathway has also been implicated in the regulation of tumour growth and angiogenesis (Fig. 3.1). IGF-mediated signalling can collaborate and interact with the TGF-β/Smad system to participate in the metastatic process. The ability of IGF-1 to promote the formation of the splice variant VEGF165 rather than the VEGF165b isoform is an attribute of much relevance in cancer metastasis. For, the isoforms resulting from exon 8 splicing at the proximal splice site promote angiogenesis, in contradistinction to the distally spliced "b" isoforms, which can bind VEGF receptors but cannot activate signalling and so are competitively anti-angiogenic (see Sherbet, 2011a for references). With these attributes and the significance of the signalling intermediates, it is hardly surprising that the biological function of the IGFs and the means by which they regulate signalling pathways have received so much attention in respect of their functional relevance as a therapeutic approach.

THE ROLE OF INSULIN RECEPTOR SUBSTRATE PROTEINS IN TUMOUR PROGRESSION

The intermediary IRS component has been shown to promote cell proliferation and inhibits apoptosis by means of three distinctive pathways. The major pathways of IGF/IGFR function in the promotion of cell proliferation and migration are shown in Fig. 3.1. The IGF/IGFR signal is transduced via the canonical pathways of ERK and PI3K/Akt. The JAK/STAT is a third mode of

Molecular Approach to Cancer Management. DOI: http://dx.doi.org/10.1016/B978-0-12-812896-1.00003-9

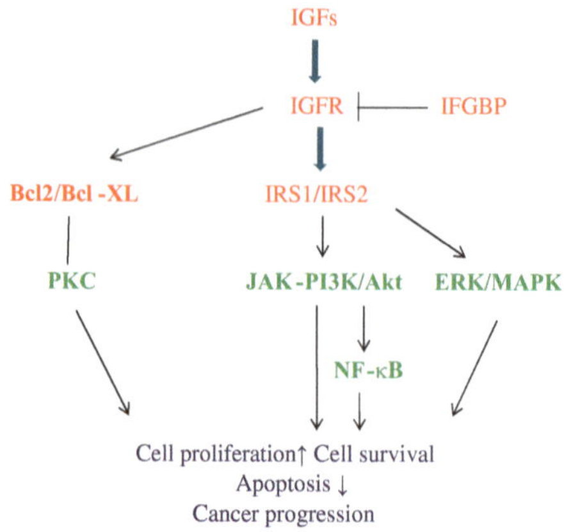

FIGURE 3.1

The signalling pathways of IGF/IGFR function in the promotion of cell proliferation and migration. The signalling takes place via the canonical pathways ERK and PI3K/Akt. The JAK/STAT is a third mode of signalling. The IRS proteins are involved in the activation of PI3K/Akt pathway. The anti-apoptosis genes Bcl2 and Bcl-XL have also implicated as influencing PI3K/Akt. IGF might promote cell survival in co-operation with other pathways of signal transduction. IGFBPs are generally inhibitory of IGF function. They interfere with the binding of IGFs to IGFRs. Some IGFBPs are said to stimulate IGF effects, which suggest a regulatory role for IGFBPs (see Sherbet, 2011a). IRS1 can be degraded via the mTORC2 pathway. This is not shown here. Often IRS1 degradation has led to the activation of PI3K/Akt pathway by other growth factor receptor signalling resulting in the promotion of cell proliferation. Resveratrol and curcumin markedly inhibit NF-κB, besides being powerful inhibitors of IGF-1-induced proliferation possibly with IRS involvement. As stated in the text, IRS function and NF-κB indeed appear to be linked. Equally, both resveratrol and curcumin are powerful inhibitors of COX-2, a promoter of tumour progression and can bring about their effects by blocking COX-2 signalling.

signalling. The IRS proteins are unmistakably involved in the activation of PI3K/Akt pathway. The anti-apoptosis genes Bcl2 and Bcl-XL have also implicated as influencing PI3K/Akt. IGF might promote cell survival in co-operation with other pathways of signal transduction. IGFBPs are generally inhibitory of IGF/IGFR function. They interfere with the binding of IGFs to the receptors. Some IGFBPs are said to stimulate IGF effects, which suggest a regulatory role for them (see Sherbet, 2011a). IRS1 can be degraded via the mTORC2 pathway. Often IRS1 degradation has led to the activation of PI3K/Akt pathway by other growth factor receptor signalling resulting in the promotion of cell proliferation. As stated in another location, growth factor/receptor signalling from another source such as the platelet derived growth factor (PDGF)/PDGF receptor (PDGFR) appears to activate PI3K/Akt signalling and IRS and promote cell proliferation. This can happen even in the absence of IRS. This aspect would need to be addressed fully in order that any attempts to target IRS are not thwarted in this way.

TARGETING IRS SIGNAL TRANSDUCTION TO CONTROL TUMOUR GROWTH

The activation of PI3K/Akt signalling so markedly correlates with aggressive growth and tumour behaviour that targeting it and subduing and suppressing its function have been seen as a viable way to control tumour growth and its aberrant behaviour. Some while ago, Reuveni et al. (2013) demonstrated in a most convincing study that NT219, a member of the so-called NT family of small molecules, led to the destruction of IRS1 and IRS2 by phosphorylating their serine residues. This effectively obliterates the activation of the PI3K/Akt pathway (El-Ami et al., 2014). NT157 inhibited IGF1R activation and reduced IRS protein expression, together with inhibition of PI3K/Akt activation in LNCaP and PC3 prostate carcinoma cells in vitro (Ibuki et al., 2014). The suppression of cell proliferation and the relevant signalling systems may require relatively long exposure to NT157 as shown for breast cancer cells. With IRS expression correlating with oestrogen receptor (ER) expression, this report has also indicated that the treatment sensitised ER+ cells to rapamycin was able to inhibit the growth of tamoxifen resistance cell (Yee D et al., 2016) a full account of which is not available at present. This could have some relevance to breast cancer management. Tamoxifen resistance can often be overcome by aromatase inhibitors and other antagonists of ER. Also one has to consider not only the balance of expression of ERα/ERβ because they exert opposing effects but also the expression of progesterone receptor (PR), which is also an important factor in the equation (see discussion later). Overall, little progress is seen concerning the utility of these compounds in the cancer context; they are said to provide protection from neurodegenerative diseases. It has been claimed that the NT compounds exert no toxic effects even at high concentrations, although no information is available in the public domain concerning the toxicity aspect.

Another candidate in the horizon seemingly able to eliminate IRS from IGFR signalling is prolylcarboxypeptidase (PRCP) and the related prolylendopeptidase (PREP). Both PRCP and PREP are said to stabilise IRS and are required for proliferation and survival of pancreatic and breast cancer cells. The depletion of PREP has led to the degradation of IRS1 and to the inhibition of PI3K/Akt activation (Duan et al., 2014). These authors have also implicated mTOR signalling in this scenario for they found that inhibition of PRCP/PREP enhanced the cytotoxic effects of rapamycin. However, none of these studies have looked into how the inactivation of PI3K/Akt signalling comes about and no attempts have been made, for instance, assessing the potential role of PTEN in the regulation of this signalling system. Neutrophil elastase (NE) has been reported to lead to the degradation of IRS1 thus suppressing the cell proliferation and survival pathways that IRS might promote.

However, the downside of this degradation of IRS is that it has led to enhanced signalling interaction between PDGFR and the PI3K/Akt pathway producing enhanced cell proliferation (Houghton et al., 2010). Indeed inhibition of NE has suppressed cell proliferation and induced apoptosis. So there is an overriding view that NE effects are generated not by the involvement of IRS but by the activation of the PI3K/Akt system by other growth factor receptors. The signalling by RTKs interacts with mTOR, Akt and MAPK (see Fig. 1.5) and so cannot be ascribed to IRS without due reckoning of the operation of other growth modulators. Overall, studies relating to the inhibition of IRSs and preventing downstream activation of signalling pathways are few and far between. The role subserved by the IRSs in cell proliferation and apoptosis most certain deserves a great deal more of attention.

CURCUMIN AND ITS ANALOGUES CAN CONTROL IRS SIGNALLING

There are many more novel avenues that can be explored. For example, resveratrol, the polyphenolic stilbene family compound, can suppress IRS1 and MAPK signalling. In vitro studies have shown that not only resveratrol inhibited the migration of vascular smooth muscle cells (VSMCs) but also that the effects correlated with the suppression of IRS1 expression (Lin YC et al., 2014). Curcumin, the active polyphenolic ingredient of turmeric (*Curcula longa*), possesses multiple biological and medicinal properties (Aggarwal et al., 2007). It markedly inhibits NF-κB as well as STAT3 (Kim et al., 2012), besides being a powerful inhibitor of IGF-1-induced proliferation of VSMCs (Youreva et al., 2013). There is also some evidence that curcumin suppresses metastases, albeit other mechanisms have been adduced for this effect from in vitro invasion and in vivo evidence derived from tumour models (Chen CC et al., 2013; Radhakrishnan VM et al., 2014). For instance, curcumin can suppress VEGF-mediated endothelial permeability and angiogenesis. Also the IGFRs are necessary for neovascularisation. Numerous clinical trials are under way (https://clinicaltrials.gov) to test and improve the bioavailability of curcumin, which is lipophilic and poorly absorbed upon enteral administration. Much work is being done to develop efficient delivery of curcumin and to assess its biological effects. These studies amply vindicate the case being made for curcumin as a suppressor of metastasis.

Resveratrol also inhibits NF-κB and possibly by this route inhibits cell proliferation and migration. The parallel incidence of the effects suggests the possible link up between IRS1 and NF-κB. In fact resveratrol and curcumin, alone or in combination seem to downregulate the activation of epidermal growth factor receptor (EGFR) and IGFR signalling (Majumdar et al., 2009). The functions of IRS and NF-κB might indeed be linked as shown by Wu SF et al. (2010). They found that IRS2 might activate PI3K/NF-κB in IGF-1-induced proliferative response elicited from breast cancer cells. Besides, curcumin has been shown to induce apoptosis in vitro by concurrent inhibition of the activations of AKT/mTOR and RAF/MEK/ERK pathways (Guo Y et al., 2014). Not less significant is that with the recognition of NF-κB as an important effector in the development of drug resistance, combining curcumin with conventional chemotherapeutic agents or other inhibitors of cell migration and proliferation would be a valuable approach that richly deserves to be explored. The drawbacks of poor solubility and bioavailability of curcumin have prompted a search of analogues of curcumin. UBS109 is one such compound, which seems to suppress NF-κB signalling. It has been shown to inhibit the growth of xenografted HNSCC cells. Plasma concentrations peaked in 30 min at 131 and 248 ng/mL following oral administration of the drug at 50 and 150 mg/kg (Zhu SJ et al., 2014). Although these figures are from animal models, it may be worth considering that curcumin was barely detectable in human subjects who had been administered curcumin at far higher dosages (Klickovic et al., 2014). The overall experience of investigators is that there are no obvious adverse effects even at high doses, but the safety needs further rigorous testing. Liu H et al. (2014) have reported that the biological effects of inhibition of cell proliferation and induction of apoptosis exerted by T63, a new 4-arylidene analogue of curcumin, were far superior to those wielded by curcumin. Meiyanto et al. (2014) have described two further analogues viz. PGV-0 and PGV-1 that enhance the cytotoxicity in vitro of MCF-7 cells exposed to doxorubicin. Of much interest is that these compounds seem to inhibit HER2 function and NF-kB activation, like the parent compound can. In fact curcumin can inhibit both EGFR and HER2 signalling (see Aggarwal et al., 2007). Whether these drugs can be delivered by taking advantage of neural stem cell, brain tropism to HER2+ metastatic lesions in the CNS is worthy of study (see Patil and Sherbet, 2015). It is worth noting here that curcumin also inhibits COX-2 signalling and induces apoptosis by that route. COX-2 promotes tumour progression by supporting cell proliferation, cell survival and the invasive behaviour of tumour. Notably, it activates EMT and the generation and self-renewal of CSCs (pp. 105–108).

IRS SIGNALLING INTERACTS WITH ER/PR AXIS

The analyses carried out some time ago of the topographical expression of IRS2 in breast cancer have revealed some interesting correlation with disease outcome. IRS2 expression in the membrane correlated with decreased overall survival. A suggestion of interactive signalling in the clinical outcome became evident when the PR status of the tumours was taken into reckoning. PR-negative tumours expressing membrane staining of IRS2 showed far worse overall survival (Clark et al., 2011). One would recall that ER/PR status is remarkably predictive of the clinical outcome of breast cancer, with PR counteracting the proliferation promoting effects of ER. That IRS signalling engages in crosstalk with ER/PR signalling axis is not new. Exposure of breast cancer cells expressing ERα induces the translocation of IRS1 to the nucleus and the IRS–ERα complex engages the oestrogen sensitive PS2 promoter and IRS1 appears to influence the ERα function (Morelli et al., 2004). Progesterone is able to regulate IRS2 but not IRS1 (Vassen et al., 1999). Compatible with this, in cells expressing the PR-B isoform, progesterone has been shown to promote IRS2 phosphorylation with associated increase in cell migration but not on cell proliferation or survival. Suppression of PR-B using siRNA suppressed this enhanced cell migration (Ibrahim et al., 2008). An analogous situation occurs in breast cancer. According to Porter et al. (2013), IRS2 levels are low in the early form of breast cancer DCIS (ductal carcinoma in situ) but high in invasive breast cancers and associated with reduced survival. In contrast, IRS1 is expressed at comparable levels in both invasive breast cancer and DCIS. So it would appear quite clearly that cell migration and proliferation do not seem to occur as similar outcomes in the response of cells to progesterone, possibly a consequence of the opposing function of IRS1 and IRS2. Indeed IRS2 itself can functionally generate positive or negative physiological outcomes. Many differences have been noted between IRS1 and IRS2. They differ in their structure and also in the fact that IRS2 interacts with IGFR through a distinct domain, which is absent in IRS1. These could constitute important differences in their signalling function and conferment of signalling specificity (Sawka-Verhelle et al., 1996).

A note of caution would not be out of place here. It is intriguing that IRS2 may be overexpressed in PR-negative breast cancer and indicate poor prognosis, for IRS was shown to be upregulated by progesterone rapidly and only when PR are also present (Vassen et al., 1999). We know that many genes are targeted by progesterone/PR and the PR-A and PR-B receptor isoforms seem to regulate different sets of target genes (Richer et al., 2002). Furthermore, given that PR is inducible by oestrogen, it would be difficult to extrapolate much information from that observation other than merely that the IRS proteins most likely engage in crosstalk with the ER/PR axis. This is presumably one of the reasons why so much controversy has surrounded the clinical value of PR in breast cancer, which is nonetheless shown by recent artificial neural network analyses to be a significant factor in patient management (Caronongan III et al., 2016).

Another important rider has to be inserted here. Progesterone signalling generates its physiological effects by the conventional canonical nuclear receptor (PR) pathway and also by the seven-pass membrane receptor (mPR). The nuclear receptor is a transcription regulator. The rapidity of some responses to progesterone has suggested the presence of extranuclear receptor, such as the membrane-associated mPRs and PGRMC1 (the progesterone receptor membrane component 1). The mPRs are GPCRs belonging to the progestin and adipoQ receptor gene family. The mPRs and PGRMC1s are encoded by different genes. It has been noted that cells seem able to respond to progesterone and produce biological effects via the mPRS and the PGRMC1s even in the absence of PR. Whilst cell proliferative signalling is modulated by them, there is a need to resolve whether mPRs and PGRMC1s work in the same phenotypic direction or exert opposing effects. Nevertheless, the recent developments make it imperative that the non-canonical mode of progesterone signalling is borne in mind while assessing the validity of PR in breast cancer management.

METFORMIN IS A VALUABLE INHIBITOR OF IGFR/IRS FUNCTION

Metformin (dimethylbiguanide, antihyperglycemic drug) used for the treatment of type II diabetes has exhibited demonstrable anti-tumour properties. There is now evidence that this might result from the activation of AMPK and the suppression of the IGFR/IRS1/Akt signalling pathway (Karnevi et al., 2013).

The AMPK is a trimeric kinase composed of the catalytic α subunit and the non-catalytic β and γ subunits, with two genes coding for the α and β subunits and three γ subunit genes (γ1, γ2 and γ3). AMPK functions with many tumour suppressor genes and interacts with several signalling systems including p53, BRCA, Wnt/β-catenin and mTOR. Thus indirectly AMPKs could provide a legitimate route for therapeutic intervention, as would metformin. Metformin is known to activate AMPKs and activation of the latter might involve binding of metformin to the γ-subunit of AMPK (Zhang Y et al., 2012e). The suppressor function of metformin/AMPK on cell proliferation and their ability to promote apoptosis are probably also mediated by other signalling systems. AMPK has been postulated to involve PI3K/Akt pathway and MAPK/p38-ERK signalling. Equally, AMPK might induce apoptosis by inhibiting mTOR signalling. The NF-κB survival pathway has also been brought into the reckoning with the recognition that metformin can inhibit NF-κB (see Sherbet, 2013 for a full discussion and references). Many clinical trials are being conducted to look at the effects of metformin in cell proliferation and apoptosis in colorectal and pancreatic tumour tissues. The outcome of administering metformin in terms of progression and disease free survival is being assessed for many forms of cancer (see https://clinicaltrials.gov).

miRNAs HAVE A ROLE IN IRS FUNCTION

Many miRNAs have been linked with the biological effects of IRS function and have recently received much attention. Zhou Y et al. (2013) reported that IRS1 is a downstream target of miR-126 and that its overexpression downregulated IRS1, together with the inhibition of Akt and ERK1/2 activation. In oral squamous cell carcinoma cells, the expression of miRNA-370 was lower than in corresponding keratinocytes and extraneous miRNA reduced cell migration and cell proliferation and so believed to possess tumour suppressor properties. The inhibitory effects of this miRNA were counteracted by knockdown of IRS1. Hence it has been suggested to be the target of the miRNA (Chang KW et al., 2013). On similar lines is the finding by Giles et al. (2013) who showed that miRNA-7-5p exerted a tumour suppressor function and that IRS2 is the target of this miRNA. Extraneous miRNA-7-5p reduces melanoma cell migration; this appears to be due to the inhibition of Akt signalling via suppression of IRS2. However, as discussed above, the IRSs do exert differential signalling effects and can contribute differently to the physiological outcome.

Much has been written expounding the potential value of miRNAs in the suppression of biological function. MicroRNAs are known to function as tumour promoter or suppressers. However, significant reservations have been expressed not only in identifying miRNAs possessing practical value but also with regard to the identification of their targets. Indeed a single miRNA species can target a multitude of genes and signalling pathways. We have hardly begun to explore the question of the possible specificity of expression, which is undeniably important in attributing specificity of function. To be meaningful in the developmental processes and in cancer progression, one has to see if miRNAs exhibit temporally sequence specific expression. Recent advances in scientific computation may offer means of accurately finding the targets and related physiological and phenotypic events, but nonetheless that is an enormous task.

CHAPTER 4

Angiogenesis in Neoplasia and Anti-Angiogenesis Strategy in the Control of Tumour Growth and Metastasis

ANGIOGENIC SIGNALLING SYSTEMS

The analysis of genetic determinants of biological features and cellular properties associated with one or more traits of cells such as proliferation, invasion, angiogenesis, and epithelial mesenchymal transition and stem cell maintenance and propagation is a major consideration in developing and evolving strategies for control of growth and secondary spread of cancer. From intensive studies of the induction of angiogenesis and increase of vascular permeability associated with tumour growth and progression have emerged distinct and discernible parallels between growth factor-related molecular events and the clinical stage of cancer progression.

Angiogenesis is an important component of many biological processes such as embryonic development, wound healing and chronic inflammation, and also a key participant in tumour growth and secondary spread. The early stage of tumour growth is avascular and so growth of the tumour is restrained. Beyond this, the tumour requires adequate vascularisation, which leads to rapid growth. Therefore the inhibition of angiogenesis is seen as a viable therapeutic strategy. Tumours induce neovascularisation and this possibly occurs as a consequence of signalling by growth factors such as vascular endothelial growth factor (VEGF), fibroblast growth factor (FGF), hepatocyte growth factor and platelet-derived growth factor, among others. They function via the agency of proteoglycans, which tether the growth factors to the membrane and facilitate their binding to their respective receptors. Other angiogenic mediators have also been identified, e.g., plasminogen activators.

VEGF/VEGFR plays a crucial role in the induction of angiogenesis. The VEGF cytokine family is composed of six members with a receptor-binding cystine knot domain, which is highly conserved. The VEGFs bind to and activate their respective receptors and several pathways downstream to transduce their

Molecular Approach to Cancer Management. DOI: http://dx.doi.org/10.1016/B978-0-12-812896-1.00004-0

angiogenic/lymphangiogenic signals. The signal transduced by VEGF/VEGFR culminates in the induction of angiogenesis integrating the regulation of endothelial cell survival, proliferation and migration. VEGF is also able to modulate endothelial cell permeability and barrier function, which might facilitate the diapedesis of tumour cells into the vasculature or extravasation from the vasculature at the metastatic sites (Fig. 4.1). Besides this, the VEGFs synergise with several other angiogenic signalling systems and that could accentuate their phenotypic effects.

The VEGFs function as homodimers and infrequently as heterodimers. VEGFA regulates angiogenesis and is highly mitogenic to vascular endothelial cells. It is a key player in tumour development. VEGFB is thought to be involved in cancer metastasis. VEGFC occurs mainly in the lymphatic endothelium and may be involved in the development of lymphatic vessels. The differences in the phenotypic outcomes of VEGFs arise from the differential activation of the receptors. The activation of VEGFR-1 and VEGFR-2 has been linked with the growth if blood vessels, and VGFR-3 with haemopoiesis and lymphangiogenesis (Iyer and Acharya, 2011).

Whilst inhibition of cell proliferation has gained much importance in the efforts to develop anti-cancer agents, it has been most prudently argued that inhibition of neovascularisation should be accorded equal importance since metastatic spread is the major cause of cancer deaths. Many naturally occurring inhibitors of angiogenesis are known. Interferons inhibit tumour growth as well as angiogenesis. Given that growth factor signalling is mediated by proteoglycans the inhibition of the latter has proved to be a useful strategy as discussed earlier. The use of heparinoids and related compounds to inhibit the heparin-binding growth factors is well documented. Thrombospondin-1 (TSP-1) is a trimeric protein involved in cell adhesion, motility and growth. TSP-1 binds with heparan sulphate mediation to cell surface proteoglycans. It was identified as an inhibitor of angiogenesis some time ago, so also were

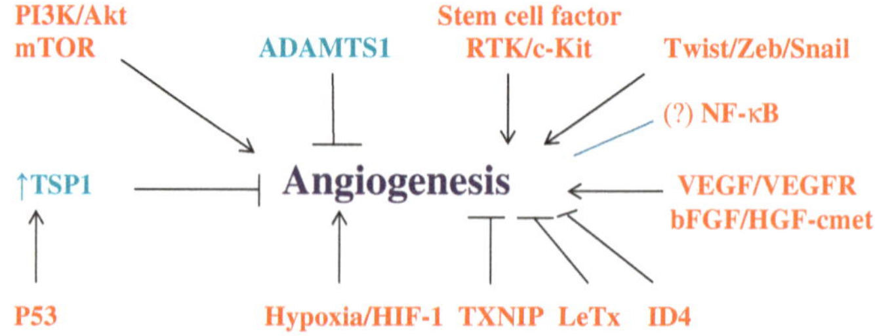

FIGURE 4.1

Some important signalling ligands and the operational pathways involved in the regulation of tumour angiogenesis. The effects of NF-κB on angiogenesis are ambiguous as discussed in the text.

ADAMTS (a disintegrin and metalloproteinase with thrombospondin motifs) proteins which possess thrombospondin repeats.

IS THERE A MOLECULAR SWITCH BETWEEN TUMOUR GROWTH AND ANGIOGENESIS?

Neovascularisation is essential for providing and maintaining an adequate supply of oxygen and nutrients for tumour growth as well as for eliminating metabolic waste products. The interior of the tumour becomes hypoxic and is deprived of nutrients and this leads to apoptosis and necrosis. The crux of the question is whether besides these environmental factors there are molecular links between tumour growth and metastasis. Interestingly there might be a link between the heterogeneous cellular elements of the tumour and their interaction with the tumour microenvironment of stromal and the extracellular matrix (ECM) components. This is an apparent provision of a switch to the initiation of angiogenesis. A case in point is basic fibroblast growth factor (bFGF) (FGF2) and the induction of angiogenesis. bFGF is synthesised by fibroblasts an endothelial cells and is found in the endothelial basement membrane and the sub-endothelial ECM. The suppressor gene p53 inhibits bFGF-mediated angiogenesis believed to be by upregulating the expression of TSP-1, synthesised by endothelial cells and fibroblasts. P53 is mutated or lost in a majority of tumours and this could result not only in loss of growth control and also allow angiogenesis to occur. In other words the link-up of the loss of control of tumour growth with a switch to the vascular phase of growth may turn out to be an important event in tumour progression. It would be in order to balance this with the view that the transcription factor NF-κB can suppress angiogenesis. This is based on reports of enhanced tumour-associated vascularisation under conditions where NF-κB is suppressed. It has also been suggested that it might protect endothelial cell integrity. If this were the case, it would be expected to inhibit metastatic dissemination. But then, it has been documented that inhibition of NF-κB inhibits tumour growth and metastasis. Also, non-steroidal anti-inflammatory drugs inhibit NF-κB and this could be read with the tumour preventive and metastasis inhibitory ability imputed to these drugs.

One does not need to dig deep to find a switch, possibly one of many switches. The transcription factor HIF-1 (hypoxia-inducible factor) targets the genes that regulate cell proliferation, angiogenesis and metastasis. However, HIF-1 can activate the expression of genes that are productive as well as counter-productive of tumour growth and progression. It can activate genes that suppress cell proliferation and also those that can promote proliferation and survival of cells. HIF-1 can induce cell motility and invasion, and promote angiogenesis and metastasis. The cell proliferation suppressor effects such as those engendered by the upregulation of the tumour suppressor gene NDRG1 (N-myc downstream-regulated gene-1) could be countermanded by the activation of genes that promote cell proliferation and survival, invasion, and angiogenesis to drive tumour progression. This can occur by a shift of the balance of opposing gene function or by a switch from counter-productive to the productive forces of tumour progression. Hypoxic conditions can operate such as a switch. As stated later, in hypoxic situations VHL (von Hippel–Lindau tumour-suppressor protein) is inactivated and HIF-1α is stabilised, accumulates and induces angiogenesis. Many ambient molecular factors can activate HIF-1. IGF is able to do that (Sutton et al., 2007) and promote angiogenesis; so can CTGF (connective tissue growth factor) activate HIF-1/VEGF and induce angiogenesis. EGF can induce HIF-1 expression and downregulate E-cadherin and in this way promote invasion (Cheng JC et al., 2013). HIF-1 can activate TGF-α and promote cell survival (Gunaratnam et al., 2003) (see further discussion below). Equally, there is a thought that HIF-1α can induce cell cycle arrest quite independently of its conventional mode of function.

ABERRANT PI3K/Akt/mTOR SIGNALLING IN CANCER

Many signalling pathways are involved in the induction of angiogenesis. These transduce angiogenic signals that integrate the function of growth factors, transcription factors and inhibitors of angiogenesis (Fig. 4.2). The mammalian target of rapamycin (mTOR) signalling pathway is pre-eminently associated with several cellular processes such as cell proliferation, growth, apoptosis, angiogenesis, cell motility and invasion. The activation of PI3K/Akt leads to the phosphorylation of mTOR. This then phosphorylates the downstream targets p70S6K and 4EBP leading in turn to cell proliferation. Aberrant PI3K/Akt/mTOR signalling features prominently in a number of human tumours. The mTOR signalling pathway is closely involved in the function of many growth factor receptors including VEGF/VEGFR. Much evidence has accumulated indicating that angiogenesis might be regulated by mTOR signalling. Inhibiting this pathway effectively suppresses angiogenesis and many inhibitors of mTOR that suppress VEGF and angiogenesis and invasion have been identified. The mTORC2 complex mediates the phosphorylation of serine-473 of Akt. Inhibitors such as PP242 inhibit both mTORC1 and mTORC2. PP242 [2-(4-amino-1-isopropyl-1H-pyrazolo[3,4-d]pyrimidin-3-yl)-1H-indol-5-ol] is a permeable pyrazolopyrimidine compound, which is a ATP-competitive reversible inhibitor of mTORC1 and mTORC2 (see Apsel et al., 2008; Feldman et al., 2009; Hsieh AC et al., 2010; Hoang B et al., 2010). PP242 inhibits cell proliferation and migration and

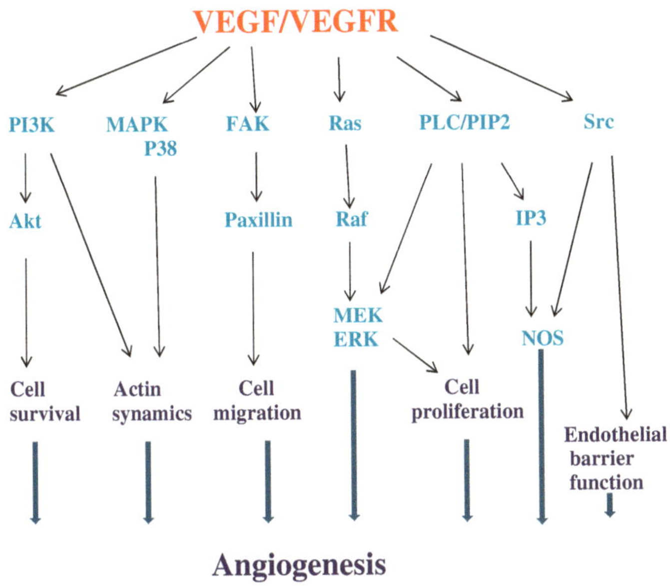

FIGURE 4.2

Pathways to angiogenesis activated by VEGF/VEGFR regulating cell proliferation, motility, endothelial barrier function possibly also including diapedesis of tumour cells, and actin dynamics.

tubule formation in vitro of human umbilical endothelial cells. It downregulates the expression of VEGF. Furthermore, extraneous VEGF counteracts the inhibitory effects of PP242 and temsirolimus. Concomitantly, the inhibitory effects have extended to suppression of PI3K/mTOR pathway (Xing XF et al., 2014; Zeng Z et al., 2012). According to Zeng Z et al. (2012), PP242 may be more effective than rapamycin in inhibiting leukaemic cells.

Many PI3K and PI3K/mTOR dual inhibitors have been assessed in clinical trials. The PI3K/mTOR dual inhibitor SAR245409 is being tested in advanced metastatic disease. Their combination with MEK inhibitors is also under study. Other candidates for PI3K/mTOR inhibition are VS-5584 and PF-05212384. Efforts are underway to check the effects of combining PI3K and PI3K/mTOR inhibitors, viz. BKM120 and BEZ235, respectively. But BEZ235 has been withdrawn from the market. Needless it is to say that many chemotherapy drugs are also being investigated in combination with mTOR inhibitors (see https://clinicaltrials.gov). As discussed in another location, the rapamycin derivative everolimus has been studied extensively on account of its ability to suppress tumour growth and inhibit angiogenesis.

An interesting study involves combination of everolimus, octreotide and metformin. One would recall that octreotide is cyclic octapeptide mimic of somatostatin and functions by binding to somatostatin receptors. It has been reported to show marked inhibition of tumour growth and to prolong the time to progression in a clinical trial of a series of patients with metastatic neuroendocrine tumours (Rinke et al., 2009). This might turn out to be significant since metformin itself has important anti-cancer properties.

HIF MEDIATED REGULATION OF ANGIOGENESIS

Hypoxia is a major regulator of angiogenesis. HIF-1α is a transcription regulator in hypoxia. Hypoxia regulates the expression of several genes including VEGF through the mediation of HIF-1. Hypoxia signals are transduced through the activation of growth factor RTK/PI3K/ PTEN/Akt and mTOR to the downstream phosphorylation of S6K1/EBP1 leading to HIF-1α expression. Some isoforms of protein kinase C may also be involved in the regulation of HIF-1 expression. HIF-1α is recognised and degraded by VHL, which is a component of the E3 ubiquitin ligase complex. The VHL gene is inactivated or lost in some tumours such as renal cell carcinoma. In hypoxic situations VHL is inactivated and HIF-1α is stabilised and accumulates. This then can activate VEGF to induce angiogenesis and the production of TGF-α and promote cell survival (Pantuck et al., 2003). Thus the VHL/HIF-1/VEGF axis would be closely linked with the progression of tumours to the metastatic state.

The ADAM proteins are Zn-dependent metalloproteinases, which release the extracellular domains of membrane-bound growth factors, cytokines and their receptors. The ADAMs have been ascribed a potential role in angiogenesis on account of their presence in endothelial cells. Inhibition of ADAMs inhibits endothelial cell migration and adhesion in vitro. The inhibition of EGFR using RTK inhibitors and the inhibition of ADAM-17 effectively block EGFR activation and downstream signalling. This suppresses endothelial cell proliferation, invasion and angiogenesis (see Sherbet, 2011a). It would be relevant to state here that HIF-1α activation and the expression of some ADAMs may be closely linked. Indeed, there is much interaction between the HIF-1α/ADAM signalling axis and some growth factors, which could influence tumour invasion, angiogenesis and metastasis.

CHAPTER 5

On the Trail of TRAIL (TNF-Related Apoptosis Inducing Ligand) in Tumour Growth and Angiogenesis

The growth of normal as well as neoplastic tissues is regulated by apoptosis. The induction of apoptosis has been used as a device for developing anti-cancer chemotherapeutic agents. Initiation of apoptosis can follow two pathways. One is the intrinsic mitochondrial pathway wherein DNA damage and other stress factors induce apoptosis. The second pathway is activated by extrinsic signals, which involve the function of death receptors located at the cell surface. Both the intrinsic and extrinsic pathways implicate caspases as the major participants of the apoptosis process. The death receptor pathway invokes the intervention of the Bcl family genes Bax/Bak/Bcl-2, which can involve regulation by p53.

TRAIL SIGNALLING TO APOPTOSIS

The death receptors are activated by the binding of specific ligands such as tumour necrosis factor (TNF), the Fas ligand of the TNF family and TRAIL (TNF-related apoptosis inducing ligand). TNF is a pro-inflammatory cytokine, which functions by binding to its receptors TNFR1 and TNFR2. TNFR1 occurs on cell surfaces and binds to soluble TNF-α, whilst TNFR2 that binds the transmembrane TNF-α shows more restricted presence on hematopoietic cells. TNFR1 that carries the death domain (DD) activates AP1, MAPK and NF-kB pathways involved in the activation of pro-inflammatory responses but induces apoptosis. The signalling by TNFR2 is less well understood and it is thought to enhance the induction of apoptosis by TNFR1. The discussion here is dedicated by design to the role of TNFR/TRAIL signalling (Fig. 5.1). The transduction of the apoptosis signal occurs via TNFR/TRADD (TNFR-associated DD) or Fas receptor (CD95) leading to the activation of caspases via FADD (Fas-associated protein with DD). TRADD can function via TRAF2 (TNF-associated factor 2) towards cell survival by NF-κB or via JNK signalling towards apoptosis (see Sherbet, 2011a). Both the intrinsic and death receptor pathways meet downstream at the initiation of the so-called executioner

Molecular Approach to Cancer Management. DOI: http://dx.doi.org/10.1016/B978-0-12-812896-1.00005-2

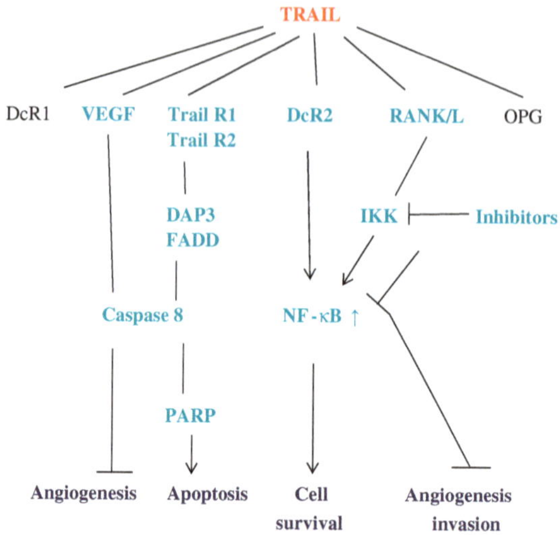

FIGURE 5.1

The induction of apoptosis by the TRAIL and death receptor pathway.
DAP3, death associated protein 3; DcR1, Trail R3 decoy receptor; DcR2, decoy receptor 2/Trail R4; FADD, Fas-associated protein with DD; IKK, IKappaB complex (subunits IKKα and IKKβ); OPG, osteoprotegerin decoy receptor; PARP, poly(ADP-ribose) polymerase involved in DNA repair and programmed cell death; RANK, receptor activator of NF-κB; TRAIL, TNF-related apoptosis inducing ligand; Trail R1, Trail receptor 1 (DR4); Trail R2, Trail receptor 2 (DR5).

caspases (caspase-3, caspase-6 and caspase-7). Apoptosis is negatively regulated by Akt as discussed at several other locations. The Akt function is in turn negatively regulated by PTEN. The PTEN/Akt pathways also involve the participation of TRAIL and the death receptors (see discussion later).

TRAIL activates the death receptors DR4 (Trail R1) and DR5 (Trail R2) containing the DD. They are proficient inducer of apoptosis. These receptors form multimeric complexes, which recruit FADD and this is followed by recruitment and activation of the caspase cascade to induce apoptosis. DcR1, DcR2 and osteoprotegerin decoy receptor (OPG) are called decoy receptors, which can bind to TRAIL but cannot induce apoptosis. The binding of TRAIL to DcR2 can in some circumstances activate the NF-κB pathway and promote cell survival and inflammation in this way mitigating the apoptosis inducing effect of DR4 and DR5. There are suggestions that RANK/RANKL (receptor activator of nuclear factor kappa-B/ligand) is able to initiate NF-κB signalling by activating IKK (IκB kinase) and promote angiogenesis. NF-κB proteins are bound and inhibited by IκB proteins. IKK phosphorylates and leads to the degradation of the inhibitory IκB and to the activation of NF-κB. So inhibition of IKK would inhibit the NF-κB-mediated path to angiogenesis. Indeed IKK is considered as a therapeutic target and small molecule inhibitors of IKK are being devised. In fact TRAIL is a robust regulator of the immune system, cell proliferation and apoptosis and angiogenesis, but resistance to TRAIL has impeded its deployment as a therapeutic strategy. Although one can identify several links in TRAIL signalling that can go functionally awry and lead to resistance, IKK inhibition could be an added asset for overcoming the resistance.

The importance of trailing the TRAIL is unambiguously emphasised by its ability to suppress angiogenesis. Na JH et al. (2014) were able to show that TRAIL inhibited VEGF-induced angiogenesis in vitro and in vivo vascularisation using chick embryo and murine models. It also inhibited cell proliferation, actin dynamics and cell motility and endothelial barrier function. The view that TRAIL might inhibit the diapedesis of tumour cells is debatable and not too well defined at present. Indeed TRAIL may enhance vascular permeability by inducing NO production by the endothelium. Also to be considered here is that PI3K activation can counter TRAIL-induced apoptosis and PI3K can also enhance endothelial permeability. Cain et al. (2010) were able to show that the catalytic subunit p110α of PI3K increased TNF-induced permeability. Anyhow, it increased caspase-8 activity and led the cells to apoptosis but suppressed angiogenesis independently of the caspase cascade. It is noteworthy that besides activating the several pathways that integrate the regulation of the many features of angiogenesis, VEGFs synergise with several other angiogenic signalling systems and this could accentuate their canonical signalling effects (see Figs 4.1 and 4.2).

TRAIL AND TUMOUR INHIBITION

TRAIL and the death receptors have long been regarded as potential targets. Most forms of interference with TRAIL signalling have resulted in tumour inhibition. In the past few years, many studies have used recombinant TRAIL to induce apoptosis. There has been a general recognition that agonistic monoclonal DR4 and DR5 antibodies might be more efficient than recombinant TRAIL in the induction of apoptosis. This may be partly due to the presence of decoy receptors diverting the function of TRAIL. Many studies are on record showing the highly effective inhibition of human tumours xenografts. Some time ago, Rahman et al. (2009) reported that TRAIL was able to induce apoptosis in some triple negative breast cancer cell lines and that only the cell lines that displayed the epithelial mesenchymal transition phenotype were sensitive, but the cells with epithelial characteristics were not susceptible to the induction of apoptosis. Earlier, Buchsbaum et al. (2003) had found that the DR5 agonistic monoclonal TRA-8 antibody, was cytotoxic to many of the breast cancer cell lines which they tested. Also it produced significant growth inhibition of breast cancer cell xenografts. Combinations of the agonist antibodies with conventional anti-cancer agents have been studied intensively. The DNA intercalating anthracycline doxorubicin, inhibitors of DNA synthesis such as gemcitabine, and the anti-mitotic microtubule stabiliser paclitaxel have been tested in combination with the agonist antibodies. The combinations have produced more pronounced growth inhibition than when they were used as single agents. There is much promise in the finding that the combined use of the DR5 agonist tigatuzumab and gemcitabine has been highly effective against pancreatic cancer stem cells (CSCs) and tumour cells (Rajeshkumar et al., 2010). This should be read in the light of the thinking that attributes the resistance to gemcitabine to CSCs.

MANIPULATION OF DEATH RECEPTOR EXPRESSION TO TARGET TUMOUR GROWTH

Whether this question can be addressed by manipulating the signalling systems involved in TRAIL function and whether the expression and activation of the receptors can be modified by manoeuvring one or more salient systems regulating cell proliferation and apoptosis has also been addressed. Apart from agonistic antibodies, it might be worthwhile looking for agents and cell proliferation-related signalling systems and their activators for upregulating the expression of the death receptors. As noted in another location, plumbagin not only controls the size of the cell population by negative regulation of the PI3K/Akt pathway and induces apoptosis, but it enhances TRAIL and DR4 and DR5 expression (Sun J and McKallip, 2011). The inactivation of PTEN with consequent-activated Akt and cell proliferation has been linked with resistance to TRAIL (Dida et al., 2008). By similar reckoning, one would expect that inappropriate activation of receptor tyrosine kinases (RTKs) would result in or potentiate TRAIL resistance and therefore might possess the potential to modulate the expression of the death receptors. Among RTKs associated with TRAIL resistance are growth factor RTKs, IGFR, c-met, etc. In fact many RTK inhibitors have been found to synergise with death receptor agonists and also sensitise the resistant cells to TRAIL-mediated apoptosis. Of considerable interest in hindsight is that inhibition of HER2 signalling increased TRAIL-induced cytotoxicity. This was reported several years ago by Kim KM and Lee (2005) without eliciting much curiosity or raising awareness of the potential significance of the finding.

Ras signalling has been implicated in the regulation of the expression of death receptors. It may be recalled here that activated Ras induces the Rafkinases to phosphorylate and activate the downstream protein kinase cascade. This culminates in the inhibition of apoptosis, induction of cell proliferation and also in drug resistance. The opposite view has been aired that the activation of Raf/MEK/ERK inhibits cell proliferation and induces apoptosis.

There are too many conflicting claims concerning Ras involvement in death receptor expression and both lines of the argument have implicated their involvement. Also, Ras signalling has been imputed with TRAIL resistance observed in some cell lines. The conflicting findings would require further elucidation of the role of Ras signalling in death receptor-induced apoptosis, so much so that the expression of these receptors would need more intensive pre-clinical studies before firm conclusions can be drawn concerning their deployment of as anti-cancer devices.

THE COX-2 LINK TO DEATH RECEPTOR FUNCTION

The isoform COX-2 (cyclooxygenase-2) is a powerful promoter of tumour progression. It supports cell proliferation, cell survival and the invasive behaviour of tumour. Whilst it is an important regulator of the cell cycle, the control exerted by COX-2 over the size of the cell population and indeed tumour growth emanates from its suppressive influence on apoptosis. COX inhibitors are known for their effects on the inhibition of cell migration and invasion, and their anti-angiogenic properties, and not least for their proficiency to promote apoptosis. COX-2 inhibitors have been employed for investigation of the possible involvement of death receptor. Liu X (2004) demonstrated over a decade ago that the small molecule selective COX-2 inhibitor celecoxib, which is putatively linked with cancer prevention, induced the expression of DR5 accompanied by the induction of the caspase cascade and apoptosis. Apoptosis was accentuated when celecoxib was combined with TRAIL. Some provisional clinical studies have indicated improvement in the response of patients with advanced NSCLC when celecoxib was combined with chemotherapy (Hou LC et al., 2016). Combination of celecoxib with other agents has offered some additional thoughts for the future of this compound.

CLINICAL CONSIDERATIONS

Many clinical trials are being carried out to assess the anti-tumour activity of recombinant TRAIL and agonistic antibodies to the death receptors. Some effort has also been directed to the manipulation of signalling systems such as the Ras/RAF/BRAF/MAPK cascade to enhance death receptor-induced apoptosis, but these have not produced tangible or unequivocal results. The potential of manipulating some signalling pathways to modify death receptor expression to target tumour growth has been discussed earlier, where one can see possible growth areas. Some of the interesting work, such as the upregulation of death receptor expression by HDAC (histone deacetylase) inhibitors (Insinga et al., 2005), has not been pursued although HDAC inhibitors have found favour in clinical trials (see also pp. 108–112 for further discussions of COX-2 inhibitors for the inhibition of angiogenesis).

CHAPTER 6

Hedgehog (Hh) Signalling in EMT (Epithelial Mesenchyme Transition), CSCs (Cancer Stem Cells) and Angiogenesis

Hedgehog (Hh) is signalling pathway of embryogenesis. It is also known to markedly influence the developmental pathway of epithelial mesenchyme transition (EMT) activation and signalling. EMT activation and the acquisition of cancer stem cell (CSC) characteristics are closely connected phenomena. Inappropriate functions of some important elements in the Hh signalling cascade and erratic functioning of the effector transcription factors have led to tumorigenesis, the inhibition of apoptosis and aberrant angiogenesis contributing in this way to the growth and metastasis of tumours. Given that Hh is activated in many forms of cancer and that high Hh expression has correlated with aggressive cancers with enhanced tumour vascularisation and metastatic spread, it follows that inhibition of Hh signalling might provide a practical path to the inhibition of CSC formation, expansion and maintenance. The highly tumorigenic subpopulation of cells characterised by the expression of CD44+/CD24+/ESA+ (epithelial specific antigen) has been found in many tumour types, although differences have also been encountered in the antigens expressed and the patterns of their expression. It may be that the defining features of CSCs might in some way are related to the histogenetic origin of the tumours (Sherbet, 2013). The CSCs of pancreatic tumours not only express these antigens but also show greatly upregulated expression of Sonic Hedgehog (Shh) as compared with normal epithelial cells. The CSCs also exhibit the characteristic feature of drug and radiation resistance. This has been correlated with enhanced tumour recurrence (Fillmore and Kuperwasser, 2008). Besides, a demonstrable link also exists between CSCs, their ability to induce aggressive tumour, and to the induction of angiogenesis (Fantozzi et al., 2014). Hence the involvement of Hh in shaping the expansion and perpetuation of CSCs has been accorded much prominence in the identification and development of drugs to inhibit Hh signalling to prevent tumour initiation, development and dissemination.

Molecular Approach to Cancer Management. DOI: http://dx.doi.org/10.1016/B978-0-12-812896-1.00006-4

THE HEDGEHOG SIGNALLING SYSTEM

The Hh family is composed of proteins called Shh, Indian Hh (Ihh) and Desert Hh (Dhh). These protein ligands bind to the 12-pass trans-membrane receptor, PTCH1 (PATCHED). The other major elements of the Hh signalling cascade are the 7-pass G-protein coupled receptors SMO (smoothened) of the Frizzled family of receptors and the effector protein Gli1. PTCH regulates SMO activity. Hh binds to PTCH and in this bound state SMO is able to activate the Kruppel family of zinc finger transcription factor Gli1. When Hh is not present, PTCH suppresses SMO and Gli1 is not activated. SMO functions through an intracellular protein complex composed of Cos2, the protein kinase Fused and the transcription factor the full-length Ci155 (Cubitus interruptus). When unbound, PTCH inhibits SMO and this leads to the cleavage of the full-length Ci155 to a truncated Ci75 repressor form. When PTCH is bound by Hh, SMO prevents the cleavage of Ci155 into the repressor form. This allows the transduction of downstream Hh signalling (Fig. 6.1). This represents the canonical signalling system. The non-canonical mode of signalling occurs with or without the mediation of SMO. SMO can function through the agency of PI3l/Akt and activate Gli. In another non-canonical route, PTCH can signal without SMO intervention via Rho/Rac GTPase and alter cytoskeletal dynamics and influence many phenotypic attributes such as cell migration (Fig. 6.2) (see Sherbet, 2013 for review and references).

POTENTIAL THERAPEUTIC TARGETS IN Hh SIGNALLING

There are clear choices for consideration to target and control Hh signalling. Hh signalling can be potentially controlled at several levels, such as the Hh ligand binding, PTCH, SMO and SUFU (suppressor of Fused) which negatively regulates Hh and Gli. The many suggested inhibitors are shown in Table 6.1. Some have been investigated in much detail and much effort has been expended to employ them strategically to inhibit Hh signalling.

SUFU negatively regulates Hh. It binds to the Gli transcription factors and regulates their expression and function. It is markedly downregulated in some tumours and this has correlated with high tumour grade and poor prognosis.

Hh INHIBITORS AND CLINICAL OUTCOME

Much interest has focused around the SMO inhibitors LDE225/sonidegib and GDC-0449 (vismodegib), which have FDA approval. Many clinical trials

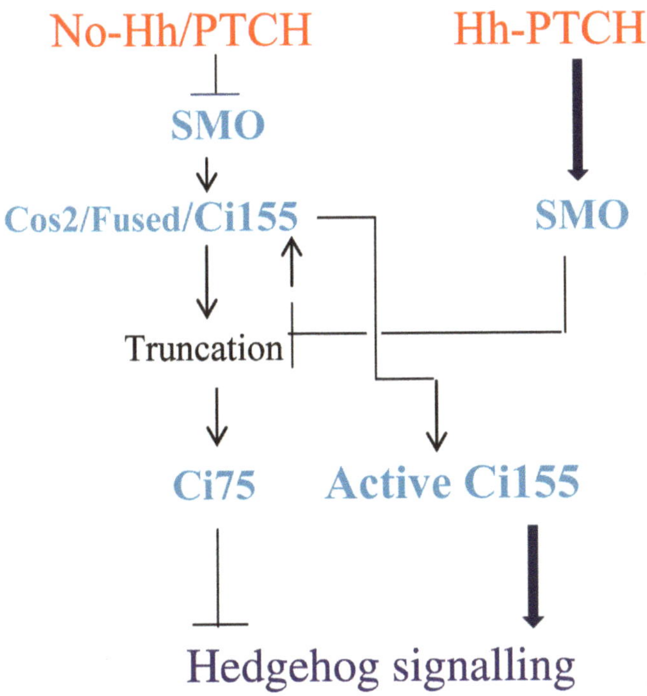

FIGURE 6.1
The mechanism of regulation of Hh signal transduction by PTCH and SMO. In the unbound state PTCH suppresses SMO. This results in the truncation of Ci155 to the suppressor Ci75. When bound to Hh, SMO is able to suppress the process of truncation so that the active form of Ci155 transduces the Hh signal downstream to the target genes. Inappropriate functioning of PTCH, SMO and Gli transcription factors would obviously lead to tumorigenesis by inhibiting apoptosis, promoting angiogenesis and in this way contribute to the growth and metastasis of tumours.

are also in hand. It is encouraging that GDC-0449 inhibits pancreatic CSCs (Singh et al., 2011), but clinical trials of patients with advanced pancreatic cancer have shown no improvement in objective response either complete or partial, progression free survival (PFS) and overall survival rates. Similarly the outcome is not encouraging in studies of other forms of cancer. In contrast, patients with basal cell carcinoma (BCC) have shown good objective responses in metastatic and locally advanced carcinomas. Another study has recorded high histological clearance rates. Adult medulloblastomas seem to be less responsive than BCC as judged from the objective response rates (see https://clinicaltrials.gov).

Cyclopamine, a naturally occurring alkaloid, was identified some time ago as an inhibitor of Hh signalling and suppressed SMO. Cyclopamine and the 5E1 antibody against Shh not only suppressed tumour growth but also

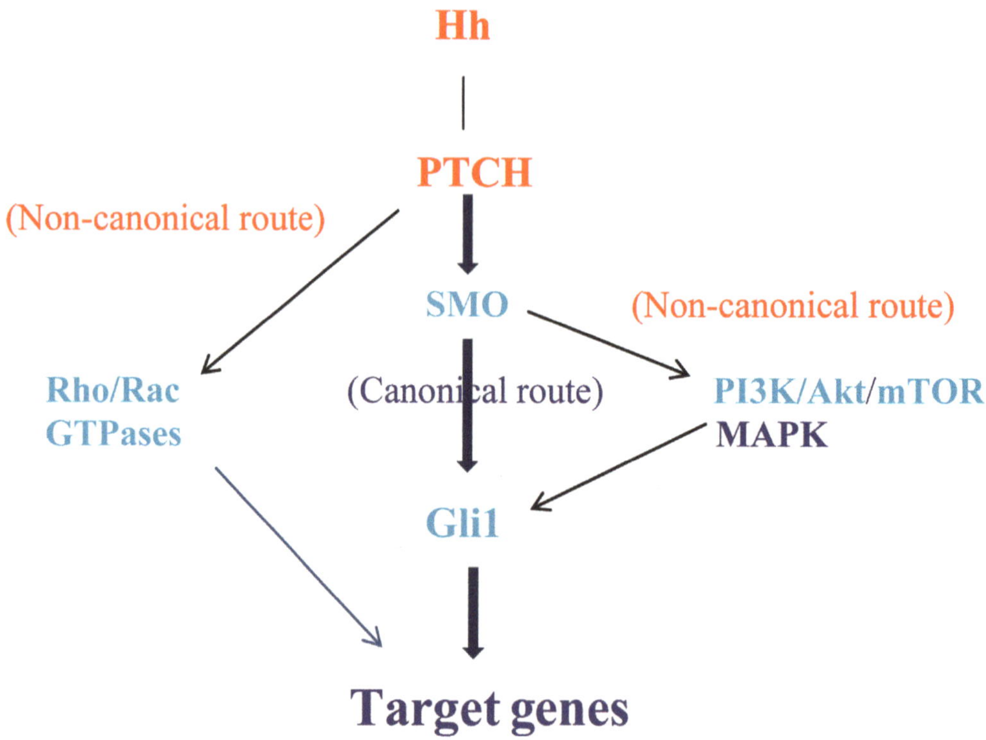

FIGURE 6.2
The canonical path and the non-canonical SMO-dependent and SMO-independent signalling routes of Hh.

Table 6.1 Inhibitors of Hh Signalling

Target Focus	Inhibitors
Hh ligand antagonists	5E1 antibody[a]; robotnikinin, BRD-6851[b]; GK 03795[c]
SMO	Cyclopamine, SANT1,[d,e] GDC-0449, IPI-926, Cur-61414[e]
Gli	Gant58 and Gant61

[a]*El Khatib et al. (2013).*
[b]*Dockendorff et al. (2012).*
[c]*Hwang S et al. (2011).*
[d]*Wickstrom et al. (2013).*
[e]*Stanton and Peng (2010).*

promoted the reverse process of EMT, i.e., the transition of cells to the epithelial phenotype by mesenchyme to epithelial transition (MET) (El Khatib et al., 2013). Qualtrough et al. (2015) have confirmed the initiation of MET. They showed that cyclopamine enhanced E-cadherin expression and downregulated the expression of the EMT-associated transcription factors Slug, Snail and Twist. These changes were paralleled by the inhibition of cell migration. Besides this, the promotion and maintenance of CSCs by Hh are also hampered by cyclopamine (Batsaikhan et al., 2014). It is well documented that this steroidal alkaloid enhances radiosensitivity and alleviates chemoresistance, which can be viewed as compatible with the loss or reduction of the CSC subpopulation. Cyclopamine has not attracted much clinical interest largely because it is a teratogenic alkaloid.

The SMO inhibitor IPI-926 is another small molecule inhibitor that has been the subject of much investigation. IPI-926 is a cyclopamine analogue (Tremblay et al., 2009), which was found to be highly effective in suppressing medulloblastoma and pancreatic tumour models. IPI-926 was later shown to be an inhibitor of SMO. Subsequent preclinical work using IPI-926 generated some optimism but this has not been borne out by clinical studies. An early investigation involving both BCC and non-BCC solid tumours supported the ground for optimism. For in the non-BCC group, stable disease was noted in 53% of 55 patients. In the BCC group, 8/28 evaluable patients achieved an objective response, 2 complete and 6 partial responses. The responses were seen in patients with locally advanced disease (Jimeno et al., 2013). BCCs are characterised by high incidence of mutations in PTCH and SMO and so they would be amenable to the treatment.

Anti-tumour activity has been noted in patients with recurrent/metastatic HNSCC (head and neck squamous cell carcinoma) administered IPI-926 after initial administration of the epidermal growth factor receptor (EGFR) inhibitor cetuximab (Bowles et al., 2016). The results were not encouraging, neither was the outcome of a phase II study in patients with myelofibrosis (Sasaki et al., 2015). Furthermore, some uncertainty has surrounded the use of IPI-926, although one phase I clinical study showed high objective response in patients with advanced pancreatic adenocarcinoma who had been given IPI-926 with FOLFIRINOX (a combination of folinic acid, 5-FU, the topoisomerase inhibitor irinotecan and oxaliplatin) and the positive effects continued even after FOLFIRINOX was discontinued. However, this study was stopped after other combinations produced adverse effects (Ko AH et al., 2016).

High expression of PTCH has been noted to reflect the potential of hepatocellular carcinoma to recur after resection. PTCH expression correlated with tumour size and TNM (tumour node metastasis) stage. But the correlation did not extend significantly to the expression of Gli (Jeng KS et al., 2013). Gant61 (2,2′-[[dihydro-2-(4-pyridinyl)-1,3(2H,4H)-pyrimidinediyl] *bis*(methylene)]bis[*N*,*N*-dimethylbenzenamine]) is a small molecule inhibitor of Gli transcription factors. Gant61 inhibits cell proliferation, induces apoptosis and suppresses cells exhibiting CSC markers thus contributing overall to tumour suppression. Gant58 (2,3,4,5-tetra(4-pyridyl)thiophene) is biologically as effective as Gant61 or perhaps even more so since it is able to inhibit PTCH, Gli and SMO.

Salinomycin has been imputed with the ability to suppress Hh signalling by downregulating PTCH, SMO and Gli. One would recall in this context that salinomycin-induced inhibition of proliferation has corresponded with the loss of CSCs in many tumour types. In vivo tumour growth in murine models has paralleled downregulated expression of genes associated with the CSC phenotype.

THE INTERLOCUTION OF Hh AND OTHER SIGNALLING SYSTEMS

This perceived ineffectiveness of the inhibition of Hh signalling has given rise to misgivings about the significance of the canonical path of Hh signalling. This has shifted the attention to the non-canonical pathways of activation of Gli involving K-Ras, c-myc, growth factors and Wnt/β-catenin, all equally capable of transducing signals that impinge upon tumour cell motility, tumour growth and spread, including the activation of Hh. So crosstalk between Hh and the non-canonical signalling systems would entangle the outcome. Equally, this could offer practical opportunities for combination therapy. This line of thought subsumes the refractoriness to chemo and radiotherapy that is often encountered in the environment of inappropriate Hh activation. This could be a consequence of the loss of integrity of the DNA damage response and repair with which the Gli transcription factors are closely involved (Mazumdar et al., 2011; Palle et al., 2015). Nevertheless, DNA damage response and repair cannot be totally dissociated from canonical Hh signalling. Arsenic trioxide is known to produce DNA damage via the generation of reactive oxygen species. It suppresses Gli and downregulates the expression of PTCH (Nakamura et al., 2013). In other words, the suppression of Hh signalling has links with DNA damage and response.

It is worthy of note that not only is there crosstalk between canonical Hh signalling and signalling by growth factors and mTOR but that this might also be integrated with the non-canonical signalling. This in essence means that even in circumstances where the inhibitors of Hh are found wanting or resistance to these inhibitors develops on account of prolonged exposure, the option would be open for the use of inhibitors of the interacting systems. Thus one can envision the integration Hh signalling with that of growth factors such as the EGF, fibroblast growth factor (FGF) and transforming growth factor (TGF)-β family members and Wnt family proteins.

Hh is said to be able to activate EGFR. Reciprocally, EGFR can influence Gli-mediated transcription of target genes by activating the Raf/MEK/ERK pathway. The signalling by TGF-β family and retinoids converges with the Hh pathway and this would profoundly influence differentiation, pattern formation, invasion and angiogenesis, and DNA replication and repair processes (Sherbet, 2011a, 2013). This wide spectrum of interaction can indeed provide vast opportunities to produce additive or synergistic outcomes to Hh inhibitors.

Active Hh signalling may operate in circumstance where inappropriate activation of EGFR signalling has occurred. The activation of EMT apparently induced by EGFR signalling could occur via Gli1. Equally, EMT and CSC generation may take place with the mediation of FOXO Forkhead box, Sox2, Sp1 and Sp3 transcription factors. However, often the arguments presented for this are somewhat indirect and convoluted. EGF does promote invasive behaviour and this is accompanied by a change from epithelial to mesenchymal morphology. The expression of EMT markers in this morphological alteration is not defined, but indeed the induction of invasive behaviour can be blocked by inhibiting Gli1. More positive evidence has been presented in this regard. HNSCC cells can exhibit EMT activation independently of or dependent upon EGFR and in both circumstances Hh is seen to function as a regulator. The EGFR inhibitor cetuximab and the Hh inhibitior IPI-926 suppress EGFR-dependent EMT (Keysar et al., 2013). Activation of Hh signalling has been found to counteract and reduce the resistance to inhibitors of EGFR signalling (Keysar et al., 2013; Della Corte et al., 2015). In fact, it is possible that Hh and EGFR signalling might mutually regulate each other. There is room for the interpretation of some of these findings from the mutual regulation angle.

An example of the non-canonical interaction between Hh and mTOR is the promotion of Gli transcription upon activation of the mTOR pathway. The downstream effector S6K1, which phosphorylates Gli, releases it from SUFU-mediated inhibition. It would be recalled that SUFU negatively regulates Hh by binding to the Gli transcription factors and regulating their expression and function. Synergistic effect of mTOR and Hh inhibitors has been reported not infrequently. These need to be read with the opposite view that S6K1 does not affect Gli1 activity. Nevertheless, since SMO can activate the PI3K/Akt/MAPK pathway, this might bypass mTOR. So in the activation of non-canonical Hh signalling, one can visualise the prospect of the synergistic use of PI3K/mTOR and Hh inhibitors.

HEDGEHOG IS INVOLVED IN ANGIOGENIC SIGNALLING BY ANGIOPOIETIN-1

In the wide spectrum of signalling mechanisms by which Hh advances cancer progression is the promotion of angiogenesis via the angiopoietin route.

Many tumour types show concurrently upregulated activation of Hh signalling and expression of Ang-1 (angiopoietin-1) and Ang-1-like proteins. This frequently occurs with the detrimental downregulation of angiopoietin-2 (Ang-2), which is thought to negatively regulate angiogenesis. Both angiopoietins bind to the endothelial receptor Tie-2. The interaction of Ang-1 with Tie-2 leads to angiogenesis. However, there is a large body of evidence that Ang-2 can promote angiogenesis independently of Tie-2 but by an alternative pathway mediated by integrin/FAK (focal adhesion kinase) (see discussion later). Here attempted is an exploration of the status of the regulators of angiogenesis and the influence of Hh on this regulation in the context of cancer progression to the metastatic state. The angiopoietin-like (ANGPL) proteins are structurally similar to angiopoietins. Several of these proteins have been identified. They display a wide range of biological activities including angiogenesis and widely implicated in the pathogenesis of cancer.

The Regulation of Angiogenesis by Angiopoietins

The angiopoietins and ANGPL proteins are important regulators of angiogenesis. Many aggressive tumours show high expression of Ang-1 and Ang-1-like proteins. High expression of Ang-1 has been reported in CSCs, which points to the association of its expression with tumour development, drug resistance and metastatic spread. The latter might be facilitated by the interaction of the endothelial receptor Tie-2 with its ligand Ang-1, which is thought to promote angiogenesis (Fukuhara et al., 2010). Compatible with this view, high Tie-2 expression is seen in CSCs. In animal tumour models these cells have shown the ability to form metastases. Furthermore, the suppression of Ang-1 results in the loss of CSC markers indicting the requirement of Ang-1/Tie-2 interaction for the maintenance of CSCs (Tang KD et al., 2016). As mentioned earlier, Ang-2 can promote tumour angiogenesis and progression independently of Tie-2. Serum Ang-2 and VEGF levels were higher in lung cancer patients than in normal subjects. Both correlated with higher tumour stage (Xu C et al., 2016). Although Ang-2 and VEGF displayed inter-correlation, one cannot establish from this that their expression was related or the correlation reflected angiogenesis.

ANGPL proteins also exert a marked angiogenesis promoting effect and high expression of these proteins has correlated with tumour growth and progression. ANGPL-2 is overexpressed in many forms of cancer. Its expression has been correlated with early recurrence of gastric cancer (Shimura et al., 2015). Metastatic progression can be attributed to the ability of some ANGPL proteins such as ANGPL-2 to activate EMT. ANGPL-2 was overexpressed in many specimens of ductal adenocarcinoma and intraepithelial neoplasia of the pancreas and its downregulation reversed EMT and inhibited cell migration (Carbone et al., 2015). The promotion of growth, the activation of EMT and metastasis could have resulted from the activation by ANGPL-2 of the ERK/MAPK cascade. Aside from the enhanced migration associated with the activation of EMT and the alterations noticed in vascular permeability, there is a paucity of information concerning how angiopoietins or ANGPL proteins might influence the effectors of the events of the metastasis cascade. One should draw attention that ANGPL-5 participates in hematopoietic stem cell (HSC) maintenance and expansion (Zhang CC et al., 2008; Khoury et al., 2011) but it is not clear at the moment if it is involved also in the genesis of HSCs.

Hh Signalling Promotes Angiogenesis Mediated by Angiopoientin-1

The role attributed to Hh signalling in the promotion of tumour progression is underscored and amplified by the association of Hh with the regulation of angiopoietins and ANGPL proteins. Ang-1 is a promoter of angiogenesis whilst Ang-2 negatively regulates angiogenesis. Shh is said to upregulate Ang-1 and suppress Ang-2 together with marked enhancement of angiogenic events. These changes are inhibited by inhibition of Hh signalling using cyclopamine. However, Ang-2 can promote angiogenesis by adopting an alternative signalling system from Hh. It is unclear at present what the prevailing genetic profile is that provides the impetus to switch to the alternative signalling. The possibility that springs to mind is the activation of integrin/FAK signalling. This has close entanglement with the appearance of CSCs and associated alterations of Hh, Wnt and Notch, which as discussed in the relevant sections do induce the generation and propagation of CSCs. Inappropriate activation of FAK signalling can occur with the formation of complex with Src and the FAK/Src kinases do activate proteinases and promote cell migration and also induce angiogenesis.

Clinical Benefits of Ang-1 Inhibition

Several anti-Ang-1 antibodies have been developed, which have shown some clinical capacity. Li XY et al. (2016) have reviewed the outcome of some clinical trials using the Ang-1 inhibitor trebananib, a recombinant peptide-Fc fusion protein, which binds to the angiopoietins and interferes with their interaction with Tie-2. These trials showed clear improvements in PFS and overall survival of patients with ovarian cancer. The benefits seemed to be superior to those observed with inhibitors of VEGF or VEGFR. However, on the negative side are the significant side effects associated with all three modes of treatment. Much work has been carried out with trebananib on other forms of cancer. Atkins et al. (2015) found some benefit from the administration of a combination of trebananib with the VEGFR inhibitor sunitinib to patients with metastatic clear cell renal cell carcinoma. The clinical outcome in patients with recurrent endometrial cancer on trebananib as a single agent was uninspiring (Moore et al., 2015). Neither have other angiopoietin inhibitors shown any clinical benefit deemed worthy of discussion.

CHAPTER 7

Hippo Signalling in Cell Proliferation, Migration and Angiogenesis

Hippo was identified as a signalling system involved in the regulation of organ size in embryogenesis. Investigation of Hippo over the past several years has revealed that it inhibits cell proliferation and promotes apoptosis and inhibits epithelial mesenchymal transition (EMT). It is also able to suppress angiogenesis albeit by an indirect mode of crosstalk with the signalling by angiogenic effector molecules such as angiomotin (AMOT) and growth factors. So the deregulation or loss of Hippo signalling would inevitably lead to unregulated growth, loss of differentiation, cell transformation and neoplastic growth and progression. The suppression of growth by Hippo signalling is mediated by the transcriptional co-activator YAP (Yes-associated protein, Yorkie of Drosophila) and TAZ (transcriptional co-activator with PDZ-binding motif). YAP and TAZ do not enjoy exclusivity as transcriptional co-activators of the Hippo system alone, as conventional wisdom has deemed it. In conformity with that wisdom here the discussions are centred round YAP/TAZ as targets to regulate the biological events accompanying tumour growth and progression.

THE HIPPO SIGNALLING CASCADE OF KINASES

The Hippo kinases of the MST (mammalian sterile20-like) family and the Lats kinases are the key regulators of the Hippo signalling system. The suppressor function of Hippo is initiated by the activation of the MST kinases by cellular stresses. The MST kinases MST1 and MST2 are in complex with and regulated by SAV1 (Salvador homologue 1, WW45) and with RASSF1 (RAS-association domain family protein) (Table 7.1)

The pro-apoptosis MST2 and MST1 complexes phosphorylate and activate Lats occurring as a complex with the regulatory protein Mob (Mps one binder) 1. The activated Lats phosphorylates and inhibits YAP1 and its translocation to the nucleus thus affecting target gene regulation. The MST kinases are characterised by the presence at the C-terminal of the SARAH

Molecular Approach to Cancer Management. DOI: http://dx.doi.org/10.1016/B978-0-12-812896-1.00007-6

Table 7.1 Signalling Components of the Hippo System

Signalling Component	Kinase Identification/Function
MST1, MST2	Ste20 family Ser/Thr kinase
SAV1 (WW45)	WW-domain adaptor
Lats1, Lats2	NDR Serine/Threonine kinases
Mats	Co-factor of Lats1 and Lats2
YAP/Yorkie/TAZ	WW-domain transcription co-factors

Lats, large tumour suppressor; MST, mammalian sterile20-like kinase; NDR, nuclear Dbf2-related family; SAV1, Salvador; YAP, Yes-associated small protein transcription co-activator.

(Salvador 1/RASSF1A/Hippo) domain that mediates interaction with other proteins. The SARAH domain binds to RASSF1 and SAV1, both SARAH domain containing proteins. SARAH possibly also mediates coupling of MST1 and MST2 to Lats culminating in the phosphorylation, inactivation and interference with its function of genetic transcription. The MST2/SAV1/RASSF1 complex is thought to control cell cycle exit. So the two vital events of the Hippo pathway are the MST1/MST2 kinases, which form a complex with regulator protein SAV1. This complex phosphorylates and activates the Lats kinases 1 and 2. The Lats kinases phosphorylate and inhibit YAP and TAZ, which act as co-activators for TEAD (TEA domain transcription factors) in the transcription of genes that promote cell proliferation and survival. The Lats2 kinase can also function via the mdm2/p53 signalling system to inhibit cell proliferation. So targeting of YAP and TAZ is an appealing prospect.

THE HIPPO IN CROSSTALK SHAPES THE CANCER PHENOTYPE

The Hippo signalling system engages and interacts with many signal transduction pathways. Among interacting signalling systems of consequence to tumour biology are the epidermal growth factor (EGF) and transforming growth factor (TGF) family growth factor, Notch, Wnt and the GPCR. Some of these are shown in Fig. 7.1. These systems interrelate and co-operate with the YAP/TAZ axis negatively or positively, and might frequently mutually regulate one another culminating in conspicuous effects on organ growth, morphogenesis, cell proliferation, EMT, the dynamics of stem cell generation and self-renewal, angiogenesis and tumour progression (Fig. 7.2). Despite the availability of a minefield of information, the signalling systems, aside from those involved in angiogenesis, have not received much attention from the point of view of devising strategies or identifying potential targets for developing new drugs. Nonetheless, given that angiogenesis is the crucial

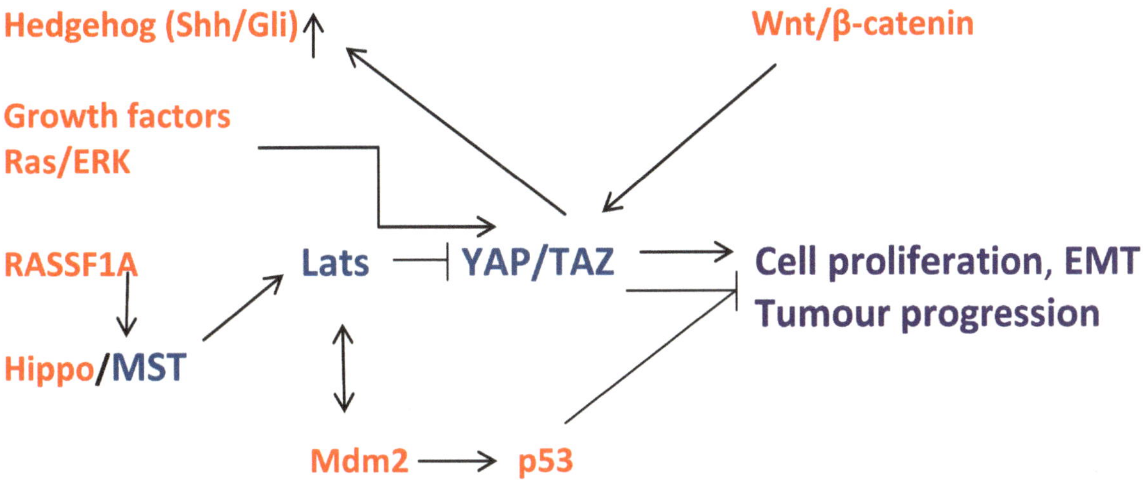

FIGURE 7.1

Signalling systems in crosstalk with YAP/TAZ axis negatively or positively determining effects on organ growth, morphogenesis, cell proliferation, EMT and tumour progression. RASSF1A activates MST and Lats to negatively regulate cell proliferation, activation of EMT and tumour progression. It functions via mdm2 to activate p53 to bring about inhibition of cell proliferation. Growth factor-mediated activation of ERK/MAPK pathway activates YAP/TAZ. Wnt/β-catenin is also able to upregulate YAP/TAZ activity. The latter is also known to upregulate the activity of Sonic Hedgehog.

determinant of metastatic spread of cancer, little needs to be said to justify the focus on the regulation of angiogenesis by Hippo.

THE YAP CONNECTION TO ANGIOGENESIS

Currently much effort has been directed towards the elucidation of the connection of YAP to angiogenesis. The supporting but indirect argument for this implicates MFAP5 (microfibril-associated protein 5) and it runs as follows. MFAPs are a component of microfibrils associated with the ECM. They tether the microfibrils to the components of the ECM providing structural stability and elasticity. The expression of MFAP5 is markedly increased in many forms of cancer. This link presumably resides in the ability of MFAP5 to induce angiogenesis-related events. It is closely associated with the progression of ovarian cancer (Spivey and Banyard, 2010; Leung CS et al., 2014). Mok et al. (2009) reported a positive correlation between MFAP5 expression and microvascular density and an inverse relationship with prognosis in a series of patients with advanced papillary serous ovarian tumours. A negative correlation with survival has also been reported in patients with HNSCC (Ceder et al., 2012). MFAP5 binds to the cell surface through $\alpha(v)\beta(3)$ integrin and promotes cell proliferation and angiogenesis. Whether

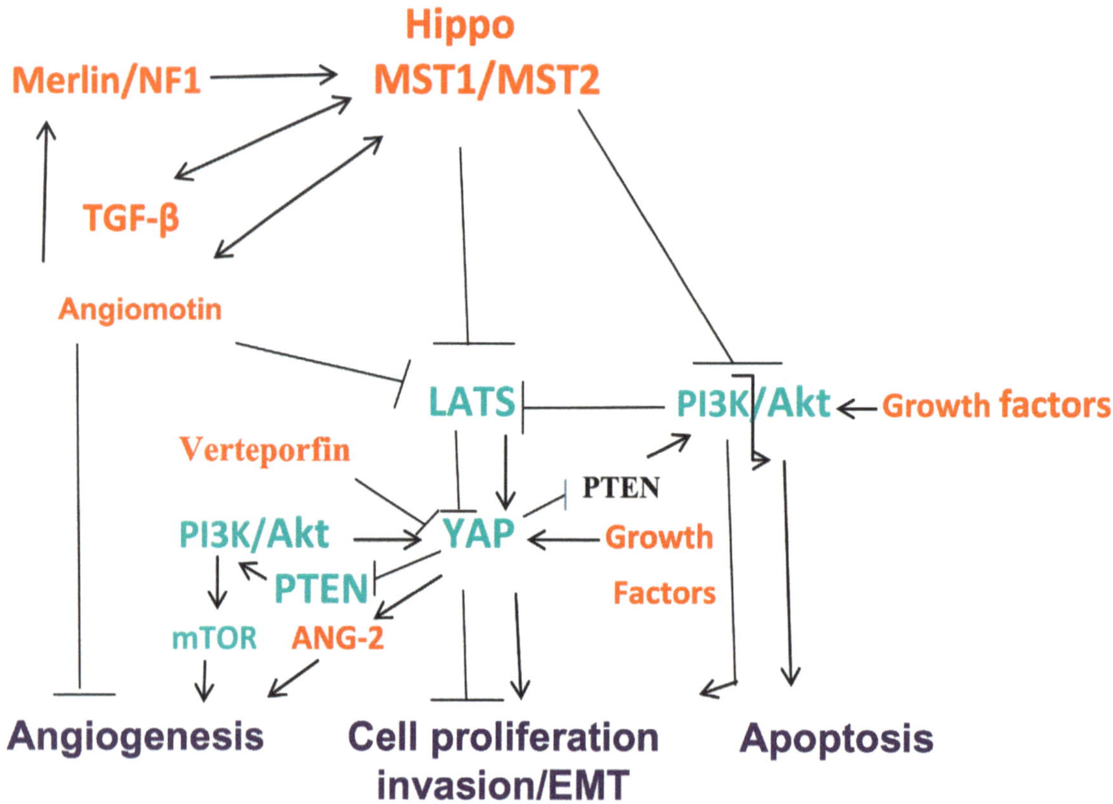

FIGURE 7.2

The regulation of Hippo signalling upstream of the core Lats kinases. AMOT can interact with the Hippo kinases and inhibit cell proliferation, etc., by the Lats route. The Hippo kinase—AMOT interaction can directly inhibit angiogenesis. TGF-β can also inhibit angiogenesis by interaction with the Hippo kinases. PI3K/Akt may be downregulated directly by Hippo-inducing apoptosis. The PI3K/Akt pathway can activate YAP to induce the expression of ANG-2 to induce angiogenesis. YAP is able to suppress PTEN, which restrains PI3K/Akt function so that the anti-apoptosis signalling by PI3K/Akt transduces unhindered to induce cell proliferation. Growth factor signalling also can induce cell proliferation by YAP activation. Equally, they can suppress Lats function and enable YAP to transcribe genes that lead to cell proliferation. These systems are discussed in the text with references.

the reduced survival reflected a consequence of metastatic dissemination is an open question, at least as far as ovarian cancers are concerned. In this form of tumour metastasis does not occur by the haematogenous route but by the release and attachment of cells to distant sites in the peritoneum or the omentum to form secondary tumours.

MFAP5 is a target of YAP and TEAD5 in cholangiocarcinoma cells. In vitro, YAP/TEAD signalling promotes cell proliferation. In the absence of YAP, the cells become susceptible to drug induced apoptosis. In tumour samples and in xenografts of cholangiocarcinoma cells, high YAP activity correlated with enhanced MFAP5. Overall the pro-angiogenic activity and the ability or MFAP5 to promote cell proliferation seem to be mediated by YAP activity (Marti et al., 2015). There are provisional suggestions that YAP might inhibit apoptosis by negatively regulating TRAIL.

It has also been claimed that YAP activation supported angiogenesis as indicated by the enhanced expression of the pro-angiogenic MFAP5 and the expression of CD31+. Both in vitro and in vivo, active YAP fully correlated with increased expression of the markers. The evidence that these events are taking place is quite convincing. However, there is no information here on the density of the vascularity associated with the tumour xenografts. Also there is no demonstrable experimental link with Hippo. This would be essential, for YAP can be activated by other signalling systems independently of Hippo. One of them is the PI3K/Akt pathway, which can and does activate YAP and can promote angiogenesis via the ANG-2 route (Choi HJ and Kwon YG, 2015). So do growth factors such as EGF. YAP is involved in a regulatory loop with several growth factor receptors. It not only induces the expression EGFR and ErbB3 but also promotes the production of EGF-like ligands such as the heparin-binding EGF-like growth factor and NRG (neuregulin)-1, which in turn activate YAP to induce tumour cell proliferation (He C et al., 2015).

On the positive aspect, a link has been established with Hippo signalling and growth factor mediation of cell proliferation. AREG (amphiregulin) is a ligand of the EGFR family and it has been shown to be a transcriptional target of YAP. YAP inspired transcription of AREG leads to the induction of cell proliferation. AREG induction is aided by the inhibition of Lats and removal of its constraint on YAP (Zhang JM et al., 2009). Fan R et al. (2013) showed that EGF treatment inhibited Hippo signalling. EGF treatment led to the nuclear accumulation of YAP and to YAP-mediated transcription of CTGF. This occurred with the mediation of PI3K-PDK1 (phosphoinositide-dependent kinase 1), which inactivated Lats leading to the activation and nuclear translocation of YAP and consequent transcription of target genes. However, there is considerable inter-regulation of growth factor function by this route with the traditional Hippo kinases (see Fig. 7.2). Further confirmation of the involvement of YAP in the function of growth factors has come from the demonstration that NRG-1-activated ErbB4 and stimulated tissue growth via transcription of YAP-regulated genes (Haskins et al., 2014). Urtasun et al. (2011) have demonstrated that there was a direct link between EGFR-mediated activation of CTGF and how it depended upon YAP. They showed that the CTGF gene proximal promoter contained elements that bound YAP and initiated CTGF expression. They also showed that CTGF suppressed DR5, which rendered the cells sensitive cytotoxic drugs and would have also promoted cell proliferation.

The PI3K/Akt/mTOR signalling axis has featured prominently in a number of human tumours. Much evidence has accumulated indicating that angiogenesis might be regulated by mTOR signalling. Inhibiting this pathway effectively suppresses angiogenesis and many inhibitors that suppress angiogenesis and invasion have been identified. Hence the importance of its association with Hippo cannot be disregarded. Hippo-YAP and mTOR pathways collaborate to regulate organ size and growth. The crosstalk between these systems is based on the fact that YAP is able to suppress PTEN, which restrains PI3K/Akt function so that the anti-apoptosis signalling by PI3K/Akt is transduced unhindered to induce cell proliferation (Fig. 7.2).

Finally, one has to allude to the suggestion that TGF-β pathway interacts with Hippo and there might be mutual modulation and a corporate phenotypic outcome for cell proliferation and angiogenesis. The significance of Hippo mediation in the suppression of angiogenesis is debatable. Hippo signalling does engage in crosstalk with TGF-β. It has been claimed that MST1 negatively regulates TGF-β. This is said to occur in a non-canonical fashion not involving Smad but via FAK and E-cadherin (Attarha et al., 2014). BMP9 does induce nuclear localisation of YAP1 in the presence of endoglin (Young et al., 2015). The interpretation of this has to be subject to the caveat that endoglin can produce sharply contrasting effects on tumour progression (see pp. 24–28). BMP9 suppresses angiogenesis by inhibiting canonical TGF-β signalling. Endoglin interacts with TGF-β receptors type II and type I and has been attributed with the ability to suppress cell proliferation, invasion and metastasis. On the other hand, it is overexpressed in tumour vasculature and specifically expressed in endothelial cells. So it could promote endothelial cell proliferation, migration and tumour angiogenesis.

PHARMACOLOGICAL TARGETING OF HIPPO SIGNALLING

The genetic changes encountered in cancers are activating mutations and the inappropriate expression of normal genes converted into the so-called oncogenes. Countermanding the inappropriate expression is one approach. In the contrasting situation suppressor genes may be rendered ineffective due to inactivating mutations or loss of heterozygosity (LOH). Therapeutic targeting to reactivate silent suppressors gene or engaging the upstream regulators of a suppressor system is the second possible therapeutic approach and in cases of genetic loss the second means of approach can envisage pharmacologically targeting the downstream effectors that would have been inactivated by the suppressor genes. The second means of approach has provided some potentially valuable information (Fig. 7.2).

VERTEPORFIN INHIBITS YAP

Verteporfin is a light-activated drug that inhibits the transcriptional activity of YAP/TEAD. Some clinical trials involving patients with brain tumours, BCCs and melanomas are taking place. However, targeted delivery of verteporfin is yet unresolved. Some success has been claimed for verteporfin loaded in cationic liposomes and administered systemically, where tangible anti-angiogenic effects were found in vivo models (Gross et al., 2013). It could be conjugated with tumour-specific proteins to enhance homing specificity. Conjugation with trastuzumab would be expected to increase targeting of the photo-activated drug to tumours expressing HER2. Savellano et al. (2005) showed over a decade ago the efficacy of targeting HER+ cells with conjugates of anti-HER2 antibodies with photo-activated drugs. They obtained a 10-fold specific targeting of HER2+ cells. Such a conjugate was prepared and tested for uptake by HER2-positive SKOV-3 cells, where the uptake was far greater as compared to HER2-negative cells (Kuimova et al., 2007). Bryden et al. (2014) constructed a verteporfin/trastuzumab conjugate. The conjugate selectively targeted HER2 expressing cells. This form of targeting would help manage not only HER2+ breast cancers but also HER+ metastasis in the brain, which HER2+ breast cancers are prone to do. Another conjugate of significance is that with EGFR antibodies. EGFR is overexpressed in many forms of cancer and is responsible for enhanced cell proliferation, activation of EMT and metastasis. Using an experimental A431 tumour model, Kameyama et al. (2011) were able to show greatly enhanced, more than ninefold, localisation in the tumour of an anti-EGFR antibody/verteporfin conjugate administered intravenously. The treatment resulted in reduced tumour size. From the viewpoint of inhibiting angiogenesis, it is worthy of note that verteporfin has been conjugated with factor VII to target the drug to endothelial cells expressing TF (receptor tissue factor). One may recall that TF, a transmembrane glycoprotein receptor for Factor VII, is involved in many pathological conditions including tumour angiogenesis. The ligand conjugate targeted TF with high affinity and specificity. In vitro assays showed that this led to the destruction of TF-expressing cells and to the inhibition of tumour growth in vivo (Hu ZW et al., 2010). However, the crucial experiments on the effects on angiogenesis, e.g., vascular density and whether the xenografted tumours showed metastatic localisation in the lungs were not carried out. This greatly limits its significance, utility and potential value. A further consideration is that although the conjugate would be expected to target tumour-associated blood vessels, TF also occurs in many other tissues. Also the conjugate would have to compete with the circulating factor VII.

BISPHOSPHONATE-MEDIATED INHIBITION OF YAP/TAZ

Bisphosphonates are a class of drugs that can prevent bone loss in pathological situations such as osteoporosis and Paget's disease. They are also administered for combating bone loss resulting from metastatic deposits occurring in breast, lung and prostate cancer and multiple myeloma. Zoledronate (zoledronic acid), a bisphosphonate, is frequently used to reduce and treat bone metastasis.

Zoledronate (ZOL) has been shown to reduce growth of tumour xenografts and this effect might be due to the induction of apoptosis. The bisphosphonate drugs have exhibited anti-tumour effects in pre-clinical tumour models and inhibit tumour cell proliferation in vitro. They also seem able to inhibit the growth of human tumour xenografts. The effects are more striking in combination with conventional cytotoxic agents. Reilly et al. (2015) have developed and tested a new compound to target the GGPP (geranylgeranyl pyrophosphate) link in the mevalonate pathway (see Fig. 7.3). The implantation of human prostate carcinoma-derived cells into SCID (severe combined immune deficiency) mice resulted in the formation of tumours in the mandible and the adrenal glands. Treatment of the tumour bearing mice with a new inhibitor of geranylgeranyl diphosphate synthase, disodium [(6Z,11E,15E)-9-[bis(sodiooxy)phosphoryl]-17-hydroxy-2,6,12,16-tetramethyheptadeca-2,6,11,15-tetraen-9-yl]phosphonate (GGOHBP), produced a marked reduction in the weight of the tumours in the adrenal gland. That the drug had targeted geranyldiphosphate was evident from the reduction in geranylgeranylation of Rap1A, the Ras family GTPase, in the adrenal tumours. However, there is no information about the status of the tumours in the mandibles, a frequent metastatic site of around 10% prostate primary tumours. Furthermore, the new drug requires more rigorous testing in determine its effectiveness as a tumour inhibitor rather than as a metastasis inhibitor. The tumours studied cannot be deemed as classic metastases, but arising from differential distribution of the injected prostate cancer cells. The authors have themselves acknowledged that prostate cancer rarely, if at all, metastasises to the adrenal glands.

Potentially useful would be the ability of these drugs to suppress angiogenesis, the obvious consequence of this would be delayed metastatic spread or its prevention, especially to extra-skeletal locations. Both ZOL and alendronate suppress the production of VEGF and ANG-1 by osteoblasts (Ishtiaq et al., 2015). Matrix metalloproteinases (MMPs), which are angiogenic, are

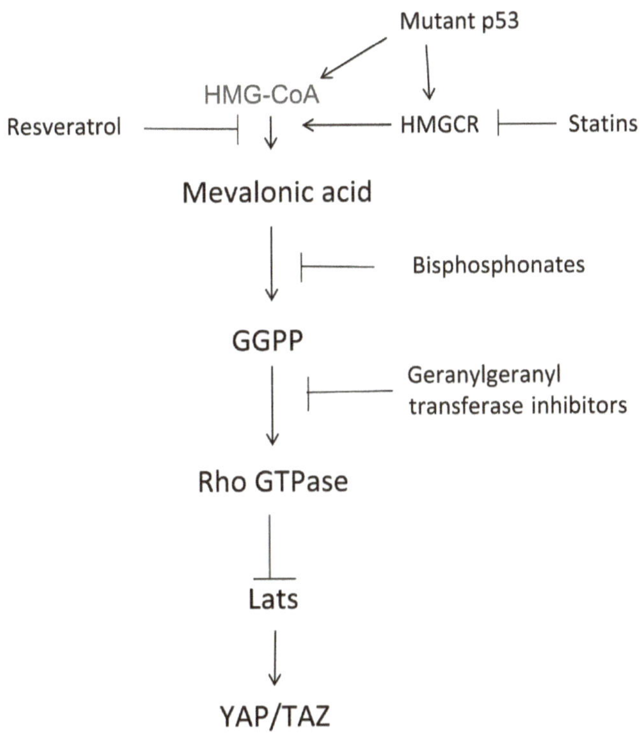

FIGURE 7.3

The mevalonic acid pathway in YAP/TAZ expression and the points where the pathway is inhibited by bisphosphophonates and geranylgeranyl transferase inhibitors. Mutant p53 upregulates both HMG-CoA and HMGCR and by that route activates YAP/TAZ.

GGPP, geranylgeranyl pyrophosphate; HMG-CoA, 3-hydroxy-3-methylglutaryl-coenzyme A; HMGCR, HMG-CoA reductase.

This figure is based on Freed-Pastor (2012), Bieging et al. (2014), Moroishi et al. (2015) and references cited in the text.

differentially affected by ZOL. ZOL downregulated the expression of MMP2 and MMP9 in PC3 prostate cancer cells, but enhanced MMP8 expression (Reel et al., 2015). But all three MMPs do enhance angiogenesis and that is well established. Reel et al. (2015) have suggested that the inhibition of MMPs could be due to downstream Ras/Raf/ERK and PI3K/Akt signalling activated by discoidin domain receptor (DDR) kinases. However, functionally the DDRs are not totally divorced from Hippo (see pp. 74–75 below). MMP expression can be differentially activated by these signalling pathways and indeed Ras can do so quite independently of PI3K/Akt involvement. Some bisphononates, including ZOL, have been found to inhibit invasion in vitro. Some of these potentially beneficial properties must be counterpoised with some serious side effects of the drugs.

A direct link with the Hippo system is seen in the demonstration that bisphosphonates block the nuclear localisation of YAP/TAZ. YAP promotes cell proliferation by physically interacting with mutant p53 and activating the functions of cyclin A, cyclin B and CDK1 genes. But when either of these effectors was deleted, the expression of the cell cycle regulatory genes was downregulated together with the downregulation of mutant p53 or YAP depletion, effectively reducing cell proliferation in vitro. Forced cytoplasmic localisation of YAP/TAZ also led to the downregulation of cell cycle regulators (Sorrentino et al., 2014; Di Agostino et al., 2016) (Fig. 7.3).

THE DDRs CONNECT TO KIBRA/HIPPO FUNCTION

At the risk of a slight digression, it might be worthwhile to briefly discuss the DDRs and their possible link to Hippo. The DDRs are important regulators of cell proliferation, cell survival and invasion. The expression of DDR1 and DDR2 has correlated with tumour development and progression. The expression of both has shown positive correlation with the expression of EMT. Gastric cancer tissue xenografts have displayed increased tumorigenesis and invasion. Activation of EMT-associated features correlated with signalling via the mTOR/Akt pathway (Wang YG et al., 2016). Some growth factors might upregulate DDRs by activating the PI3K/Akt, without engaging mTOR (Mata et al., 2016). It should be appreciated that it is difficult to make such exclusions because in several cancers the mTOR/PI3K/Akt signalling axis plays many prominent roles.

How do the DDRs relate to Hippo and signalling? That is through Kibra which is an upstream regulator of Hippo signalling. Kibra suppresses cell proliferation and is silenced by hypermethylation in leukaemias and so regarded as a tumour suppressor. It is a cytoskeletal protein possessing two amino-terminal WW domains. These WW protein domains recognise proline-rich peptide motifs and phosphorylated-serine/threonine-proline sites of proteins and mediate their interaction and facilitate the formation of a physiologically important network.

Now Kibra binds to DDR1 and releases it to interact with its ligands activating the MAPK/ERK-mediated proliferation signalling pathway (Wilson et al., 2016). Equally, the DDRs released by Kibra could interact with YAP, itself a WW-domain protein. If such an interaction were to localise YAP to the cytoplasmic compartment that would result be the suppression of biological processes involving YAP. However, there is no evidence of the DDRs being the targets of WW-mediated interaction with YAP. Nonetheless, YAP binds many biological important proteins by its WW domains. YAP/TAZ interacts through the WW domain with apoptosis promoting proteins, pro-apoptosis transcription factors as well as proteins linked with tumour progression. YAP expression has often correlated with the stem cell phenotype with the characteristic expression of transcription factors such as Oct4, Sox2 and myc among others associated with the reprogramming of differentiated cells into stem cells. YAP expression is higher in stem cells of NSCLC. The interaction of YAP with Oct4 and Sox2 has been suggested to be a basis for the maintenance of stem cells (Bora-Singhal et al., 2015). In contrast, BMP2 inhibits the proliferation of mouse embryonic NSCs. This occurs with the mediation of YAP (Yao MH et al., 2014) and the direct interaction of YAP with Smads, which are WW-domain proteins.

AMOT is another YAP-binding partner. The significance of AMOT in the present context is that it stimulates migratory ability and angiogenesis in tumours (see pp. 127–128). Chan SW et al. (2011) found that AMOT and AMOTL1 interact with YAP/TAZ via the WW domain. The overexpression of the AMOTS localises YAP/TAZ to the cytoplasmic compartment and in this way invalidates its function. How this affects the induction of angiogenesis by AMOTs is unclear. That could happen with the intervention of angiostatin. Possibly, angiostatin is anti-angiogenic because it binds to and suppresses AMOT-mediated angiogenesis. It is possible that YAP/TAZ binding might prevent the anti-angiogenic effect of angiostatin, quite independently of the canonical function of YAP/TAZ.

It has been acknowledged that the outcomes of the protein interactions might vary greatly since the WW domains within the same protein might possess different binding specificities to other proteins, thus providing for differential recognition of targets. Hence the practical value of modulating these interactions to influence the signalling by Hippo or the interacting systems of signal transduction is noticeably nebulous at present.

THE RASSFs IN THE REGULATION OF HIPPO

The RASSF family genes are upstream regulators of Hippo signalling. Two subgroups have been identified in the RASSF family. The RASSF1–RASSF6 (the C-terminal family) carry the RA (Ras-association domain) domain at the C-terminus whilst that domain occurs at the N-terminus in N-terminal family of RASSF7–RASSF10. The RA domain mediates RASSF binding to GTPases. The SARAH domain is also an important motif of the RASSFs. SARAH occurs immediately C-terminal to the RA domain in RASSF1–RASSF6. The RASSF7–RASSF10 lack the SARAH domain. The SARAH domain promotes the heterodimerisation of the RASSFs with the MST1 and MST2 kinases.

The RASSFs are hypermethylated and inactivated in many tumours and the frequency of the incidence of methylation can vary greatly. Indeed, the RASSFs act as suppressors of tumorigenesis, cell proliferation, regulate the cell cycle and induce apoptosis. Some members may be involved with the stabilisation of cytoskeletal structures. They display localised distribution with microtubules and the mitotic spindle. This association could account for the ability of the RASSFs to inhibit cell motility. This is also related to the methylation status. The function of the RASSFs is regulated by the phosphorylation of the RA domain. RASSF signalling takes four important paths of pro-apoptosis Bcl-2 genes/caspase or inhibition of the anti-apoptosis PI3K/Akt pathway. Akt may also phosphorylate and activate the Hippo kinases. Equally, the Hippo kinases can act independently of Akt. The RASSFs are also known to inhibit Wnt/β-catenin and NF-κB signalling. Not much advantage has been taken of the operation of these signalling pathways, especially of Wnt/β-catenin and NF-κB signalling. Under conditions where the RASSFs are suppressed or depleted, both these signalling systems are manifestly hyper-activated (Lock et al., 2010; Song H et al., 2012). Given that the RASSFs are silenced in many human neoplasms, there is a case to be made for the inhibition of these pathways. Many inhibitors of these signalling systems are available and these might accentuate the suppressor effects of the RASSFs.

It is needless to state that the effects of demethylating agents have been studied from time to time. However, since these produce a global demethylating effect, their clinical value would be limited. The reactivation of silenced suppressor genes has long been sought as a potential path in the treatment of human disease. Targeted demethylation of silenced suppressor genes has to be a preferred option over global demethylation where inhibitors of DNA methylation such as 5-azacytidine and 5-aza-2′-deoxycytidine are employed. Similarly, the use of histone deacetylase (HDAC) inhibitors would have generalised effects on suppressor genes, oncogenes and essential transcription factors.

At this point, genetic reprogramming would seem worthy of a brief reference. Targeting of specific gene loci is achieved by using DNA-binding proteins such as zinc-finger proteins, transcription activator-like effectors (TALEs) and clustered regularly interspaced short palindromic repeats (CRISPRs). These are constructed to target the required genetic sequence. Gene manipulation is achieved by forming a fusion complex with the appropriate effector domain. The activation of suppressor genes silenced by hypermethylation has been achieved at least at the laboratory level by designing fusion complexes made up of demethylases such thymine/DNA/glycosylate (TDG) and TET (ten-eleven translocation family enzymes) bonded with DNA-binding domains of zinc-finger proteins or the TALEs. This technology of genetic engineering is also employed to alleviate effects of inherited genetic defects and DNA repair (Moore et al., 2014; Falahi et al., 2015). So far as clinical practice is concerned, the use of this technology is not yet in the realm of reality.

MERLIN/NF2 IN HIPPO SIGNALLING

Merlin/NF2 (Neurofibromatosis 2) and the protein known as Expanded of *Drosophila melanogaster* of which the human homologue FRMD6 (FERM four-point-one protein, ezrin, radixin, moesin) domain containing protein are cytoskeletal proteins of the ERM family. Merlin is a tumour suppressor. The suppressor attribution flows from its participation in several cellular functions such as contact inhibition of growth, intercellular and cell–substratum interaction and adhesion, regulation of cell proliferation and apoptosis. Merlin integrates ECM receptors such as CD44, the integrins and the actin cytoskeleton. Besides influencing the invasion mechanism in this way, Merlin is reputed to regulate growth factor signalling and cell survival. Historically, it has been identified as a regulator of organ size and the loss of Merlin enhances organ growth with eventual tumorigenesis. Consistent with this is the activation of EMT with the loss of the Merlin homologue FRMD6. The deregulation of growth arrest and cell–cell adhesive interactions that occur in the wake of the loss of Merlin enhances cell motility. The suppressor function might accrue from the suppression of other signalling systems such as the Ras/Rac pathway involved in cell transformation by modulating the disposition or suppressing the functions of downstream effectors of the Ras cascade. Merlin signalling may be suppressed by LOH or by inactivating mutations, which have been encountered in many forms of cancer.

Merlin is an upstream regulator of Hippo signalling. It regulates the activation of MST1 and MST2, activation of Lats and the inactivation of YAP. The inactivation of the transcription co-activator leads to the suppression of many cellular attributed charactering tumour development and progression (see Sherbet, 2013 for a detailed discussion of the biology of Merlin).

ADAPTING TO THE LOSS OF MERLIN FUNCTION FOR TUMOUR SUPPRESSION

The loss of suppressor genes by inactivation or LOH has to be tackled in one of two ways. The suppressor would need to be reactivated or reinstated. Gene therapy of common parlance would involve the reinstatement of vector- borne suppressor gene. If there were genetic defects, the replacement of the defective genes are aspects of genetic engineering regarded as viable propositions. Whilst these still lie within the ambit of experimental options, but are technically feasible, these approaches may not be pragmatic or expedient approaches. Realistically one has to consider if adapting to the loss of the repressor function by engaging alternative modes of signalling which in the normal course of events would have interacted with or influenced by the suppressor function.

Garcia-Rendueles et al. (2015) noted the activation of Ras signalling when Merlin is not functioning. This has raised the possibility that in the event of Merlin inactivation and the Ras system operating one can achieve the phenotypic effects of cell transformation by resorting to the inhibition of the secondary signalling route. In fact, Garcia-Rendueles et al. (2015) have been able to show that verteporfin blocked RAS signalling and inhibited cell growth. Given that Merlin is an upstream regulator of Hippo, probing how the loss of Merlin would have affected Hippo signalling might provide valuable clues as to how verteporfin, which inhibits YAP, might function in the background of Merlin inactivation. For one can legitimately ask how would the 14-3-3 proteins discussed later and CTGF would perform in such a situation. CTGF and CYR61 are YAP-regulated proteins closely linked with endothelial cell proliferation, migration and angiogenesis.

DO 14-3-3 PROTEINS INFLUENCE HIPPO SIGNALLING?

To recapitulate, the TAZ is the transcriptional co-activator possessing the PDZ protein interacting domain. Upon being negatively regulated by Lats-mediated phosphorylation, TAZ and YAP lead to the manifestation of the suppressor effects of the Hippo pathway on cell proliferation and induction of apoptosis and inhibition of angiogenesis. TAZ is a 14-3-3 binding protein and legitimately therefore the role of 14-3-3 proteins demands discussion.

The 14-3-3 proteins are ubiquitously expressed proteins and associated with signalling of cell proliferation, apoptosis, cytoskeletal dynamics and play crucial roles in tumour development and dissemination. Some are tumour suppressors and others promoters. The 14-3-3s operate by binding to phosphorylated-serine/threonine motifs on their target proteins and modulate their function. They influence several signalling pathways in this way and positively or negatively regulate cell motility and invasion, and cell proliferation and apoptosis, EMT and metastasis. A prominent aspect of 14-3-3 activity is that they bind to important signalling proteins and regulate their intracellular translocation and localisation and disposition with serious consequences to signal transduction.

The mode of action by which 14-3-3 proteins influence Hippo signalling is the subject of some investigation. The alterations in the subcellular localisation of effector molecules brought about by interactions with 14-3-3 proteins have been focused on. Nuclear translocation of the Merlin homologue FRMD6, which is an upstream regulator of Hippo, is hampered by binding of 14-3-3 (Meng FB et al., 2015). Since Merlin regulates the activation of MST1 and MST2, activation of Lats and the inactivation of YAP, inhibiting the movement into the nucleus of FRMD6 would shut down the suppressor function of Hippo.

Another suggested mechanism is that the translocation of YAP into the nucleus might be impeded by binding to 14-3-3 proteins such as 14-3-3σ to YAP. When such binding is prevented, the inhibitory effects of 14-3-3σ on cell proliferation are blocked (Sambandam et al., 2015). Earlier Lei QY et al. (2008) reported that Lats phosphorylation created 14-3-3 binding sites in TAZ and that TAZ then seemed to be sequestered by 14-3-3 and retained in the cytoplasm, which led to an effective inactivation of TAZ. It would not be out of context to point out here that 14-3-3ζ, which promotes cell proliferation and tumour aggression, downregulates 14-3-3σ. This has been suggested as a mechanism involved in the dual function of TGF-β as a suppressor effect in early stages of tumorigenesis and as a promoter of progression in the later stages of tumour development. The downregulation of 14-3-3σ seems to be linked with alteration of Smad signalling partners and to the switching TGF-β from its tumour suppressor function to a tumour promoter mode (Xu J et al., 2015).

The 14-3-3 proteins engage YAP and this complex links up with vascular endothelial-cadherin, which occurs at endothelial cell junctions effectively preventing subcellular translocation of YAP (Giampietro et al., 2015). As noted earlier, verteporfin inactivates YAP and this occurs through the upregulation of and binding to 14-3-3σ. This effectively sequesters YAP to the cytoplasmic compartment and targeted for proteasome-mediated degradation (Wang C et al., 2016).

The 14-3-3 protein might be able to influence Hippo by interfering with the function of Lats kinases. The phosphorylation of YAP does create binding sites for 14-3-3 proteins. The Lats phosphorylation site of the CHO1 isoform of kinesin is also binding site for 14-3-3 (Fesquet et al., 2015) and this might be a relevant consideration in the function of the kinesin isoforms in the process of cytokinesis. Dephosphorylation of TAZ and the prevention of its binding 14-3-3 facilitate its nuclear localisation. Canonical Wnt signalling has been shown to activate TAZ in this way (Byun MR et al., 2014). Similarly, dephosphorylation of YAP2 results in its accumulation in the nucleus and to transcriptional activity (Wang P et al., 2011).

CLINICAL VALUE OF 14-3-3 INHIBITION

The 14-3-3 isomers interact with many signalling systems. Among therapeutic approaches being attempted are the development of 14-3-3 inhibitors that might directly attenuate or inhibit the cell proliferation and tumour promoting activity of these proteins. Conceivably, 14-3-3 inhibitors could act synergistically with established inhibitors of the affected signalling systems. In either case the inhibition of 14-3-3s would be expected to sensitise tumour cells to conventional therapeutic agents. Such amenability to inhibition requires the identification of their reputedly numerous target proteins. Nonetheless, much attention has been devoted to this aspect.

A comparatively more easily manageable approach would be to focus on the suppressor isoform 14-3-3σ, which is silenced by CpG methylation in many forms of cancer. It was suggested some years ago that it would be possible reactivate it by demethylation using methyltransferase inhibitor 5-aza-2-deoxycytidine and HDAC inhibitors (Mhawech et al., 2005). Schultz et al. (2009) were able to show that combining the use of the HDAC inhibitor 4-phenylbutyric acid contributed to the overexpression of 14-3-3σ induced by 5-aza-2′-deoxycytidine as a single agent. This drug combination was highly effective and resulted in the total inhibition of cell proliferation. A complicating factor of this approach is that overexpression of 14-3-3σ has been linked with the acquisition of drug resistance. Furthermore, selecting cells for drug resistance has led to the overexpression of the isoform by demethylation (Qin L et al., 2014).

In the context of Hippo, there does not appear to be much scope in pursuing the combination strategy. Verteporfin is said to upregulate the expression of 14-3-3σ. The latter interacts through the mediation of WW-binding sites to complex with YAP. This leads to its sequestration in the cytoplasm and targeted for proteasome-mediated degradation (Wang C et al., 2016). Also noteworthy is that Lats-mediated phosphorylation of AMOT 130, the 130 kDa isoform of AMOT, leads to the formation of a 14-3-3 binding site. The 14-3-3 may be involved here albeit indirectly in the suppression of CTGF, for suppressing AMOT 130 prevents Lats from inactivating YAP and leads to upregulated expression of CTGF (Adler et al., 2013). CTGF is a target gene of YAP involved with the promotion of endothelial cell proliferation, migration and angiogenesis. So, one can adduce some evidence of the integration of 14-3-3 with Hippo suppressor signalling of cell proliferation, cell migration, angiogenesis and tumour progression.

CHAPTER 8

Notch Signalling in Carcinogenesis

Notch is a developmental signalling pathway transducing signalling of normal processes of morphogenesis and growth. It is a key signalling element in neuronal differentiation, mesoderm segmentation, in the formation of new blood vessels, haemo- and lymphopoiesis and the determination of cell fate. The deregulation of the Notch pathway leads to pathogenesis and developmental abnormalities. On account of the kinship between embryonic systems and neoplasia, it was reasonably expected and in fact proven to be closely linked with the generation of the cancer phenotype.

The Notch receptors Notch 1–4 are transmembrane glycoproteins. The binding of ligands, Delta-like ligands (DLL) 1, 3 and 5 and Jagged-1 and -2, to its extracellular domain activates Notch and leads to the cleavage of the Notch ICD (intracellular domain), which translocates into the nucleus and binds the transcription factor CSL (CBF1/RBP-Jk, Suppresser of Hairless, Lag-1). CSL can repress or activate target genes by associating with co-repressor complexes or co-activator complexes. When the Notch ICD is not released CSL binds with co-repressor complexes and suppresses transcription. But Notch ICD dissociates the CSL/co-repressor complexes and promotes the CSL/transcription activating complexes. The latter in turn regulate the appropriate target genes. Besides this, the Notch signalling pathway intersects and co-operatively functions with other signal transduction systems controlling stem cell maintenance and propagation, cell proliferation, epithelial mesenchymal transition (EMT) activation and induction of angiogenesis. A consequence of the operation of this interacting signalling network is the extensive influence on the biological behaviour of tumours.

NOTCH SIGNALLING ACTIVATES EMT AND THE STEM CELL PHENOTYPE

The activation of EMT is an important distinguishing feature of cancer progression to the metastatic state. Its status and substance is highlighted by

Molecular Approach to Cancer Management. DOI: http://dx.doi.org/10.1016/B978-0-12-812896-1.00008-8

the attendant generation of the pluripotent cancer stem cells (CSCs) with the ability for self-renewal. The activation of EMT has strong associations with the function of a family of transcription factors that include Snail, Twist, Zeb and TCF3 (transcription factor 3, E47). Many of these transcription factors have been linked with cell migration, proliferation and apoptosis and angiogenesis, which are definitive outcomes of EMT activation. This could involve reprogramming of gene activation and conceptually might link EMT with the generation of CSCs. Direct evidence for this is still not available barring that CD24 and CD44 are regarded as CSC markers for some forms of tumour. CD44 and EPCAM (epithelial cell adhesion molecule) are concurrently upregulated with Notch in pancreatic CSCs. CD44 determines several CSC features notably initiation and self-renewal of CSCs phenotype. Besides, both CD44 and Notch signalling systems may be regulated by γ-secretase.

Much evidence has accumulated that Wnt and growth factor signalling might interact with Notch and forge a link. It has been noted in many studies that the activation of EMT and the activation of Notch signalling go hand in hand. The downregulation of E-cadherin expression is an obvious link with EMT and acquisition of invasive potential. Zeb-1 is upregulated upon Notch activation with the loss of E-cadherin expression. It has been established now with certainty that Hh and TGF-β, and Wnt pathways may operate together with Notch in the activation of EMT. Both Zeb and TCF3 are closely involved with Wnt signalling. Signalling via RTK, mTOR, NF-κB and PTEN/PI3K/Akt pathways has been deeply implicated in EMT activation and the appearance of CSCs, as discussed already in several locations. So if a common factor was to operate downstream of these pathways that might turn out to be a suitable target. The Sox transcription factors of the high mobility group (HMG) box family come to mind. They participate in stem cell generation and propagation in development and differentiation and are deregulated in pathogenesis. Sox proteins are active downstream of many EMT/CSC signalling systems including Notch. It is needless to say that one can implicate other factors such as the MAPK cascade. A critical caveat has to be inserted here that is that EMT has been claimed to have no link with CSC generation but that the reverse process of mesenchymal epithelial transition has. The crux of arguments in either direction must depend upon the choice of markers utilised for christening CSCs because their expression would qualitatively differ and vary by reason of degree of transition and cell lineage.

NOTCH INDUCES ANGIOGENESIS

Induction of angiogenesis is essential for the growth and metastatic dissemination of cancer. The inhibition of Notch signalling has been viewed as a means of inhibiting both tumour growth and progression. But some Notch ligands promote and others inhibit angiogenesis. Notch has been shown to regulate vascular endothelial growth factor (VEGF) function and induce angiogenesis. Not only this, VEGF can induce the expression of Notch and its ligand Delta4 in human arterial endothelial cells. Interestingly, Delta4 is highly expressed, besides some normal tissues, in the vasculature of human tumour xenografts and in breast cancer. HIF1-α (hypoxia-inducible factor) is induced in MCF7 breast cancer cell lines transfected with constitutively active Notch1. The signalling circuitry is strengthened by the fact that HIF1 not only mediates VEGF-induced angiogenesis, but also upregulates Delta4 expression. Indirectly, angiogenic agents such as platelet-derived growth factor might stimulate Notch to signal via VEGF and matrix metalloproteinases (MMPs).

Xu ZB et al. (2016) have employed a monoclonal antibody raised against Delta4 to inhibit the activation of Notch. The overexpression of Delta4, which is in the tumour vasculature, promotes the formation of organised vascular structure. The antibody induced the formation of abnormal vasculature with reduced vessel dimension effectively making the structures dysfunctional. This inhibited the in vivo growth of tumours. The authors claim that the generation of CSCs was also suppressed. The reasoning behind the induction of angiogenesis is based on the idea that Delta4-Notch signalling pathway acts as a negative regulator of vascular morphogenesis and remodelling by preventing VEGF-mediated angiogenesis. Interference with the constraint imposed by Delta4, for instance, by using anti-Delta4 antibodies, could induce defective vascularisation and consequent suppression of tumour growth. Undeniably, this is compatible with the development of defective vasculature, increased vascular density with reduced vessel size in haplo-insufficiency of Delta4 (Gale et al., 2004; Krebs et al., 2004). Nonetheless, Notch ligands can have demonstrably opposing functions, so the conclusions drawn seem too premature. One needs to know if the immature vasculature had altered permeability and had resulted in reduced diapedesis of tumour cells. It would be relevant to draw attention here that HIF-1α/Notch signalling induces both EMT together with the generation of CSCs and angiogenesis. Endothelial Jagged-1 also a Notch ligand is markedly pro-angiogenic in function. The effects seem to be mediated by the upregulation of VEGFR-2 whilst negatively regulating VEGFR-1 (Pedrosa et al., 2015). Delta4 and Jagged-1 do exert opposing effects on angiogenesis as Benedito et al. (2009) showed some time ago, who have also suggested that the final angiogenic outcome would obviously depend upon the balance of the activation of Notch by these ligands.

NOTCH AND CELL PROLIFERATION

The induction of the CSC phenotype, invasive ability and proliferative potential are the inalienable attributes of EMT and hence also of Notch activation.

It is well established that inhibiting Notch profoundly suppresses these phenotypic features of EMT. The HDAC inhibitor TSA (Trichostatin A) modulates proliferative signalling by influencing the Akt as well as MAPK/ERK1/2 pathways. In parallel, TSA suppresses EMT with concurrent inhibition of Notch signalling. These findings provide some indirect evidence that Notch could be functioning via the MAPK signalling in the induction of cell proliferation that accompanies the activation of EMT (Xiao W et al., 2014). So does the γ-secretase inhibitor DAPT (*N*-[*N*-(3,5-difluorophenacetyl)-L-alanyl]-(S)-phenylglycine t-butyl ester) suppress cell proliferation as discussed in detail in another location. DAPT possibly also suppresses invasion and is capable of targeting EMT and CSCs (pp. 87–88). It may be recalled here that DAPT has been associated with the inhibition of Notch signalling (Layden and Martindale, 2014; Marlow et al., 2013) by inhibiting the release of the Notch ICD.

Notch functions with other angiogenic growth factors such as FGF, BMP and IGF. The collaboration with these growth factors and Wnt family proteins has implications for not only for angiogenesis but also for tumour growth. One would recall that Wnt proteins are closely associated with cell proliferation and migration and yet capable of modulating the expression of β-catenin-linked cadherins and regulates intercellular adhesion. The tie-up of Notch with the Wnt system would inevitably have marked repercussions on tumour cell behaviour. This alignment with invasive ability may be compounded by the activation of EMT. The interactive connection of Notch with other signalling systems also extends to the generation and propagation of CSCs as evidenced by the fact that these events are erased upon Notch inhibition. Furthermore, the promotion of the CSC phenotype occurs virtually invariably with the promotion of cell proliferation in general.

NOTCH SIGNALLING IS LINKED TO DRUG RESISTANCE

The activation of EMT and the generation of CSCs have frequently been linked with the development of drug resistance. The faculty of resistance to drugs exhibited by CSCs can be attributed to abnormalities of ABC (ATP-binding cassette) transporters involved in the transport of molecules across the plasma membrane, endoplasmic reticulum and membranes of the cell organelles. The deregulation of signalling systems such as NF-κB and PI3K/Akt and of apoptosis-associated gene function also results in the development of drug resistance.

It was inevitable that given its participation in the EMT/CSC phenomenon Notch should be associated with the development of drug resistance. The downstream effector Hes1 is actively involved in CSC maintenance and propagation, tumour progression and also in the development of drug resistance.

Sethi et al. (2010) showed that rabconnectin-3α *encoded by DMXL2* is an important activator of Notch signalling. The silencing of rabconnectin-3 markedly disrupts Notch and V-ATPase activity. The inhibition of the V-ATPase attenuated Notch signalling. This could be because V-ATPase is involved in the cleavage and the release of the Notch ICD by γ-secretase.

Recently, Notch activation by rabconnectin-3 has been reported to result in the development of drug resistance. The DMXL2 protein is overexpressed in some breast cancer cell lines resistant to endocrine treatment and this leads to the activation of Notch signalling by V-ATPase (Faronato et al., 2015).

SUPPRESSION OF NOTCH SIGNALLING AS A THERAPEUTIC APPROACH

The well-established ability to activate EMT and promote CSCs delivers Notch as an accessible target for therapeutic intervention. The presence of signalling systems that function synergistically or additively with Notch underscores its status as a target to manipulate and manoeuvre for treatment.

The intramembrane protease γ-secretase, which cleaves Notch upon activation by ligand binding and releases the Notch ICD, has been a major focus of attention. Several inhibitors of γ-secretase have been investigated for their efficacy for the inhibition of Notch as a means to the inhibition of HMG box family proteins to suppress tumour development and progression. Several clinical trials are underway testing the efficacy of RO4929097, a small molecule inhibitor of the enzymatic function of γ-secretase, in several forms of cancer.

The postulated outcome of the inhibitory effects exerted by RO4929097 has included the suppression of angiogenesis and the induction of apoptosis. As yet, here is no consensus in the findings in relation to angiogenesis. However, PF-03084014 a γ-secretase inhibitor also has been reported to reduce microvessel density (see discussion later). Nair et al. (2013) found that apoptosis occurred only when PTEN was expressed and the expression of Akt was suppressed. These authors also noticed an enhanced susceptibility of PTEN expressing tumour cells to temozolomide. These are likely additive outcomes but the findings are nonetheless significant for they underline the importance of taking the ambient molecular environment into consideration. On the other hand, Jin et al. (2013) found that and the selective Akt inhibitor MK-2206 suppressed Akt phosphorylation but the γ-secretase inhibitor MRK003 inhibited Notch as well as Akt phosphorylation. Both were effective in inhibiting cell proliferation and invasion, but in combination these agents produced a far greater inhibition of invasion than proliferation, possibly indicating a preponderance of the effects of MRK003. Excessive proliferative pressure can lead to invasive behaviour. Indeed some growth factors can actively induce cell migration. So to overview, the significance of this in practice has to be further studied, perhaps in preclinical tumour models to check whether the combination suppresses metastasis more effective than as single agents.

The preclinical studies recorded so far concerning the effects on xenografts of gliomas and the in vitro effects have been ambivalent and the early results are not very encouraging. The effects of combining the Notch inhibitor with mTOR inhibitors on glioma xenografts were also equivocal (Dantas-Barbosa et al., 2015). Even at minimum tolerated dose, mTOR inhibitors seem to have exerted significant side effects (Piha-Paul et al., 2015). The clinical level also the findings were variable. In a study of high-grade ovarian cancer resistant to platinum-based therapy, the best outcome was stable disease and no objective responses had been noted (Diaz-Padilla et al., 2015). The clinical response was poor in metastatic melanoma (Lee SM et al., 2015). No objective response was noticed in metastatic colorectal cancer even when Notch signalling was seen to be suppressed. Six of 33 patients in this series showed stable disease (Strosberg et al., 2012).

PF-03084014 and MK-0752 are also receiving some attention. Both have similar patterns of biological effects. In vitro studies have indicated that PF-03084014 reduces cell migration and proliferation and suppresses angiogenesis (Shang H et al., 2015; Lopez-Guerra et al., 2015). MK-0752 in a similar vein inhibits cell proliferation and induced apoptosis in vitro and in tumour xenografts. MRK003 and MK-2206 are also said to be effective in inhibiting cell proliferation and invasion (Jin RH et al., 2013). It would be relevant to state here that modulation by PF-03084014 of the Wnt/β-catenin signalling pathway might have compounded its effects on migration. Zhang CC et al. (2014) used xenografted MDA-MB-231Luc tumours and have shown that the Notch inhibitior suppresses tumour-associated angiogenesis. This suppression was accompanied by reduced expression of VEGFR and HIF-1α. Cui D et al. (2015) have made all-compassing sweeping claims that tumour inhibition occurs in parallel with the suppression of cell survival and cell proliferation pathways and activation of apoptosis signalling. The non-malignant desmoid tumours that resemble fibrosarcomas seem to respond well to the Notch inhibitor.

The clinical outcome of a preliminary study was somewhat encouraging in a study of patients with advanced solid tumours. One patient with a thyroid carcinoma had complete remission. Desmoid tumours showed partial remission in five out of seven patients. The responses occurred in parallel with Notch inhibition (Messersmith et al., 2015). Of considerable potential interest is that PF-03084014 combined with Gemcitabine induces the regression of xenografted pancreatic ductal adenocarcinomas and suppressed metastatic dissemination. But Gemcitabine on its own did not suppress xenograft growth or the numbers of CD24(+)CD44(+) and ALDH(+) stem cells (Yabuuchi et al., 2013). Clinical evaluation has not been carried to a perceptible level. Neither does MK-0752 seem to offer much promise. An early study of high-grade gliomas one patient showed objective complete response and 10 others stable disease over a 4-month period (Krop et al. 2012), not remarkable by any means. Even for glioblastomas far better PFS outcome has been recorded in historical perspective and recently with other forms of treatment.

A preliminary study of patients with HNSCC investigating the effects of combining Notch inhibition with mTOR inhibition (Piha-Paul et al., 2015) has provided little ground for optimism. However, an earlier report indicated that MK-0752 suppressed the generation of breast cancer CSCs in xenografted tumours and in serial tumour biopsies from patients. The adverse effects of treatment with the Notch inhibitor and docetaxel did seem manageable (Schott et al., 2013; NCT00645333).

Some recent work using in vitro systems and tumour xenograft model has studied the effectiveness of DAPT for Notch suppression. DAPT seems to inhibit EMT, cell proliferation in general and probably also CSCs. Treatment of gastric cancer cell lines with DAPT enhanced the expression of epithelial markers together with the downregulation of mesenchymal ones. Perhaps one needs to address the question whether DAPT targeted CSCs, by looking at CD44 expression, efficiency of treated cells in colony formation and if there was a significant reduction tumorigenic ability of the cells following DAPT treatment. There is a report that the suppression of Notch by DAPT suppressed MMP function (Tian Q et al., 2015). Possibly, this might be reducing the invasive ability of treated target cells. Potentially, this could also suppress angiogenesis and reduce metastatic spread of xenografted tumours noticed by these authors. However, HIF-1α was employed here for primary treatment, which did lead to enhanced invasion together with the activation of Notch. Notwithstanding, one should be mindful that the effects could have occurred quite independently of Notch, since HIF-1α is not only angiogenic but also capable of promoting invasion via MMP action.

An important provision in the designing of clinical studies should be the state of expression of the Notch ligands. The DLLs and the Jagged differ in their domain structure. Jagged possess a cysteine-rich domain, which is absent in DLL. As noted earlier, DLL and Jagged have opposing effect on the induction of angiogenesis. They can also differentially affect the expression of membrane proteins associated with cell adhesion interactions and could possibly modulate cell motility. The differential expression of these ligands has been described as being able to affect tissue differentiation. Furthermore, the expression of ligands may be related to the prevailing molecular environment in the cell. Zhang S et al. (2014) found that suppression of c-met, the RTK linked with the function of HGF and cell adhesion and motility, leads to the downregulation of DLL but to the upregulation of Jagged. Besides, the efficacy of the inhibitor is likely to depend upon its binding to plasma proteins. This was suggested a while ago (Wu JM et al., 2012), but studies on the pharmacokinetics and dynamics are few and far between. These issues and circumstances would inevitably influence the outcome of Notch inhibition.

CHAPTER 9

Canonical and Non-Canonical Activation of NF-κB in Tumorigenesis

The activation of NF-κB in apoptosis, cell survival, cell proliferation, angiogenesis and migration occurs along two pathways viz. the canonical and the non-canonical pathways. The process of activation involves the removal of its inhibition by IκB (inhibitor of NF-κB) by degradation of the latter. This depends upon the activation of the IKK (IκB kinase) complex constituted of IKKα and β catalytic subunits and the regulatory IKKγ (NEMO/NF-kappa B essential modulator). This results in the generation of p65/p50 transcription factors in the canonical pathway. In the non-canonical system, NIK (NF-κB inducing kinase) activates IKKα and leads to the phosphorylation and processing of p100 by a proteasome complex to produce RelB/p53 dimeric transcription factors (Fig. 9.1).

The engagement of these pathways is not mutually exclusive in the expression of features of cell proliferation and apoptosis and cell migration. Both canonical and non-canonical systems are activated in some forms of cancer, but the emphasis has to be placed on the activation of NF-κB non-canonically. Interleukins and tumour necrosis factor (TNF) appear to activate the canonical pathway, whilst GPCRs can employ both, as evident from their synergistic function with growth factors such as EGF and PDGF and also in being activated by interleukins. NF-κB has been well established as an efficient integrator of the PI3K/Akt/mTOR and JAK/STAT signalling pathways.

TGF-β/Smad canonical signalling and TAK (TGF-β-activated kinase) activation by TGF-β are obvious opportunities of crosstalk between TGF-β function via the canonical route and NF-κB signalling. One would recall here that the binding of TGF-β to the receptors RI and RII results in the activation of the Smad signalling pathway and regulation of genetic transcription. However, Smad6 and Smad7 inhibit the activation of the Smad route by a negative feedback self-regulation. Freudlsperger et al. (2013) have taken the cue from the ability of TAK1 to promote NF-κB. The canonical Smads upregulate Smad7, which negatively regulates TGF-β/Smad and TGF-β/TAK activation. Furthermore, they show that in HNSCC cells TAK1 activates NF-κB, but

Molecular Approach to Cancer Management. DOI: http://dx.doi.org/10.1016/B978-0-12-812896-1.00009-X

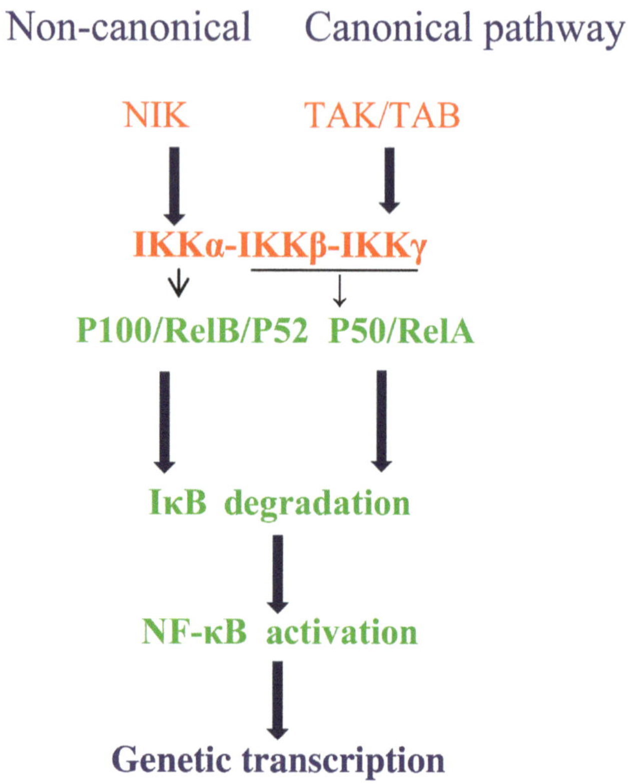

FIGURE 9.1

The non-canonical and canonical pathways of NF-κB activation leading to the transcription of responsive genes in tumorigenic processes of apoptosis, cell proliferation and migration and several other biological phenomena such as inflammation and innate and acquired immunity. IκB, inhibitor of NF-κB; IKK, IκB kinase; NIK, NF-κB-inducing kinase; TAK/TAB, TGF-β-activated kinase/TAK-binding protein.

Smad7 inhibits both canonical and non-canonical TGF-β signalling. The inhibitory Smad7 would also suppress canonical Smad signalling impinging upon the epithelial mesenchymal transition (EMT)-inducing activity of TGF-β (see also Sherbet, 2011a). Thus the crosstalk between the two systems would influence the expression of the malignant phenotype. No specificity of association of either or both pathways is evident at present but the potential of such an approach should not be underrated. It would worthwhile checking the importance of tackling NF-κB signalling by targeting specific components such as the NIK and TAK. An alternative would be taking advantage of the crosstalk between the two systems with the possibility that some growth factor/receptor system might enable the switching of pathways. EGF and some inflammatory cytokines can promote the positive Smad effects and at the same time enhance the expression of the inhibitory Smads, in this way they might alter the balance of signalling. It is needless to add this would be dependent upon and determined by the prevailing molecular environment.

NIK IS A TARGET IN THE CONTROL OF NF-κB ACTIVATION

NIK, which is highly expressed in tumour-associated endothelia as well as in rheumatoid arthritis, activates NF-κB non-canonically and this process is inhibited by the inhibition of NIK using siRNAs directed against NIK. NIK (−/−) mice display normal angiogenesis and are unaffected by TNF or VEGF exposure; also in this animal model induction of angiogenesis by non-canonical activation of NF-κB is markedly curtailed (Noort et al., 2014). Consistent with this is that silencing of NIK inhibits in vitro growth of ovarian cancer cells and has led to the suppression of tumour formation by xenografted cells (Uno et al., 2014). Interestingly, the expression of matrix metalloproteinase 9 (MMP9), which is able to promote tumour invasion and angiogenesis, was also suppressed. However, Uno et al. (2014) made no attempt to look at whether tumour-associated angiogenesis had been affected or possibly had affected metastatic spread. Although NF-κB can so strikingly sway tumour growth and angiogenesis with implication of distant spread, attempts at regulating the aberrant growth and behaviour of tumours by inhibiting NF-κB are not too numerous.

Radhakrishnan P et al. (2013) have come up with a quinoxaline urea analogue 13-197, which inhibits NF-κB as well as mammalian target of rapamycin (mTOR) signalling in vitro. The compound showed good bioavailability without obvious cytotoxic effects. In vivo xenografts of pancreatic cancer cells showed inhibition of growth and metastasis. The analogue inhibited cell cycle progression together with the downregulation of anti-apoptosis proteins. It also inhibited microvessel density. Consistent with these effects, the compound reduced metastatic deposits in lymph nodes, intestine and spleen, but there was a greater than twofold increase in peritoneal tumour nodules; there was no liver involvement. One ought to remark here that peritoneal metastases are found in around half of patients with pancreatic cancer and liver is a major metastatic locus. Peritoneal metastatic cascade is distinct from the classical spread of tumours in that in peritoneal spread the cells liberated into the peritoneal cavity from the primary tumour have to adhere to the mesothelium, invade and then develop neovascularisation for the disseminated nodules to grow. So the findings of Radhakrishnan P et al. (2013) are somewhat intriguing.

One ought to be circumspect in theorising about NIK as a target in the control of NF-κB activation in cancers. Paradoxically, NIK is ubiquitinated by cellular inhibitor of apoptosis proteins (cIAP) 1 and 2 and targeted for degradation, but the cIAPs are frequently overexpressed in cancers. In this setting one has to consider the possibility that cIAP-mediated degradation of NIK might be counteracted by the activation of the canonical path of NF-κB signalling, which growth factors, cytokines and other stimuli are known to be able to do and so regulate cell survival, proliferation and migration. Indeed cIAP antagonists are being considered for anti-cancer therapy. Targeted depletion of cIAP could be expected to supplement tumour necrosis factor-related apoptosis-inducing ligand (TRAIL)-induced apoptosis and enhance the efficacy of cytotoxic agents. From this view point, investigations are afoot on cIAP antagonists such as LCL161. Preliminary studies in patients with advanced solid tumours show that LCL161 is well tolerated. There were no severe side effects. There was no objective response but clear indications that cIAP was degraded in tumour tissue as well as other tissues and circulating cytokines increased with treatment indicative of activation of NF-κB (Infante et al., 2014). Circulating inflammatory cytokines do activate NF-κB, and Smad signalling, among other physiological events, to apoptosis. The overall effects need to be balanced with the activation of the canonical pathway as stated above. Albeit subject to several caveats, many cIAP inhibitors, which share their mechanism of action with LCL161, have been identified.

REGULATION OF NF-κB BY A20

NF-κB function is regulated by A20, the intracellular ubiquitin-editing protein, also known as TNF-α induced protein 3 encoded by the TNFAIP3 (TNF-α-induced protein 3) gene. The A20 zinc-finger protein inhibits NF-κB activation and inhibits the cell survival pathway. It is inactivated by mutation, deleted or silenced by methylation in some neoplasms such as B-cell lymphomas. Upon introduction into cells carrying the inactivated gene, it induces apoptosis and growth arrest (Compagno et al., 2009), thus act as a tumour suppressor. A20 inhibits TNF-induced NF-κB activation and suppresses cell survival and tumour growth. But it is also responsive to NF-κB and thus involved in negative feedback regulation of NF-κB signalling (Coornaert et al., 2009). It may be that the deubiquitinase function of A20 may not be an imperative for NF-κB regulation (De A et al., 2014). However, in the general context of cell survival or apoptosis, one ought to note that A20 can be anti-apoptotic via a different mode of actin. It can suppress TNF-induced apoptosis by suppressing JNK/ASK1 signalling (Won M et al., 2010). Sohn KC et al. (2014) have implicated A20 in the induction of apoptosis by imiquimod, of squamous cell skin carcinoma cells. When A20 was overexpressed, imiquimod-induced apoptosis was inhibited, and A20 knockdown enhanced apoptosis induction by imiquimod. This has been suggested to result from regulation of JNK activity by A20.

It may be recalled that imiquimod, the synthetic imidazoquinoline, is an active inducer of cytokines that can improve antiviral and anti-tumour immune responses (see pages 235, 238 and Fig. 26.4 for a detailed discussion of TLRs). Although it is thought that the immunity is acquired in response to imiquimod via TLR7, imiquimod can function independently of TLRs. Imiquimod is an approved form of treatment for human papilloma virus-linked genital warts and has been used also for superficial and nodular basal cell carcinoma over the past decade. Several clinical trials are underway in patients with advanced breast cancer, CIN (cervical intraepithelial neoplasm) grade 3 and persistent CIN 2. In a small series of breast carcinoma patients (NCT00899574) with recurrent chest wall disease and skin metastases, topical application of imiquimod cream seemed to be well tolerated with patients showing some low-grade side effects. A partial response was seen in 2 out of 10 patients and there was evidence of tumour regression attributable to immune mediation as indicated by lymphocyte infiltration and local production of cytokines. The disease was static in 5 out of 10 patients. No response was noticed in one patient and two patients showed progressive disease (Adams et al., 2012). The study also revealed that two patients with static disease showed complete systemic remission with the ER antagonist fulvestrant. Although interesting per se, this is hardly surprising since A20 was shown to be an ER responsive gene some time ago (Vendrell et al., 2007). Also endometrial cancer cells experimentally engineered to express PR-B showed induction of A20 and ABIN-2 (A20 binding inhibitor of NF-κB activation-2) and the A20/ABIN-2 complex inhibited NF-κB consistent with the known ability of progesterone to inhibit growth and promote apoptosis (Davies et al., 2004).

Finally, it would be of great interest to see a report that inhibition of expression of A20 using interference RNA inhibited tubule formation and the length of tubules formed in Matrigel of HUVEC (human umbilical vein endothelial) cells (Chng HW et al., 2006). However, it ought to be recognised that the length of tubules was measured by manual segmentation of images, which is not totally free of bias. Supporting evidence from in vivo work would have helped the case being made for angiogenesis. Also no corroborative evidence has emerged in over a decade, which is rather surprising. As regards the cellular distribution of A20 is concerned, it should be noted that its expression is not exclusive to the vasculature accompanying tumours, it is expressed in tumour cells, infiltrating lymphocytes and mesenchymal stem and progenitor cells as well as in endothelial progenitor cells. Indeed endothelial progenitor cells transduced to overexpress A20 did not differ much from un-transduced control cells in respect of tubule formation.

Furthermore, both transduced and parental cells showed similar levels of angiogenic factors (Liu JW et al., 2010). Nonetheless, one cannot underrate the potential importance of A20 in the angiogenic process. For one would recall, ABIN-2 can interact with the endothelial receptor Tie2, which is an essential participant in blood vessel formation and survival of endothelial cells. It is actively involved in tumour angiogenesis as well as inflammatory conditions of arthritis. As discussed in another location (pp. 170–172), NF-κB has been implicated in thalidomide action. Keifer et al. (2001) demonstrated this over a decade ago. Thalidomide inhibited IKK and NF-κB target genes IL-8, TRAF1, and c-IAP2. Indeed both thalidomide and the derivative lenalidomides may block NF-κB activation. Liu WM et al. (2004) noted inhibition of NF-κB together with marked increase in Bax/Bcl-2 ratio and that the effects on the apoptosis family genes were more prominent than NF-κB inhibition.

PLUMBAGIN AND VITAMIN K IN TUMOUR SUPPRESSION

Plumbagin (5-hydroxy-2-methyl-1,4-napthoquinone) is a quinoid extracted from the roots of the *Plumbago zeylanica*, the wild leadwort plant and analogue of vitamin K. The vitamins K3 (menadione; 2-methyl-1,4-naphthoquinone) and K2 (menaquinone) have been shown to be powerful anti-tumour agents and transduce their signals by similar routes and generate similar phenotypic changes.

Inhibition of the NF-κB/Akt/mTOR Signalling Axis by Plumbagin

NF-κB/Akt/mTOR is a major signalling axis involved in the function of growth factors, activation of EMT, cell survival, proliferation, tumorigenesis, invasion and eventual metastatic deposition. The anti-tumour properties of plumbagin are thought to occur as a consequence of the suppression of the NF-κB/AKT/mTOR signalling axis. NF-κB integrates the PI3K/Akt/mTOR and JAK/STAT signalling. It may also indirectly signal through the JAK/Src/STAT pathway. Ras/Raf/MEK/ERK can interact with the PI3K/Akt system and regulate cell proliferation. So the inhibitory activity of plumbagin also extends to these signalling systems (Bin Hafeez et al., 2012, 2015; Sandur et al., 2010; Yan W et al., 2013).

The biological consequences are suppression of cell proliferation and promotion of apoptosis. Inevitably, these inhibitory influences will involve alterations in the expression of the pro- and anti-apoptosis genes of the Bcl-2 family. Whether PTEN, the negative regulator of PI3K/Akt is involved with plumbagin function may be deemed as not fully established. Besides controlling the size of the cell population by inducing apoptosis by inhibiting the PI3K/Akt pathway, plumbagin may achieve the same result via TRAIL/death receptor signalling. It induced apoptosis of leukaemia cells K562. This was associated with reactive oxygen species (ROS). Furthermore, enhanced expression of TRAIL and the death receptors DR4 and DR5 was encountered (Sun J and McKallip, 2011). Plumbagin does also seem to inhibit cell proliferation by functioning via the FOX M1 protein, which is an associated transcription factor overexpressed in many tumours. It has been found to downregulate its targets viz. cyclin D1 and the cdc25B phosphatase, which activates cdc2 kinase, and upregulate the expressions of p21 and p27 (Niu MS et al., 2015).

Plumbagin Disturbs the ROS/Antioxidant Equilibrium and Induces Apoptosis

A major growth inhibitory mechanism of action of naphthoquinones as a class and, in the present context, of plumbagin is by generating ROS in cells exposed to its action. Tumour cells produce both ROS and antioxidants to protect them from the deleterious effects of ROS. A state of equilibrium is maintained between these two entities in the cancer cell. Plumbagin can tip this balance towards ROS. ROS is a most important mediator of apoptosis. This seems to occur by the agency of Nrf2. *Nrf2* is a basic leucine zipper transcription factor involved in the regulation of the expression of antioxidant proteins. Nrf2 occurs in a dormant form and upon activation enters the nucleus, where it transcribes the production of antioxidant enzymes. This weighs in favour of a reduction in the ROS status. Plumbagin has been shown to suppress Nrf2 and thus restore the ROS-mediated induction of apoptosis. Pan ST et al. (2015) were able to show that the suppression of cell proliferation and inhibition of EMT and the generation of cancer stem cell (CSCs) by plumbagin occurred as a result of the suppression of entry of Nrf2 into the nucleus. This would have prevented Nrf2 from activating the production of antioxidants.

Suppression of Invasion and Angiogenesis by Plumbagin and Vitamin K

The actual mechanics of suppression of invasion and metastatic spread of cancer by plumbagin and vitamin K are yet to be fully unravelled. Suppression of invasive behaviour in vitro of prostate cancer cells was demonstrated some time ago (Aziz et al., 2008). Some evidence has been adduced for the suppression of the conventional signalling pathways in the inhibition of invasion by plumbagin. Plumbagin has been found to inhibit invasion by downregulating Wnt signalling and β-catenin expression

(Raghu and Karunagaran, 2014). This would be expected to upregulate the expression of E-cadherin and reduce invasive ability. STAT3-mediation has been suggested as a mode of the suppression of invasion by plumbagin. TGF-β is an established promoter of invasion and metastasis. It was downregulated together with lowering of the expression of MMPs in the suppression of invasion. Also noted in this series of experiments was the downregulation of IL-1α, which is also known to promote invasion by upregulating MMPs (Yan W et al., 2013).

Much of the information about plumbagin and invasion is of recent origin. However, there is some early but indirect evidence that vitamin K3 and K2 may suppress invasive ability. In fact, it was reported over a decade ago that administration of vitamin K2 suppressed the growth of hepatocellular carcinoma (HCC) cells inoculated into nude mice. The inhibitory effects extended also to in vitro invasion of HCC cells and were apparently brought about by the activation of protein kinase A (Otsuka et al., 2004). Even earlier, this group revealed that administration of the vitamin to HCC patients prevented the invasion of the carcinoma into the portal vein (Koike et al., 2002). Indeed, HCC has shown more frequent vascular invasion and intrahepatic metastasis in the absence of vitamin K (Miyaaki et al., 2007). This has been confirmed in another study where absence of the vitamin correlated with VEGF expression (Amaoka et al., 2007) with obvious links to angiogenesis.

Surprisingly, scant is the attention devoted to the angiogenic effects of plumbagin considering that its effects of suppression of cell proliferation and invasion have been known for quite some time. Plumbagin has suppressed angiogenesis in vitro and in vivo experiments. It reduced the growth of ovarian cancer cell xenografts and this seemed to be a result of reduced angiogenesis as indicated by reduced immunohistochemical staining using anti-von Willebrand factor antibodies (Sinha et al. 2013). It is rather surprising that most studies of this kind have not had a look whether the xenografts had metastasised and if metastasis had been reduced. The VEGFR-activated Ras/MAPK angiogenic signalling is suppressed by plumbagin (Lai L et al., 2012). Most of such investigations have employed in vitro assays such as Matrigel or CAM (chorioallantoic membrane) angiogenesis. Furthermore, on the angiogenesis front the finding that plumbagin-mediated activation of AMP-activated protein kinases (AMPKs) gains some significance, since AMPK is a known suppressor of angiogenesis. AMPK has been implicated also in the inhibition of cell proliferation, and the generation of CSCs by suppressing several signalling systems which regulate these events (see citations below, and Table 20.1).

The analogue vitamin K2 suppresses cell migration and angiogenesis in the same manner as plumbagin. The vitamin K effects have been confirmed in a few studies (Samykutty et al., 2013). Some studies have used the vitamin K-dependent glycoprotein called protein S as a marker and have shown that the circulating protein S inhibited VEGFR2-mediated angiogenesis in Matrigel assays and inhibited endothelial cell migration and proliferation. The MAPK/ERK/Akt pathway was inhibited in parallel with the anti-angiogenic effects (Fraineau et al., 2012).

Plumbagin Suppresses CSC Development

In respect of tumour development, there are clear indications that plumbagin can target CSCs in BRCA1 defective breast cancer cells. BRCA1/BRCA2 defective cells were susceptible to plumbagin-induced apoptosis (Somasundaram et al., 2016; Reshma et al., 2016). Obviously, these effects are due to the inability of the defective cells to repair double-strand DNA breaks (DSBs). The induction of ROS would explain the DNA-strand breaks and the induction of apoptosis. Whether stem cells are prone to the induction of DNA-strand breaks has to be debated. The survival and propagation of stem cells would depend on their ability to repair DSBs and they would possess protective mechanisms against DSBs and oxidative damage (Nagaria et al., 2013). Stem cells do repair DSBs more efficiently. BRCA1 deficiency leads to the impairment of DSB repair. So the targeting of BRCA deficient stem cells using plumbagin is indeed a viable proposition given the significance of BRCA genes in breast cancer susceptibility. As stated in a previous section, the suppression of CSC by plumbagin-mediated activation of Nrf2 can occur by the alteration in the balance of antioxidants/Nrf2. Indeed the suppression of EMT and CSCs by this means might make plumbagin a powerful tool for tumour suppression.

Combinatorial Strategies Using Plumbagin

Combination therapy with synergistically functional drugs and biological response modifiers has been an important arm of treatment strategy. Ramentaceone, a naphthoquinone derived from the Sundew Droseraceae family plants, can induce apoptosis by inhibiting PI3K/Akt signalling in parallel with reduction in the expression of the anti-apoptotic Bcl-2 and enhancement of the pro-apoptosis Bax and Bak (Kawiak and Lojkowska, 2016). Plumbagin can function by activating AMPK and the pro-apoptosis ASK1/JNK/p38 signalling (Chen MB et al., 2013). Zoledronate (ZOL) can inhibit tumour growth by inducing apoptosis. The bisphosphonates are attributed with the ability to inhibit YAP/TAZ of the Hippo system. They block the nuclear localisation YAP/TAZ and suppress cell proliferation by the downregulation of cell cycle regulators.

Plumbagin does indeed upregulate p53 suppress G1 phase regulators cyclins D1 and E (Zhang XQ et al., 2016). Plumbagin and ZOL can synergistically target the MAPK/JNK/ERK system (Qiao H et al., 2016). Plumbagin can inhibit VEGF-induced MEK, ERK and JNK. ZOL is also able to target ERK/JNK signalling and influence endothelial cell adhesion. It reduces the expression of the highly potent inducer of vascular growth VEGF-A in some systems. Interestingly, ZOL may suppress angiogenesis and inhibit invasion in vitro. It suppresses the production of VEGF and ANG-1 and also downregulates MMPs (see discussion below). Thus the synergy extends also to the suppression of invasion and angiogenesis, with both plumbagin and ZOL being able to influence angiogenic outcome.

New avenues of approach to the use of plumbagin in therapy have emerged. Hwang GH et al. (2015) were able to show that thioredoxin reductase was a target of plumbagin. The latter suppressed the proliferation of HepG2 HCC cells by enhancing apoptosis. This suppression of cell proliferation occurred with reduced expression of thioredoxin reductase (Hwang GH et al., 2015). One may recapitulate here the participation of the thioredoxin system in protecting cells against oxidative stress and DNA damage repair. Thioredoxin reductase activates thioredoxin, which binds ROS and protects cells oxidative injury. It has important functions in the operation of the immune system. Notable here is that thioredoxin promotes cell proliferation and inhibits apoptosis and promotes angiogenesis. Hence inhibiting thioredoxin reductase has been much espoused for the control of tumour growth and progression. As discussed in another location, PX-12, which inhibits thioredoxin reductase, has been shown to inhibit cell proliferation and induce apoptosis and it has been evaluated in clinical trials (p. 103; Epilogue Table 2). In the light of the finding that plumbagin targets the reductase, studying the synergy between PX-12 and plumbagin would be well worth the effort.

Other options are also opening up for the combinatorial use of plumbagin. Its inhibitory effects of suppression of the PI3K/Akt/mTOR and the MAPK pathways are said to be accompanied and accentuated by the activation of AMPK signalling (Zhou ZW et al., 2015). As noted in another location, metformin possesses marked anti-tumour properties. Significantly, a major effector of metformin is AMPK. The involvement of AMPK here is significant since it collaborates with several tumour suppressor genes and interacts with several signalling systems, inhibiting the anti-apoptosis PI3K/Akt/mTOR and activating the pro-apoptosis ASK1/JNK/p38 pathways. This suggests a viable and legitimate basis for combining plumbagin with metformin in therapeutic intervention. It might be worth making a note here that flavonoids can inhibit cell proliferation, induce apoptosis and suppress angiogenesis; they can produce these effects via AMPK activation. As discussed in another location, quercetin suppresses angiogenesis by inhibiting COX-1 and downregulating HIF-1, besides activating AMPK (pp. 152–153).

A mode of function quite distinctive from the deregulation of signal transduction systems has been suggested for plumbagin. Liu XJ et al. (2014) have postulated that CRM1 (chromosome region maintenance 1; exportin 1), which is involved with the nuclear transport of proteins, is a target of plumbagin. Apparently plumbagin interferes with the interaction of certain suppressor proteins with CRM1 and inhibits their function by obstructing nuclear transport. The translocation of YAP to the nucleus is an crucial step in YAP function. This is regulated by CRM1. Blocking CRM1-despendent nuclear translocation using the Streptomyces antibiotic leptomycin B suppresses YAP function. Leptomycin B binds CRM1 and prevents its normal function (Kudo et al., 1998). This would provide a good adjunct to the suppression of YAP by leptomycin and plumbagin in combination.

The anti-tumour effects of plumbagin seem to be enhanced upon administration by its binding to serum albumin (Gou Y et al., 2015). This is not unexpected, since the interaction of drugs with serum albumin is well established. Drugs interact with albumin at specific binding sites and this effectively enhances the efficacy of drugs and their pharmacokinetic features (Yamasaki et al., 2013).

Concluding Thoughts on NF-κB Suppression in Carcinogenesis

The discussion mentioned previously has highlighted the positive aspects of plumbagin and related compounds of their ability to suppress invasion, angiogenesis and to block the development and propagation of CSCs. The signalling pathways are also reasonably well elucidated and some efforts are afoot to test combination therapy. These potential areas of interest are evident from the varied description of the phenotypic influences exerted by these compounds and from the signalling systems, which they influence and bring them to fruition. Nonetheless, much more well-structured and planned experimental and pre-clinical work is necessary to underscore the latent and conceivable biological benefits. So it is unsurprising that although the vitamin K and plumbagin were recognised as significant mediators of biological functions, they have aroused little clinical interest.

CHAPTER 10

Tumour Suppression and Inhibition of Angiogenesis by TXNIP (Thioredoxin Interacting Protein)

ARRESTINS IN THE REGULATION OF ANGIOGENESIS

Arrestins are important signalling regulators. The arrestin family consists of arrestin 1 and arrestin 4 (the visual arrestins found exclusively in the retina) and β-arrestin 1 and β-arrestin 2 (also known as arrestins 2 and 3) occur in many tissues and regulate the signalling initiated by G-protein coupled receptors (GPCRs). Upon activation of the arrestins, GPCRs, and G-receptor kinases (GRKs) can regulate many signalling systems. β-Arrestin for instance is involved with the regulation of ERK/p38/JNK, Akt, RhoA and NF-κB pathways. With GRK mediation, β-arrestin can activate MEK1 (MKK1/MAP2K1, mitogen-activated protein kinase kinase), RKIP/Raf1, PI3K/Akt and the mdm2/p53 pathways. β-Arrestin generates a wide array of phenotypic effects, which include apoptosis, cell proliferation and possibly also cell motility. It acts as an adaptor protein; its structural features enable it to bind simultaneously to several protein components that are involved in signal initiation or cessation (Milano et al., 2002). Thioredoxin interacting protein (TXNIP), an arrestin family protein, is a powerful inhibitor of tumour growth and angiogenesis.

THE THIOREDOXIN SYSTEM

The thioredoxin (TRX) system, which includes TRX, TRX reductase (TRXR) and NADPH, subserves many important cellular functions. This is an invaluable system, which provides protection against oxidative stress. It plays key roles in DNA and protein repair, genetic transcription, function of the immune system and in cell proliferation and apoptosis. TRXR is an important ingredient of the redox function of TRX. It activates TRX, which binds ROS and protects cells from oxidative injury. Notable in the present context is that TRX is involved with the promotion of cell proliferation and with inhibition of apoptosis. It promotes angiogenesis as evidenced by its ability to induce hypoxia-inducible factor (HIF)-1 and vascular endothelial growth

Molecular Approach to Cancer Management. DOI: http://dx.doi.org/10.1016/B978-0-12-812896-1.00010-6

factor (VEGF). TXNIP inhibits the active reduced form of TRX, and can promote apoptosis by blocking the binding to and inhibition of the apoptosis signal regulating kinase 1 by TRX.

TXNIP, an arrestin family protein, is an endogenous inhibitor of the TRX system, which is strongly implicated in the angiogenic process. TRX is represented by two isoforms TRX1 and TRX2. Both actively engage signalling systems that promote cell proliferation, inhibit apoptosis and induce angiogenesis. TXNIP interacts with the catalytic site of both TRX1 and TRX2 and inhibits these functions. TXNIP is downregulated in many tumours and has been regarded as a tumour suppressor.

THE TUMOUR SUPPRESSOR FUNCTION OF TXNIP

The tumour suppressor function of TXNIP seems to derive from its ability to control cell proliferation and induce apoptosis. It has also been attributed with suppression of metastatic behaviour, which seems to be related to the suppression of cell motility and adhesion-dependent phenomena. TXNIP engages many signalling systems to bring about these phenotypic outcomes (Fig. 10.1). The suppression of metastasis would be aided by the inhibitory effects of TXNIP on angiogenesis. TXNIP inhibits endothelial cell migration and angiogenesis. The molecular circuitry involving TXNIP in angiogenesis has been unravelled reasonably well. Possibly, TXNIP could inhibit angiogenesis by suppressing Akt activation and the Akt-mediated upregulation of VEGFs and the enhancement of microvessel density. TXNIP also inhibits the NF-κB survival pathway and promotes apoptosis. Rather more importantly, TXNIP inhibits EMT, which is the driving force of tumorigenesis and tumour progression. With this background and also in hindsight, it is hardly surprising that there have been some early efforts to find other inhibitors of the TRX system. Undeniably, the biological action of TXNIP that would provide

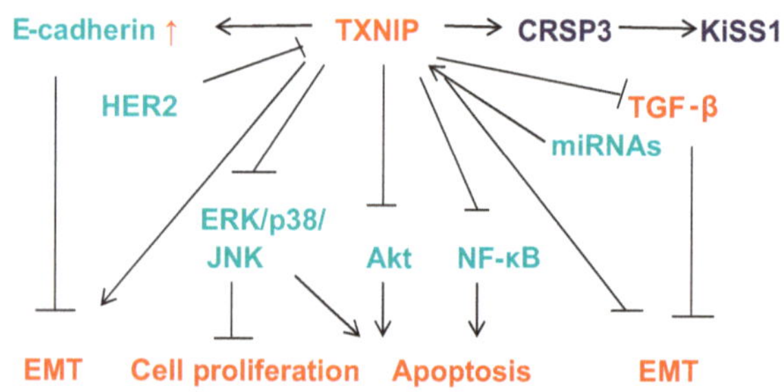

FIGURE 10.1
The pathways of TXNIP signalling systems in exerting its suppressor effects. *From Sherbet, 2013. Therapeutic strategies in cancer biology and pathology, Elsevier; ISBN: 978-0-12-416570-0.*

is an open opportunity for identifying endogenous or synthetic agonists of its function in cancer control.

INHIBITION OF TRXR BY PX-12 AND THE EFFECTS PX-12 ON TUMOUR GROWTH

Some while ago pleurotin, a reversible inhibitor of TRXR, and the TRX inhibitor 1-methylpropyl 2-imidazolyl disulphide (PX-12) were shown to inhibit HIF-1 and HIF-induced VEGF production (Welsh et al., 2003; Baker et al., 2006). Recent reports have shown that PX-12 inhibited TRX1 and in parallel inhibited cell cycle progression at G2/M transition, induced apoptosis and inhibited migration of colorectal carcinoma cells migration in vitro (Wang F et al., 2015). It also induced caspase-mediated apoptosis in AML (acute myeloid leukaemia) and in A549 cells in a dose-related manner (Tan YX et al., 2014; You BR et al., 2014).

CLINICAL OUTCOME FROM PX-12 TREATMENT

PX-12 has been tested in the clinical setting but the results have not been very encouraging. Early studies did indicate some potential benefits. Kirkpatrick et al. (2005) claimed enhanced patient survival. But later studies have held out little promise. Baker et al. (2013) noticed no clinical activity in patients with advanced gastrointestinal cancers who had been administered PX-12 at the tolerated dose of 300 $mg/m^2/24$ h intravenously once a week, although PX-12 bound irreversibly to plasma proteins. No changes were seen in plasma TRX1, VEGF or FGF-2. Earlier, Ramanathan et al. (2012) had reported stable disease in one patient with colorectal cancer. There was no clinical activity in pancreatic cancer. The disease was stable in two patients, but without corresponding anticipated changes in TRX1 or the commonly employed marker CA 19-9 (carbohydrate antigen 19-9).

Despite the high expression of TRX in tumours and its link with cell proliferation, apoptosis, cell migration and the perceived parallelism with tumour progression, no TRX inhibitor has achieved the benchmark that justifies further evaluation in the laboratory or the clinic.

CHAPTER 11

Cyclooxygenase-2 Inhibitors Suppress EMT, CSCs and Angiogenesis

The cyclooxygenases (COXs) are enzymes involved in the biosynthesis of prostaglandins. Of the three COX enzymes, COX-1 is the commonly expressed form and COX-2 is the inducible isoform and COX-3 is a splice isoform of COX-1. COX-2 promotes tumour progression by supporting cell proliferation, cell survival and the invasive behaviour of tumour. Whilst it is an important regulator of the cell cycle, the control exerted by COX-2 over the size of the cell population and indeed tumour growth emanates from its suppressive influence on apoptosis. COX-2 inhibition induces apoptosis by the mitochondrial pathway as well as by tumour necrosis factor-related apoptosis-inducing ligand (TRAIL)/death receptor signalling. Indeed it has been well established over the years as a major regulator of tumour cell behaviour modulating cell motility, angiogenesis and tumour progression. Enhanced expression of COX-2 has been encountered in many tumour types and most importantly its expression has links with cancer stem cells (CSCs) with its implication in the self-renewal of CSCs and in drug resistance.

COX-2 SIGNALLING, CSCs AND CANCER PROGRESSION

COX-2 expression is altered by many growth factors and cytokines. COX-2 can activate the signalling systems involved in the induction of cell proliferation, suppression of apoptosis, activation of epithelial mesenchymal transition (EMT) and the generation and self-renewal of CSCs. This is a most significant relationship, which accounts for the promotion of tumour initiation, growth and metastatic spread. It is controlled and manoeuvred by many modes of signal transduction by COX-2.

The link of EMT with tumour initiation, growth and metastasis encompasses the generation of CSCs and their evolution to the tumour initiating and invasive phenotype and as active inducers of angiogenesis. These are prerequisite elements in the dissemination of the tumour cells and the development of overt metastases. A large body of evidence has accumulated showing the

Molecular Approach to Cancer Management. DOI: http://dx.doi.org/10.1016/B978-0-12-812896-1.00011-8

initiation of EMT by COX-2 signalling. This is reversed by the non-steroidal anti-inflammatory drug celecoxib. Most of these are in vitro observations but there is much indirect evidence that this relationship subsists in tumour tissues too.

Huang MS et al. (2016) have looked at this on hepatocellular carcinoma (HCC) tissues from patients before and after TACE (transcatheter arterial chemoembolization) surgery. In the heightened hypoxic environment that results from TACE treatment, HIF-1α expression is altered. In the HCC tissue after TACE, HIF-1α was upregulated together with enhanced expression of COX-2. This correlated with enhanced expression of EMT markers. These features also correlated with vascular invasion and the state of intrahepatic metastases. Compatible with the marked reduction of E-cadherin expression in hypoxic condition and the COX-2 upregulation is that inhibition of COX-2 has led to the restoration of E-cadherin levels in HNSCC cells (Fujii et al., 2014).

Bocca et al. (2012) exposed colon cancer cells to EGF and to hypoxia and recorded an increase in cell proliferation and the activation of EMT. Again these effects were reversed by celecoxib. A reversal of EMT also took place when HT colon carcinoma cells were exposed to the COX-2 inhibitor apricoxib (Kirane et al., 2012; St John et al., 2012). Indeed apricoxib has been claimed to be more efficient in reversing the EMT phenotype than celecoxib (St John et al., 2012). One should point out here it is essential that the activation or reversal of EMT should be shown to be accompanied by alterations in COX-2 levels, for there is a thought that some COX-2 inhibitors might influence EMT regardless and independently of COX-2 expression. Apricoxib is said to be able to sensitise tumours to conventional chemotherapy and is being evaluated at the clinical level, but the studies carried out so far do not seem to suggest any significant benefit in disease control.

The suppression of CSCs could be the single most important element in the control of cancer growth and metastasis. It is now beyond reasonable doubt that CSCs are generated by a COX-2-dependent mechanism, although the actual mode of signalling is yet to be elucidated. Pancreatic CSCs are seen in the early stages of the development of ductal carcinoma and they increase in number with disease progression. The enhanced CSC marker expression is also accompanied by the expression of inflammation-related genes. Ablation of COX-2 from genetically engineered pancreatic cancer models has led to the reduction of the CSC marker expression. The expression of EMT markers occurs also in experimentally induced pancreatitis (Mohammed et al., 2015). These findings underscore the significance of combating COX-2 signalling not only as a potential preventive measure against cancer initiation but also for the suppression of the progression of overt disease. In an HCC cell line, Guo Z et al. (2015) have identified a subpopulation of cells with CSC characteristics. These cells overexpress COX-2 and show enhanced cell migration and proliferation activity. They found that this was accompanied by the suppression of PDCD4 (programmed cell death 4) and PTEN. Both genes are tumour suppressors; PDCD4 restrains CSC generation and maintenance and in fact promotes them to differentiate and PTEN suppresses PI3K/Akt proliferative signalling. The EGF/EGFR/Akt signalling cascade has also been implicated in the generation and maintenance of the CSC population.

An illuminating set of findings is that breast cancer CSCs can resist TRAIL-induced apoptosis by the downregulation of the death receptors. Breast cancer cells grown in vitro as spheroids are said to contain a high number of CSCs with reduced expression of DR4 and DR5. Treatment of these spheroids with COX-2 inhibitors rendered them susceptible to TRAIL-mediated apoptosis. This correlated with the upregulation of the expression of the death receptors (Chandrasekaran et al. 2014). One should add a caveat here that resistance to TRAIL can result also from activation of NF-κB survival signalling as shown some while ago (Keane et al., 2000). Furthermore, the formation of spheroids is based on intercellular adhesion and the dictates of adhesion-mediating ECM components and cell proliferation signalling. Whilst stem cells grown as spheroids might exhibit enhanced anti-inflammatory and drug resistance characteristics, the converse cannot be held as fully substantiated. In other words, although in some situations, they might show a preponderance of CSCs, no obvious signalling mechanisms have been linked with the appearances of CSC in spheroids. Most spheroids are derived from adult cells, not from pluripotent embryonic cells. So, one must assume that they contained pre-existing CSCs or that adult cell had dedifferentiated and acquired CSC features. Acquisition of enhanced proliferative potential does not bestow CSC features but would enable propagation and maintenance of CSCs. Nevertheless, as a positive aspect one can envisage a role for ECM components in spheroid formation and the putative appearance of CSCs.

Other mechanisms have been sought and postulates constructed to explain the generation of CSCs. Matrix metalloproteinases (MMPs) are regarded as a driving force. CSCs may bind MMPs at their surface, which would aid invasion but the thought that MMPs induce the generation of CSCs is not thoroughly sustainable. Celecoxib is said to suppress STAT3 phosphorylation and this is held to suppress the formation of CSCs (Yang MY et al., 2014).

The promotion of cell proliferation and invasion induced by COX-2 should not be uncoupled from its putative ability to generate CSC and promote their propagation. As stated earlier, COX-2 reduces the expression of PDCD4 and PTEN (Guo Z, 2015), whilst inhibition of COX-2 activates PTEN (Meng Z and Gan, 2015). COX-2 expression is often higher in cancers than corresponding normal tissues and is linked with the production of VEGF and angiogenesis. Celecoxib would induce S-phase arrest and apoptosis and also downregulate the expression of MMPs (Zhou X et al., 2015). The latter findings offer clear scope for its use for inhibiting invasion and angiogenesis. Equally, it has been appreciated that these modes of COX-2 signalling might be related to the generation and propagation of CSCs, rather than represent a mere means of expanding the cell population.

Among other possible ways evoked in this regard is the deregulation of the actin cytoskeletal dynamics without the involvement of β-catenin participation (Behr et al., 2015). However, Wnt/β-catenin signalling pathway is intricately linked with actin cytoskeletal dynamics in intercellular adhesion and also in EMT activation. Furthermore, Wnt can induce MMPs and this would affect cell motility. The involvement of E-cadherin and MMP has been suggested in respect of the action of another COX-2 inhibitor, viz. meloxicam, also a non-steroidal anti-inflammatory agent. HCC cells have been found to respond to meloxicam treatment with reduced cell proliferation and invasion in vitro. This seemed to be an outcome of the inhibition of MMPs and upregulation of E-cadherin expression (Li T et al., 2016). Indeed, it has been suggested that manipulation of the Wnt/E-cadherin pathway might provide a potentially powerful means to inhibit EMT. Besides, there is evidence of extensive crosstalk between Wnt/β-catenin signalling and the Ras pathway and NF-κB pathway (see Sherbet, 2013). The factors would impinge upon the manifestation of invasive and angiogenic phenotypes. It would be well to reiterate that CSCs are intrinsically resistant to radiation and chemotherapy and represent a highly invasive phenotype, the very properties that contribute to the initiation, development and secondary dissemination of cancer.

COX-2 INHIBITORS IN CANCER CONTROL

In the light of the involvement of many signalling pathways that drive the metastatic cascade and their susceptibility to modulation by COX-2, the idea of employing COX-2 inhibitors to control these neoplastic processes has gained ground. The use of extraneous inhibitors and of naturally occurring COX-2 inhibitors has been the subject of intense study. Among naturally occurring COX-2 inhibitors of interest are curcumin, resveratrol and quercetin. The synthetic non-steroidal anti-inflammatory drugs like celecoxib and apricoxib were alluded to before. They are small molecule selective inhibitors of COX-2. Apricoxib is comparable to celecoxib in the potency in respect of PGE2 (prostaglandin E2) inhibition, but there are reports that it reverses the EMT far more efficiently than celecoxib.

The application of combination therapy has gained currency because of the reported inefficacy of COX-2 inhibitors as single agents to produce favourable outcome in clinical trials. A recent meta-analysis of nine randomised trials with NSCLC patients on COX-2 inhibitors has proved rather discouraging. Whilst there were increases in the overall response rate, no tangible improvement was seen in overall survival, 1-year survival rate or progression free survival. There were also concerns about toxicity (Zhou YY et al., 2016).

Vandetanib (ZD-6474) is an inhibitor of VEGFR2 kinase and suppresses endothelial cell proliferation and vascular permeability. Together with the inhibition of EGFR, vandetanib suppresses cell proliferation and angiogenesis. It has shown clinical benefit in patients with advanced medullary thyroid carcinoma in a phase III trial (NCT00322452). In a phase III study, vandetanib as single agent showed no improvements over the EGFR RTK inhibitor erlotinib in the clinical outcome of advanced NSCLC (Natale et al., 2011). Nevertheless, combining vandetanib with celecoxib produced markedly greater inhibition of proliferation of osteosarcoma cells in vitro and tumour growth from cells xenografted in vivo (Liu JN et al., 2015). Similar additive suppression of proliferation has been encountered when celecoxib was combined with rapamycin (Cao YB et al., 2015), which suggests the potential benefits of combination with mTOR inhibitors. HT-29 colon cancer cells treated with celecoxib exhibited reduced cell viability roughly equal to that observed with imatinib, a RTK inhibitor, but there was no remarkable change in combination treatment. The reduction in viability was accompanied by the inhibition of COX-2 and increase of caspase-3. The caspase increase was similar to that encountered with imatinib and celecoxib. But the latter combination resulted in a substantial reduction in COX-2 (Atari-Hajipirloo et al., 2016). One would get an overall impression here that imatinib and celecoxib are operating via disparate signalling pathways.

As discussed in another location, the clinical value of COX-2 inhibitors is vastly enhanced by their implicated role in death receptor function. COX-2 inhibitors have been employed with death receptor inhibitors to investigate whether any additional benefits would accrue from the combination. Liu X et al. (2004) demonstrated over a decade ago that celecoxib, which is putatively linked with cancer prevention, induced the expression of DR5 accompanied by the induction of the caspase cascade and apoptosis. Apoptosis was accentuated when celecoxib was combined with TRAIL. Zuo CH et al. (2015) employed IFN-α to target TRAIL and demonstrated the possible involvement of the death receptor in the induction of apoptosis. IFN-α treatment of cells in vitro produced a moderate inhibition of growth, but celecoxib was more effective. Although as a single agent IFN-α was less effective, it did work synergistically with celecoxib providing an overall growth inhibition that was superior to their effect as single agents. The growth inhibition was a result of the induction of apoptosis. Combined treatment was more effective in inducing apoptosis, but the increase was not remarkable. However, it is intriguing that IFN-α upregulated the expression of TRAIL and as single agents slightly reduced the expression of DR4 and DR5. Nonetheless, in combination the treatment increased the expression of both the receptors and TRAIL. This differential upregulation is attributed with the observed synergy (Zuo CH et al., 2015). One ought to qualify this by saying that TRAIL expression in the tumours was not remarkably greater after combination therapy as compared with celecoxib alone. There is also some insufficiency in the information concerning tumour weight and volume.

CG100649 (polmacoxib) is a dual COX-2 and carbonic anhydrase (CA) inhibitor, which has received some but not overwhelming attention. Many isoforms of CA have been identified. The isoforms CA I, II and VII are cytosolic and CA IX and CA XII are transmembrane isoforms. Two isoforms have been studied in relation to tumour growth. The isoform CA IX is a hypoxia-inducible isoform and promotes tumour growth. CG100649 has been found to induce cell cycle arrest and inhibit the growth of xenografts of colon carcinoma cells (Kim SH et al., 2014; Woo JK et al., 2015). The inhibitor upregulated DR4 and DR5 but reduced the expression of the decoy receptors (Woo JK et al., 2015).

CA IX is regulated by HIF-1, which promotes angiogenesis and is overexpressed in many cancers. The level of expression of CA IX correlates with Gleason grade of prostate cancer (Ambrosio et al., 2016). It may be associated with aggressive neuroblastomas and disease prognosis. High levels of expression correlated with reduced survival, possibly attributable to metastatic disease (Ameis et al., 2016). This may imply the possible promotion of angiogenesis. Unfortunately no experimental evidence is currently available to put this postulated relationship on an assured footing. An isolated finding is that the inhibition of the isoform CA II also similarly suppresses the proliferation of the NSCLC cells H727 and A549 in vitro. The cells in which CA II had been silenced produced tumour xenografts with reduced growth rate and importantly with much reduced tumour vascularisation as indicated by CD31 staining (Zhou YX et al., 2015). One does not know if the suppressed vascularisation of the xenografts had any effect on metastasis. No attempt was made to inspect the animals for metastases; assessments of the biological effect of treatment were restricted merely to the measurement of the tumour volume.

In spite of the deficiencies and shortcomings of the data currently on record, there could be some benefit in inhibiting CA together with the inhibition of COX-2. In the hypoxic environment, inhibition of the isoform CA IX has been reported to potentiate the inhibitory effects of rapamycin in murine tumour models (Faes et al., 2016).

The efficacy of celecoxib has been tested in combination of docetaxel and the bisphosphonate zoledronic acid (ZOL) in a phase II clinical trial of a series of patients with prostate cancer. No improvement in overall survival was noticed (Kattan et al., 2016). ZOL is used to reduce bone metastasis and combat the loss of bone associated with the metastasis of breast, lung and prostate cancer. So the outcome of this trial is somewhat discouraging. However, other investigations have shown that it inhibits tumour cell proliferation in vitro. Pre-clinical work has shown that ZOL is able to inhibit the growth of human tumour xenografts, apparently by the induction of apoptosis. The effects were more striking in combination with conventional cytotoxic drugs (see pp. 72–74). ZOL does improve bone mineral density and would counteract the loss of bone density occurring from androgen deprivation. It has been found to increase the time to progression in a series of hormone resistant prostate cancer patients (Nagao et al., 2016). Satisfactory modes of treatment of hormone-refractory metastatic prostate cancer are still sought, because the mechanisms of hormone resistance are not well understood, but androgen deprivation does induce apoptosis. Hence further studies aimed at accentuating the apoptosis process may be warranted.

Meloxicam, another COX-2 inhibitor, was shown some time ago to be able to inhibit tumour growth. Goldman et al. (1998) had noticed that meloxicam did inhibit the growth of COX-2+ colorectal tumour cell xenografts. Furthermore, meloxicam inhibited in vitro growth of COX-2+ but not COX-2 negative cells. The response of COX-2 positive and COX-2 negative NSCLC cells was similar to that of colorectal cancer cells and pancreatic cancer models confirming the inhibitory effects on tumour growth (Tsubouchi et al., 2000). The signalling systems involved are yet to be fully elucidated but upregulation of E-cadherin expression and the suppression of MMPs has been suggested as a mechanism by which it inhibits in vitro invasion (Li T et al., 2016).

Among other COX-2 inhibitors of note are resveratrol and indomethacin. Resveratrol does inhibit COX-2 signalling but it does, however, induce apoptosis by other means also. We showed some time ago that it induces apoptosis by three different pathways. It can activate the pro-apoptosis p53/p21waf/Bax pathway. It can also inhibit cell survival by inhibiting Notch signalling and also the PI3K/Akt pathway (Cecchinato et al., 2007). This does not detract from the merits of combining resveratrol or Notch inhibitors with COX-2 inhibitors, but might indeed enhance them. This is supported by the perceived crosstalk between the signalling systems. As mentioned earlier, COX-2 does reduce the expression of PDCD4 and

PTEN. We also know that the Notch2 intracellular domain binds to the COX-2 promoter and induces COX-2 expression (Tseng YC et al., 2012).

A finding of much potential interest is that HER2 seems able to activate COX-2 signalling and promote cell proliferation (Chi F et al., 2016). If this were confirmed, it might be a valuable means of targeting COX-2 inhibitors to tumours overexpressing both COX-2 and HER2. The COX-2 inhibitors can be tagged to anti-HER2 antibodies to deliver the drug to the target and indeed one might see a composite tumour suppressive effect by the inhibition of both HER2 and COX-2 signalling. Not only does COX-2 expression presage poor prognosis for breast cancer, but a majority of breast cancer also overexpress HER2. Besides this, HER2 + tumours have a greater propensity to metastasise to the brain. These facts are persuasive and compelling arguments for testing the efficacy of COX-2 inhibitors conjugated with anti-HER2 antibodies in breast cancer management.

CHAPTER 12

Endogenous Inhibitors of Angiogenesis

Endogenous inhibitors of angiogenesis were identified many years ago. The practical implication of employing their derivatives and agonists and naturally occurring substances that can mimic their function was simultaneously appreciated in the context of treating pathological events involving neovascularisation. The anti-angiogenic effects of thrombospondins (TSPs), endostatin and angiostatin recognised by many laboratory and pre-clinical studies have led to the elucidation of the signalling pathways involved in the suppression of angiogenesis. The TSPs and endostatin have been described as endothelium-specific inhibitors. The overexpression of endostatin in the endothelium correlates with marked inhibition of tumour growth (Sund et al., 2005). TSP-1 is also overexpressed in the endothelial cells but it is also expressed in stromal fibroblasts and immune cells. Although the inhibitory effects of TSP-1 are predominantly due to direct effects on endothelial cell proliferation and migration, to describe them as endothelial-specific inhibitor appears rather artificial. TSPs and endostatin have shown a biphasic concentration-related effect on angiogenesis. Given the wide spectrum of signalling operating in the regulation of angiogenesis by these inhibitors, it could be that the biphasic effects are also compounded by the contribution from other factors. This would explain the synergistic enhancement of inhibition often described for these inhibitors. That is not an unusual situation in biological events or with angiogenesis in particular. More than one system of signalling can combine to generate a given phenotype in a collaborative assurance rather than by double assurance of an outcome; so it is more than a matter of semantics.

TSPs IN CANCER DEVELOPMENT AND PROGRESSION

TSPs are extracellular proteins and are actively involved in intercellular interactions and interaction with the extracellular matrix (ECM) and retained as an ECM protein. The role of TSPs in cancer progression is still being debated fiercely. Indeed, evidence has often been proffered, some indicating

Molecular Approach to Cancer Management. DOI: http://dx.doi.org/10.1016/B978-0-12-812896-1.00012-X

promotion and others indicating inhibition of progression. The mode of action of TSPs shown in Figs 26.2 and 26.3 makes compatible reading with these comments. Tumour cells may display reduced expression of TSPs, which might eliminate binding to adhesive glycoproteins and promote tumour invasion. This role in cell invasion is still a subject of some controversy. An enhanced induction of TSP-4 has been described in the stromal component of invasive breast tumours (McCart-Reed et al., 2013), which could possibly reflect the activation of the stromal component akin to inflammatory response to suppress tumour progression. More important are the claims that TSPs promote cell proliferation and promote epithelial mesenchymal transition (EMT) activation and thus they may be conducive to tumour growth and dissemination

Contrasting with this is the general recognition that TSP might inhibit cancer progression, possibly by altering the adhesion-related properties of the tumour cells. This is a more persuasive thought. Much evidence can be found in the literature now which confirms that TSPs do indeed inhibit cancer progression. TSP-1 expression is totally or partially downregulated in a majority of breast cancers and this has been allied with enhanced risk of disease recurrence. High TSP-1 expression has been linked with loss of tumour spread to sentinel and regional lymph nodes. TSPs have also been credited with suppression of cancer stem cells (CSCs). Furthermore, genetic inactivation of TSP by hypermethylation has been seen in high-grade invasive tumours and has also correlated with poor disease prognosis. TSPs are often downregulated in carcinomas with lymphatic spread. The suppression of tumour spread is compatible with their ability to inhibit angiogenesis. This view has gained much ground and practical prominence.

The Domain Structure and Molecular Interactions of TSPs

The TSP family comprises of five members divided into two groups, the trimeric group with TSP-1 and TSP-2 and the pentameric TSP-3, TSP-4 and TSP-5. They possess a characteristic domain structure with a shared signature domains, viz. the C-terminal epidermal growth factor (EGF) repeat domain, TSP type 3 domain and L-lectin domain. Towards the N-terminus from the EGF repeat domain are the TSR (TSP repeat) domain, the von Willebrandt factor C domain and the Laminin G-type domain. TSPs bind to ECM components such as fibronectin, laminin, type V collagen and integrins $\alpha V/\beta 1$, tenascin syndecan-1 and fibrinogen; the interactions occur through their RGD (Arginine-Glycine-Aspartic acid sequence) domain and may be implicated in the regulation of cell adhesion and migration. The RGD domain is also concerned with the retention of TSPs as an ECM protein. The TSR (thrombospondin type 1) domains mediate the interactions with TGF-β,

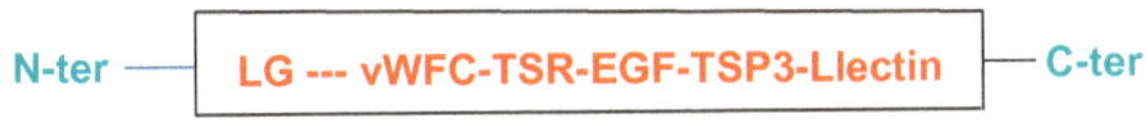

FIGURE 12.1
The domain structure of TSP-1 and TSP-2. LG, laminin G like domain; vWFC, von Willebrandt factor type C; TSR, TSP repeat domain; EGF, EGF-like repeat domain; TSP-3, TSP type 3 domain; L lectin: L type lectin module (see Adams and Lawler, 2011).

VEGF/VEGFR1 and metalloproteinases (Adams and Lawler, 2011). A C-terminal lectin-line module is involved in cellular adhesion and aggregation mediated by the 4N1 peptide. The latter mediates the interaction of TSPs with CD47. It is able to act as a CD47 agonist. The TSR-1 domain probably contains the CD36 binding site (Febbraio et al., 2001). TSP binds to the receptors CD36 and CD47 and inhibits the angiogenic signalling of VEGF/VEGFR-2. The binding to CD47 also inhibits eNOS signalling besides actuating immunological function and promoting apoptosis by activation of the fas/CD95 route (Fig. 12.1; see also p.229; Fig. 26.2).

Suppression of Angiogenesis by Thrombospondin

TSP was spotted as an endogenously occurring inhibitor of angiogenesis over two decades ago. Good et al. (1990) reported the secretion of a protein by a suppressor gene in hamster cells, which was biochemically and immunologically akin to TSP. Both proteins shared the ability to suppress angiogenesis and endothelial cell migration in vitro. The TSP domains occur in in many molecules such as connective tissue growth factor (CTGF) the ADAMTS (a disintegrin and metalloproteinase with thrombospondin motifs) proteins, CCN family members, and WISPs (Wnt inducible signalling pathway protein), among others. The notion that TSP domains may offer interacting sites for angiogenically active molecules derives from the well-established anti-angiogenic properties of TSP and to its participation in cell–ECM interaction and cell-to-cell signalling. These are considerations that have inevitably led the investigations to focus on the relevance of TSPs and macromolecules harbouring TSR domains in cancer invasion and metastasis. TSPs are not only anti-angiogenic but they also inhibit cell proliferation and cell migration. The inhibition of cell proliferation might be an intrinsic ability of TSPs, which conceivably a consequence of being able to control cell cycle via p53 function or by Ras/myc signalling.

TSPs use a variety of receptors; among them are CD36, CD47, proteoglycans and integrins. The anti-angiogenic effects of TSP are attributed to the TSRs, which activate CD36. The inhibition of angiogenesis has been ascribed to the induction of apoptosis of endothelial cells and to the downregulation of VEGF function. TSP interacts with HGF, EGF, TGF-β and FGF-2, besides

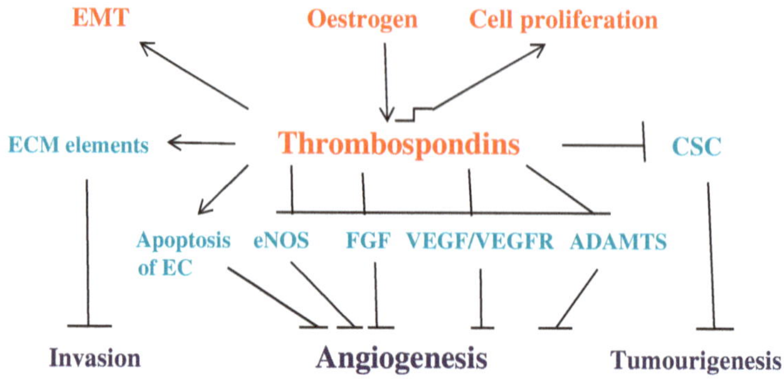

FIGURE 12.2

The signalling pathways that generate the phenotypic effects of inhibition of angiogenesis, inhibition of invasive faculty and suppression of tumorigenesis. The figure also shows the postulated flipside of TSP effects of promotion of cell proliferation and activation of EMT. Also shown here is the stimulation by oestrogen of cell proliferation and of TSP-1 expression in non-conformist fashion in vitro. The interaction of oestrogen with TSP is supported by the detection of an ERE in promoter region of TSP-1. But one has to be mindful that oestrogen effect would depend upon a balance of the function ERα or ERβisoforms and the PR expression status.

CSC, cancer stem cells; ECM, extracellular matrix; eNOS, endothelial nitric oxide synthase; FGF, fibroblast growths factor; VEGF/VEGFR, vascular endothelial growth factor/VEGF receptor.

VEGF. Hence much pre-eminence has been ascribed to TSPs in cancer development and progression (Fig. 12.2).

TSP Suppresses EMT Activation and CSCs

The generation of the CSCs is a follow-up event of EMT. So the function of TSP as a common denominator is of interest. A further thought is that TSPs might suppress stem cell characteristics and make tumour cells liable to destruction. The suppression of the emergence of CSCs would render tumours vulnerable to conventional and immune therapy. Zheng YH et al. (2015) carried out experiments based on this premise using Lewis lung carcinoma (LLC) cells, HCT116, A549. They found the cells surviving photodynamic and immune therapy showed enhanced expression of stem cell markers, viz. CD44, CD133, and CD34. TSP-1/CD47/SIRP-α signalling largely prevented the emergence of the CSC phenotypes. Indeed there is much documented evidence that the TSP-1/CD47 signalling axis suppresses CSC formation and by implication possible also suppresses the activation of EMT. One has to consider other possible modes of signalling. TSP-2 also inhibits angiogenesis and this may be mediated by the suppression of matrix metalloproteinases (MMPs) and the latter finding ties in with the possible suppression of EMT. The loss of E-cadherin, which is a feature of EMT, may occur by the action of MMPs, also promoting cell invasion in the event.

Suppressing MMP function inhibits EMT activation. Conversely, cancer cells that display features of EMT do exhibit enhanced MMP expression.

One has to accord credence to the many claims that TSP-1 activates EMT as indicated by the expression status of E- and N-cadherin and induction of the invasive phenotype. Inhibition of TSP using anti-TSP antibodies or siRNAs inhibited invasion of melanoma cells (Jayachandran et al., 2014). The activation of EMT could be an indirect effect initiated by the activation of EGFR signalling. TSP-1 is able to do this by virtue of the EGF modules it possesses. To contrast with this, TSP-1 seems to act as an antagonist of BMP4 (bone morphogenetic protein) (Sallon et al., 2015) and interestingly the effects of this binding with BMP4 are quite the opposite of EGFR activation. Tsuchida et al. (2014) had noticed that BMP4 inhibited tumour-associated vascularisation by suppressing the expression of VEGF and this was mediated by the induction of TSP-1. In the growth factor milieu relevant in the context of tumour growth that might influence TSP function is oestrogen.

Oestrogen stimulates cell proliferation and tumour growth. It was shown some years ago by Hyder et al. (2009) that it induces TSP-1 expression in breast cancer cell lines and cell proliferation. Suppression of TSP-1 using antibodies inhibited the proliferation of oestrogen/ER dependent MCF-7 cells lines. Hyder et al. (2009) also demonstrated the presence of an ERE (oestrogen-response element) in promoter region of TSP-1. But in the context of oestrogen receptor function, one has to take into account whether ERα or ERβ was involved. The outcome of oestrogen signalling depends upon a balance of the function of the two receptor isoforms, which have markedly different biological functions. Also it is imperative to know the status of PR expression, which has profound effects on the biology of ER function. Nonetheless, the p38/MAPK signalling pathway has close links with growth factor function. Suppression of the MAPK signalling pathway has been associated with increase in apoptosis, reduced cell proliferation and suppression of HER2 and EGFR signalling. Now TSP-1 inhibition has been shown to suppress p38/MAPK signalling and inhibit invasive behaviour (Radziwon-Balicka et al., 2014). There is also an increasing awareness that TSPs can engage immune mechanisms, which lead to the perceived therapeutic effects and that the levels of TSP expression in immune cells might determine the degree of the immune response.

To indulge in a minor digression, some comments concerning ADAMTS proteins are relevant here. From the view of practicability is the fact that many ADAMTS proteins, which possess TSP motifs, can and do inhibit angiogenesis and function as tumour suppressors (Kumar et al., 2012). The basic organisation of ADAMTS proteins is exemplified by ADAMTS4, which contains from N-terminal end a signal peptide, a pro-region of variable length essential for stabilisation, secretion and biological functioning, an MMP domain, a disintegrin domain, a central TSR, and cysteine-rich domain. Other members have the same basic organisation but differ in the C-terminal region downstream of the central TSR and contain a variable number of TSR motifs. MMPs cleave TSP-1 and TSP-2 and generate fragments, which are anti-angiogenic or capable of sequestering angiogenic factors. MMP-independent activity of ADAMTSs has been attributed to the TSR motifs (Kelwick et al., 2015). However, some ADAMTS proteins can suppress both angiogenesis and tumorigenesis. Others can be ambivalent in the sense that they either suppress or promote both angiogenesis and tumorigenesis, probably dependent upon the tumour type and the prevailing conditions, especially the potential interaction with other signalling systems. Therefore, TSR-dependent activity cannot be linked exclusively with anti-angiogenesis.

MicroRNA and the Function of TSPs

MicroRNAs (miRNAs) can modulate many angiogenic pathways, such as those activated by VEGF and HIF, among others. Inevitably this has led to the suggestion of altering the signalling systems by altering the functional miRNAs. That certain miRNAs can suppress TSP-1 and suppress angiogenesis was reported over a decade ago. miRNAs have long been implicated in the activation of EMT and the promotion of invasion and metastasis. Some miRNAs overexpressed in cancers promote TGF-β-mediated activation of EMT. Hypoxia/HIF-1 signalling is known to downregulate TSP-1 by miRNA mediation. It has also been found that miRNAs can suppress cell migration and experimental metastases by inhibiting the transcription factor Sox4, an activator of EMT. Conversely, the expression of some miRNAs is induced by the transcription factors associated with EMT activation. This is highly significant given that miRNAs can accentuate and augment angiogenic signalling. MicroRNAs of the miRNA-17-82 family suppress TSP-1 and CTGF. The CCN family members CTGF and Cyr61 induce angiogenesis by activating HIF-1/VEGF signalling. They can do that via bFGF and the MMP/TIMP system. The influence on CTGF is thought to be due to the interaction between specific miRNA with binding sites in the 3′ UTR of CTGF. Many miRNAs are also known to interact with 3′ UTR of TSP-1 and influence its function. In fact, the TSR module is one of the functional modules of CTGF. The TSR of CTGF is required for its inhibitory effect on invasion and possibly also angiogenesis since TSRs can bind angiogenic factors such as VEGF. Whether this module might take part in the regulation of CTGF by miRNAs is unclear at present. Interestingly, Let-7f directly targets and binds to the 3′ UTR of MYH9 (myosin-9 also known as cellular myosin heavy chain, type A) gene, and thus provide functional role in the regulation of the invasive process by influencing the cytoskeleton dynamics. Compatibly, MYH9 modulates cell motility and invasion. However, given the numeric abundance therapeutic use of miRNAs does not appear to be a viable proposition. The Let-7 family members are also able to suppress the expression of HMGA2 and suppress cell motility and EMT activation.

The Therapeutic Potential of Thrombospondin Mimetic Drugs

The discussion mentioned previously clearly underlines the importance of ascertaining the molecular environment before one can assess the potential of TSPs as a treatment modality. Whether activation of the TSP-1 signalling axis has beneficial effects or could be counterproductive in outcome may be debated. Treatment of epithelial ovarian carcinoma cells with recombinant TSR repeats (3TSR) is said to lead to apoptotic cell loss. In a xenografts model of ovarian cancer, pre-treatment with TSR repeats has resulted in tumour regression and normalisation of tumour-associated vasculature. Combination of 3TSR with chemotherapy has accentuated the inhibition of tumour growth together with inhibition of VGFR phosphorylation (Russell et al., 2015). The same group of workers have shown that glioblastoma cells also exhibit a similar outcome of induction of apoptosis by the upregulation of death receptors (Choi SH et al., 2015). This is largely compatible with the established anti-angiogenic effects of TSPs. In contrast, high TSP-2 and FGF-2 levels abode poor prognosis in NSCLC patients (Naumnik et al., 2015). Whilst appraising the effects of TSR repeats in apoptosis, one has to recognise that the cell-binding domain also binds the IAP (inhibitor of apoptosis protein) and participates in the inhibition of apoptosis.

Many pre-clinical and laboratory studies have been described concerning the effectiveness of TSR repeat peptide mimetics of TSP-1. Among them is ABT-510. A clinical evaluation of ABT-510 was made in advanced head and neck cancer and the trial (NCT00113334) noted in 2009 stable disease in two out of three patients and progressive disease in one out of three patients evaluated. Hasina et al. (2009) employed a murine model of chemically induced HNSCC and have noticed a decrease in the incidence of tumours and delayed tumour development in host animals that had been administered ABT-510. The decreased incidence was statistically significant but not substantial. Early studies showed little promise. In a study involving stage 4 melanoma, only 3 out of 20 patients were found to be progression free after 18 weeks of treatment, despite decreases in VEGF-A and VEGF-C levels, and CD146 and CD34/133 counts (Markovic et al., 2007). Very little clinical benefit was claimed in a phase II study of renal cell carcinoma patients. In the group of patient on 10 mg/per day of the mimetic, a 4% objective response was noted and only two cases of partial response at 100 mg. Progression free survival (PFS) of 4.2 and 3.3 months was noted in 39% and 32% of patients. However, the toxicity profile seemed favourable (Ebbinghaus et al., 2007). Neither was the clinical outcome particularly encouraging in the study reported by Baker et al. (2008) of patients with soft tissue sarcoma. The response to the administration of 20 and 200 mg of the mimetic was stable disease in roughly half the number of treated patients. Overall survival was 341 days in the 20 mg administered group and 295 days in the group given 200 mg of the drug. Consistent with other studies, the drug seems to be well tolerated and safe.

The efficacy of combining ABT-510 with the anti-VEGF-A monoclonal antibody bevacizumb has been tested recently in a phase I study of solid tumours. Although the combination was well tolerated (Uronis et al., 2013), there seemed to be no significant gains in clinical outcome. It may be that combination with immune activation regimes might be more effective in therapy, as the findings of Schadler et al. (2014) would suggest. To-date, the best outcome of 3TSR repeats from treatment of animal tumour models of ovarian cancer has been described by Russell et al. (2015), who reported a greater than sixfold decrease in tumour size when the treatment with TSR in combination with chemotherapy began at an advanced stage of the disease. NO/NOS (nitric oxide/nitric oxide synthase) promote angiogenesis and are targets of TSP-1 and inhibitors of NO/NOS may provide a means of accentuating the anti-angiogenesis effects of TSP-1.

ABT-898 is another TSP-1 mimetic described in animal models to have suppressed and induced the regression of ovarian tumours with reduction in tumour vasculature and VEGF expression. The drug was said to be effective and enhanced the disease free survival of host animals even when administered at late stage disease (Campbell et al., 2011). Judging by the success or lack of it over the past decade or so, the TSP mimetics do not appear to hold much promise, whether used as single agents or in combination with other angiogenesis inhibitors.

ANTI-ANGIOGENESIS BY COLLAGEN FRAGMENTS CANSTATIN, ARRESTEN, TUMSTATIN AND TETRASTATIN

Many fragments of ECM components of interest in terms of anti-angiogenesis are known, notably fragments of collagen IV and collagen VIII. Canstatin, arresten, tumstatin and tetrastatin are examples of collagen-derived anti-angiogenic factors known to decrease growth of experimental tumours (Monboisse et al., 2014). Arresten and canstatin are derived from collagen IV A1 and A2 chains, respectively. Arresten was shown some time ago to inhibit invasion in vitro and suppress cell proliferation and angiogenesis of xenografted human carcinomas (Aikio et al., 2012). Canstatin also exerts marked inhibitory effect on growth of gastric tumour xenografts (Xing YN et al., 2014). Apart from promoting apoptosis, canstatin seems also able to suppress the VEGFR pathway of angiogenic signalling in vitro systems as well as in tumour xenografts (Hwang-Bo J et al., 2012).

Tumstatin is another collagen IV-derived 28 kDa fragment, which has been described as an endothelial-specific angiogenesis inhibitor and a promoter of apoptosis. Its expression is downregulated in many tumour tissues. Fragments of tumstatin as well as peptides with specified amino acid sequences of tumstatin have been synthesised and have been shown to be anti-angiogenic. These efforts were possibly intended to help tumstatin deployment in gene therapy, but it might indeed be helpful to focus the angiogenic activity to defined domains or regions of tumstatin. One can perceive some advantages in identifying short sequences of tumstatin with the inhibitory properties. In reflective thought molecular size would be an important consideration for many reasons. It is imperative that immune responses to the transgene product are obviated in order that they do not diminish its biological effect. The duration of transgene expression has to be reconciled with plasma half-life of the product. Furthermore, its clearance rate would markedly relate to molecular size. The biodistribution of and targeting the product to the tumour might be determined by the molecular size of the product and the relative unbound state of the product and the quality of the vector. Wang W et al. (2015) have shown that apoptosis inducing ability was associated with tumstatin 185–191 fragment and the inactivation of Akt signalling. The treatment sensitised tumour cells that were refractory to chemotherapy. This is in accord with the practical advantages inherent in small molecule-based transgene therapy.

The presence of $\alpha v\beta 3$ integrin on the blood vessels is an essential requirement for the biological effect of tumstatin. This integrin is highly expressed in both resting and active endothelial cells. Circulating endothelial cells are found in higher numbers in cancer patients. They might participate in the restitution of vascular damage and possibly also in angiogenesis, but their precise role in cancer is not fully understood. Tumstatin was thought to function via interaction with $\alpha v\beta 3$ integrin with imputed signalling via several systems, e.g., FAK, PI3K and mTOR (Maeshima et al., 2002). Zan et al. (2012) believe that many tumstatin-binding sites might be present in $\alpha v\beta 3$ integrin. Tetrastatin was identified as a derivative of collagen IV some time ago (Karagiannis and Popel, 2007). This is also anti-angiogenic and shares the features of functioning by binding to $\alpha v\beta 3$ integrin (Brassart-Pasco et al., 2012).

There is consensus that the inhibition of angiogenesis by these collagen fragments occurs as an outcome of the inactivation of VEGF/VEGFR signalling.

Hwang-Bo J et al. (2015) have implicated Fas-mediated signalling in the promotion of apoptosis and inhibition of tumour growth. This confirms the earlier reports that two fragments of tumstatin promoted apoptosis by Fas/FasL mediation (Li YJ et al., 2009). Assadian et al. (2012) have linked p53 with the release of arresten from the ECM by an MMP-dependent action. This correlated with the inhibition of angiogenesis and tumour growth. They also showed that the expression of p53 correlated with that of arresten in prostate tumour tissues. This is a plausible correlation. Mutant p53 proteins do induce the secretion of enzymes that can degrade the components of the ECM. MMPs are often expressed in parallel with mutated p53 in tumours.

INHIBITION OF ANGIOGENESIS BY ENDOSTATIN

Endostatin was identified as an endogenous inhibitor of angiogenesis nearly three decades ago (O'Reilly et al., 1997). It is a 20 kDa C-terminal fragment of collagen XVII of the subfamily of ECM proteins called multiplexins (proteins with multiple triple-helix domains and interruptions) (Oh SP et al., 1994). The effect of inhibition of endothelial cell proliferation, inhibition of angiogenesis and suppression of cell motility flows from the ability of endostatin to bind to many ECM components including $\alpha 5\beta 1$ and $\alpha v\beta 3$ integrins, heparan sulphate proteoglycans and cell surface receptors such as VEGFR1, VEGFR-2, VEGFR-3, TSP-1, SPARC (secreted protein acidic and rich in cysteine; osteonectin), nucleolin and uPAR (urokinase-type plasminogen activator receptor) involved in angiogenesis (Fig. 12.3).

Whilst the mechanisms of action of VEGFRs and TSP-1 are well established, the mode of nucleolin mediation in angiogenesis is worthy of discussion at the risk of some digression, for it is seen as a target to suppress tumorigenesis and angiogenesis. Nucleolin is the major nucleolar protein of growing eukaryotic cells, but occurs also on endothelial cells. Functionally, it is implicated in angiogenesis, inhibition of apoptosis and positive regulation of cytokines such as tumour necrosis factor and interleukins. Synthetic ligands for nucleolin have been devised and these have shown anti-angiogenic and anti-tumour potential. The ligand known as HB19 and its analogue N6L not only inhibited invasive behaviour of tumour cells in vitro, but also inhibited tumour growth and angiogenesis. The aspect of much significance here is that this seemed to be a consequence of the upregulation of TIMP-3 (Destouches et al., 2011, 2012), although Krust et al. (2011a) reported no effect on TIMP-1. One would recall here that TIMPs are inhibitors of metalloproteinases, which are markedly pro-angiogenic. Equally, it is possible that MMPs, which break down collagen, might release the surface bound nucleolin and the TIMPs would prevent this. Nucleolin antagonists have been postulated to exert differential effects dependent upon the tumour cell type, with

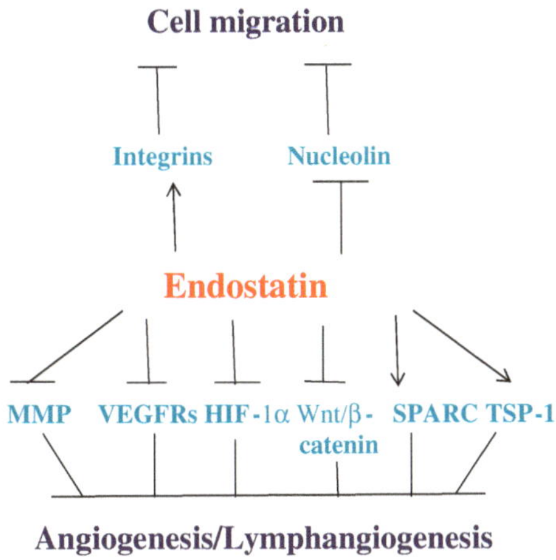

FIGURE 12.3

The signalling pathways by which endostatin suppresses angiogenesis/lymph-angiogenesis and cell migration. SPARC (osteonectin) is a matrix protein, which inhibits cell proliferation, cell adhesion interactions and also suppresses pro-angiogenic PDGF, VEGF and FGF-2. This figure is based on references cited in the text. Endostatin may bring about its phenotypic effects by additive or synergistic collaborative signalling.

adhesion-related effects on carcinoma cells but induction of apoptosis in leukaemic cells (Krust et al., 2011b). But one cannot see a clear rational basis or the display of distinction in the signalling that resulted in these differential effects, most certainly not an outcome related to MMP types, which this group of workers had reported. Selective downregulation of MMPs does occur and has been reported. It is postulated that nucleolin is relocated to the cell surface by the cytoskeletal machinery with VEGF mediation and functions as a receptor of endostatin. The non-muscle myosin heavy chain 9 binds to nucleolin and may be involved in its translocation from the nucleus to the cell surface (Huang et al., 2006; Shi H et al., 2007).

VEGF induces the localisation of nucleolin at the cell surface and this induce surface expression may be associated with endothelial cell migration. This could be a direct effect of VEGF or mediated by myosin heavy chain 9/cytoskeletal involvement. The downregulation of expression of cell surface nucleolin has led to the inhibition of endothelial migration and capillary formation (Huang Y et al., 2006). Possibly, this could have occurred by the binding to endostatin. Equally, nucleolin functions as a receptor for cell adhesion molecules as well as growth factors and their receptors. So the nucleolin involvement in the angiogenic process cannot be an exclusive attribute of endostatin. Nucleolin is said to interact with CXCR4 and seems able to suppress phosphorylation of ERK and Akt (Dai CX et al., 2015). This would have obvious effects on proliferation of endothelial cells. Furthermore, the chemokine receptors CCR and CXCRs are active promoters of angiogenesis and tumorigenesis. CXC ligand chemokines also show higher expression in some cancers. Higher expression of CXCL1 and CXCL5 expression has been associated with colon cancer as compared with adenomas (see Sherbet, 2011a). Compatible with this, there is some evidence that endostatin is able to downregulate CXCL1 and inhibit tumorigenesis (Guo LF et al., 2015a,b).

The route adopted by endostatin to bring about its anti-angiogenic effects was studied by Ling Y et al. (2007) using the recombinant endostatin Endostar. Endostar negated the effects of VEGF on the proliferation, migration and tube formation of HUVEC cells. Furthermore, they were able to demonstrate the suppression by Endostar of VEGFR-2 phosphorylation and also the suppression of the ERK/p38/MAPK and Akt signalling pathways. However, Okada et al. (2015) have reported stimulation of cell proliferation and cell migration by endostatin via activation of PI3K/Akt but no ERK/p38 MAPK signalling. Among other putative signalling systems are the Wnt/β-catenin pathway which also been implicated with endostatin function (Xu X et al., 2014).

Endostatin Expression Relates to Disease Prognosis

Given the wide spectrum of anti-angiogenic effects, it is hardly surprising that the expression of endostatin would correlate with disease activity. Pre-clinical studies using animal tumour models have confirmed the effects of endostatin. A recombinant endostatin effectively reduced the growth of xenografts of lung cancer A549, hepatocellular carcinoma QGY-7703 and breast cancer Bcap37 cells. The inhibition was more pronounced when it was administered peritumorally. In B16 melanoma experimental metastasis assay, B16 melanoma cells were injected intravenously and endostatin administered a day later. This resulted in reduced lung colonisation (Ren ZH et al., 2014). Quite possibly this is due to loss of adhesion of tumour cells to the substratum of lung tissue. The authors did induce tumours by subcutaneous implantation of some tumour cell types. For these experiments, the incidence of metastasis or the effects of endostatin thereon are not available. Also no effort was made to check the microvascular density of the subcutaneous tumours. Wang HB et al. (2014) have produced a chimeric peptide containing MMP-2/9 inhibitory sequence, and anti-angiogenic endostatin mimic and kringle 5 (see later). They have demonstrated that this chimeric product is highly effective as a tumour inhibitor in experimental tumour models. It inhibited MMPs, endothelial tubule formation, cell proliferation and migration. In murine models the chimeric peptide inhibited angiogenesis.

The incidence of experimental metastases was reduced and the survival time of the host animals increased. The recombinant peptide was not perceptibly toxic.

At the clinical level, the expression of VEGF was noticeably higher with Endostar than endostatin in NSCLC patients and this correlated with poor prognosis (Hu Y et al., 2014). Combination of Endostar with chemotherapy and concurrent radiotherapy of stage III NSCLC patients has resulted in favourable survival and control of local progression (Bao Y et al., 2015). In patients with locally recurrent nasopharyngeal carcinoma, a similar treatment programme produced complete response in 20 and partial response in 2 or 22 patients (Guan Y et al., 2015). Combination therapy administered whether by the intravenous or by arterial route has had the effect of enhancing PFS and overall survival of patients with advanced NSCLC (Jiang X et al., 2015). However, understandably a phase II study of the aggressive extensive-stage SCLC patients treated with Endostar alone or in combination with etoposide/carboplatin has been described by Lu S et al. (2015). The results of this have not been encouraging. No improvements were noted in the response rate, PFS or overall survival. Numerous clinical trials are in progress wherein the intervention has been mostly of Endostar/endostatin in combination with chemotherapy.

One ought to recognise that increase in circulating endostatin has also often been reported. The salient features of endostatin are inhibition of neovascularisation, suppression of oedema and inflammation, which are peritumoral effects actuated by the presence of appropriate receptors in the cell periphery. Therefore the significance of circulating endostatin in relation to tumour growth and progression is unclear in comparison with the expression in intra or peritumoral locations.

Whether genetic polymorphism leading to impairment of function might be a reason for the perceived infrequent correlation of high endostatin levels with poor prognosis is still an open question. Li HC et al. (2005) had found no support for this view. But Bi WZ et al. (2015) found that D104N polymorphism might indeed be a factor associated with a high risk of developing osteosarcoma. These authors reported that patients with the homozygous p. D104N (p. 104NN) genotype carried higher risk than control subjects.

ANGIOSTATIN IN THE CONTROL OF ANGIOGENESIS AND TUMOUR GROWTH

Angiostatin was identified as a circulating endogenous angiogenesis inhibitor derived from the primary tumour, also capable of suppressing endothelial cell proliferation. It is an internal cleavage product of plasminogen and represents a 38 kDa N-terminal fragment (O'Reilly et al., 1994, O'Reilly, 1997). The so-called kringle domains are found in many proteins, e.g., plasminogen, thrombin, uPA (urokinase-type plasminogen activator) and tPA (tissue plasminogen activator). Kringle domains are units of conserved sequences. They fold into large loops that are stabilised by three disulphide bonds. The kringle repeats of 80 amino acid residues occur together with other motifs such as the EGF motifs. These domains are involved in protein–protein interaction and molecular recognition. The plasminogen heavy chain contains five kringles (Castellino and McCance, 1997). The kringles 1–3 and 8 of the plasminogen fragment are thought to possess tumour inhibitory ability (MacDonald et al., 1999). Kringle 5 inhibits tumour progression and angiogenesis. Ansell et al. (2010) have shown that kringle 5, which is anti-angiogenic, can bind the c-met receptor of HGF and suppress the pro-angiogenic growth factor. Human plasminogen contains kringles 1–5 and the proteolytic fragment containing these kringle domains as well as recombinant kringles 1–5 are inhibitory of angiogenesis. They are known to interact with fibronectin and laminin of the ECM (Moser et al., 1993) in this way influence cell faculty of adhesion and motility.

Pre-Clinical Evaluation of the Biological Properties of Angiostatin

Much new effort has been made at the pre-clinical level to devise new means to inhibit tumour growth and angiogenesis using angiostatin in conventional approaches, after earlier efforts seemed to have failed to make a mark apparently as a result of the short half-life of angiostatin upon administration. Kuo CH et al. (2015) seems to have achieved long-term expression of angiostatin kringles 1–5 incorporated into the adeno-associated virus vector. The transgene was expressed for 567 days after a single injection of the recombinant virus, and inhibited lung colonisation in experimental metastases assays using the B16 melanoma model and suppressed xenografts of LLC as well as the human melanoma A2058. The adeno-associated virus is a satellite virus that cannot replicate without a helper virus. The advantages of using this vector are its long half-life of expression and its safety. The vector elicits low immune response. These positive features have prompted investigations of using recombinant forms for therapeutic genes transfer. However, tissue-specific targeting of the vector needs much constructive design. Vectors encoding specific monoclonal antibodies such as trastuzumab have been designed and tested in animal tumour models with some success.

Another approach to achieving long-term sustainability of expression of potential suppressors is the use of stem cells. Prolonged expression of kringle 5 has been achieved by introducing an adenovirus vector carrying kringles 1–5 into human placental mesenchymal stem cell (MSC). The MSCs expressed kringle proteins both in vitro and in vivo. Upon administration, the infected MSCs were detected within 2 weeks in vivo and there was marked inhibition of microvessel density in vitro (Chu Y et al., 2014). The practicalities of targeting MSC to the tumours are a major factor that needs to be addressed in the use of MSC-directed cancer therapy (Patil and Sherbet, 2014).

Angiostatin Binds to Angiomotins: The Anti-Angiogenesis Credentials of Angiostatin

The angiomotin (AMOT) family has attracted much attention on account of its members being important targets of angiostatin. AMOTs are expressed in endothelial cells as well as other tissues with associated angiogenesis such as in tumours. AMOTs enhance the migratory ability of endothelial cells and stimulate angiogenesis, but this is suppressed upon binding with angiostatin. AMOT activity is also suppressed in the tumour cell environment. The anti-angiogenic effects of angiostatin are well established since its discovery, but the molecular mechanisms of its function are still not fully defined. The inhibitory functions of angiostatin flow from its binding to and regulation of the motin family proteins. The putative pathways by which angiostatin signals anti-angiogenesis and suppresses tumour progression are shown in Fig. 12.4.

THE MOTIN FAMILY: THE ANGIOMOTINS

The motin family members are AMOT together with AMOTL1 (AMOT like protein) and AMOTL2. AMOT was originally identified by its ability to bind to angiostatin. The three AMOT proteins share much sequence homology and many structural features. AMOTL1 and AMOTL2 share the same biological features. Another member of the family AMOT-p130 is generated by alternative splicing of the AMOT gene. Two important and characteristic domains occur at the C-terminal regions. These are the conserved CC (coiled-coil) domain and the C-terminal PDZ-binding domain. The CC domain subserves many biological and structural functions and the PDZ domain is involved in interaction with other proteins especially in signalling function. The angiostatin-binding domain is located between the CC and PDZ domains and occurs in AMOT and AMOT-p130 but not in AMOTLs. The AMOTs are differentially expressed in different tissues and might indeed subserve dissimilar functions dependent upon their location (Bratt et al., 2002; Moleirinho et al., 2014). Possibly differential functions could arise from differences in

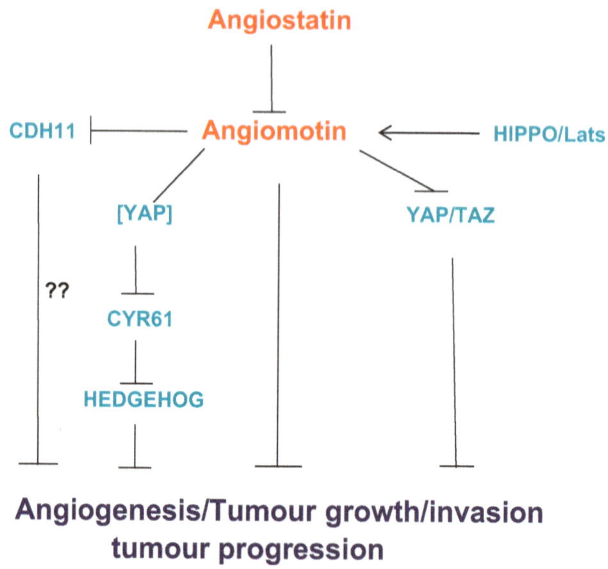

FIGURE 12.4

Putative signalling pathways functional in the suppression of angiogenesis, growth, invasion and progression of tumours by angiostatin/AMOT. AMOT can also suppress angiogenesis and tumour growth independently of angiostatin. Like CYR61, Gli is also a target of YAP/TAZ but not shown here. See text for references. AMOT is said to suppress CDH11 (type II cadherin-11), which unlike E-cadherins, is believed to promote cell invasion and metastatic spread of tumours.

the ability of the AMOTs to bind angiostatin and activate the appropriate signalling pathway. This might also be dictated by the PDZ-binding partner proteins in the molecular environment of the cell.

Hippo Signalling in Angiomotin Function

Besides being neutralised by angiotensin, AMOT might also be able to suppress tumour progression independently of angiostatin by recourse to the Hippo signalling system. The Lats gene homologues Lats1 and Lats2 constitute a major component of Hippo signalling and the Lats are known to be tumour suppressors. Lats kinases inhibit cell proliferation and promote apoptosis. The kinases MST2/STK3 (serine/threonine kinase 3) and MST1/STK4 are in complex with and regulated by Sav1 (human WW45, Salvador family WW domain containing protein 1), which in common with other WW domain containing proteins, is able to regulate many cellular activities. The pro-apoptosis MST2 and MST1 phosphorylate and activate Lats occurring as a complex with the regulatory protein Mob (Mps one binder) 1 phosphorylates and inhibits YAP1 and its translocation to the nucleus thus affecting target gene regulation (see Sherbet, 2013). AMOT and other members of the AMOT family activate the Lats2 kinase (Paramasivan et al., 2011). The Lats kinase then phosphorylates and suppresses the tumorigenic YAP and in this way suppresses cell proliferation and tumour progression. Equally, YAP inhibition may occur as a direct interaction with AMOT (Zhao B et al., 2011). On the other hand, in breast cancer tissues and cell lines, the downregulation of AMOT besides decreasing cell proliferation and invasion, also downregulates YAP and Lats1 (Lv M et al., 2015).

Several pathways intersect with the Lats/YAP axis in determining phenotypic effect of morphogenesis, cell transformation, cell proliferation and EMT. Hippo signalling is modulated by many upstream elements, which have themselves been attributed with tumour suppressor function. NF2/Merlin localises Wnt/β-catenin at the cell membrane, which renders the proliferative signalling by Wnt ineffective. Merlin is an upstream regulator of Hippo signalling. Suppression of Merlin leads to enhanced organ growth and eventually to tumorigenesis. It regulates the Hippo kinases MST1 and MST2, activation of Lats and inactivation of YAP (see Sherbet, 2013). The involvement of AMOT in Merlin mediation of Hippo activation has recently been highlighted (Li YJ et al., 2015). The role of Hippo signalling in angiogenesis is discussed in greater detail in another location. The Hippo signalling is also regulated by atypical cadherins. Furthermore, the function of AMOTs may be influenced by the classical cadherins.

Type II Cadherins in Angiomotin Function

The cadherin family is composed of the classical cadherins, protocadherins and the atypical cadherins. The cadherins Fat, Dachsous (Ds) and Flamingo are atypical cadherins involved in the maintenance of cell polarity and probably also in cell proliferation. Fat has been implicated in the regulation of Hippo signalling. The cadherin Fat is a cell adhesion molecule and is mutated in many tumours, possibly resulting in the deregulation of Hippo signalling. Unlike the classical cadherins, Fat and Dachsous do not bind β-catenin in spite of the fact that they share sequence homology in their cytoplasmic domains (reviewed by Halbleib and Nelson, 2006). So they might not function in the canonical fashion of the classical cadherins. Although E-cadherins are notable invasion suppressors, the classical type II cadherin-11 (CDH11) is believed to promote cell invasion and metastatic spread of tumours. The type II classical cadherins differ from type I cadherins in that they lack the specific cell adhesion recognition sequence of type I cadherins, viz. the HAV (histidine alanine valine) sequence (www.ncbi.nlm.nih.gov/gene/1009). The HAV sequence is required for the inhibition of cell invasion (Noe et al., 1999). But then this might be cell-specific outcome. For in other tumour systems, CDH11 has been found to be silenced by methylation. Forced expression of CDH11 has suppressed tumorigenicity and promoted apoptosis. Compatible with this, it inhibited Wnt/β-catenin and Akt/Rho pathways (Li L et al., 2012). Ortiz et al. (2015) have shown that AMOT interacts with CDH11 in this process and that it is a component of the β-catenin/catenin δ1 complex that is involved in the migratory function of cells. However, there is no need to totally dissociate Hippo signalling from actin-mediation of cell migration in that AMOT proteins do bind actin as Chan SW et al. (2013) have been able to demonstrate.

Angiomotins Interact With Hedgehog Signalling

Interactions of AMOT with the pro-angiogenic Hedgehog signalling are also a factor that needs to be taken into consideration. CYR61 (cysteine-rich angiogenic inducer 61, CCN1) is downstream contributor target of Hedgehog signalling. It has been implicated in the development of pancreatic tumour and is able to activate EMT and promote stem cell features. CYR61 is a regulator of the Sonic hedgehog signalling pathway (Haque et al., 2011, 2012; Harris et al., 2012). Its expression has been linked with the aggressive behaviour of osteosarcomas and compatibly its downregulation reduces tumour vasculature and microvascular density (Habel et al., 2015).

It is of interest in this context that expression of AMOT has been described to be significantly reduced in lung cancer specimens. In vitro, suppression of AMOT has resulted in enhanced cell proliferation, migration and invasion, and activated EMT in CL1-0 lung cancer cell line. AMOT sequesters YAP and decreases Cyr61 expression and in this way suppresses cancer progression (Hsu YL et al., 2015).

CHAPTER 13

Stem Cells in Cancer Therapy

The association of genetic instability with stage-specific gene function has provided a mechanistic relationship between genetic instability and cancer progression. Alterations in the expression of these key genetic determinants have allowed the construction of a model of tumour progression. The molecular concept of cancer progression has delivered a solid basis for the cancer stem cell (CSC) hypothesis, which is indeed inextricably entrenched in and closely allied with the postulate of temporal acquisition of stem cell characteristics. Importantly, the acquisition of stem cell features goes hand in hand with activation of epithelial mesenchymal transition (EMT) and tumour progression.

One has to distinguish three major types of stem cells (Table 13.1). Focusing here on CSC, it would be reasonable to suggest that on account of epigenetic links, CSCs might resemble embryonic stem cells. CSCs share stem cell features with adult stem cells but differ with regard to homoeostatic regulation, survival and perpetuation. These differences would indeed flow from the different pathways operating in their generation and are bound to impinge upon the function of modulators of stem cell biology (Sherbet, 2013).

THE RATIONALE FOR STEM CELL THERAPY

The advocacy of deployment of stem cell therapy is founded on two important attributes of stem cells viz. cellular reprogramming leading to the activation of EMT and selective tissue tropism that they display. Many tumour suppressor genes and crucial developmental signalling systems have been linked with EMT and with endowing CSCs with their specialist survival and maintenance character. EMT itself a developmental pathway and signalling pathways such as the Hedgehog, Wnt and many microRNAs (miRNAs) are notable for their association with and recognition as stem cell pathways. So targeting of stem cells and negating or mitigating their resistance to therapy, focused inhibition of EMT and possibly also the promotion of the reverse

Molecular Approach to Cancer Management. DOI: http://dx.doi.org/10.1016/B978-0-12-812896-1.00013-1

Table 13.1 Stem Cell Types

Embryonic stem cells
ES (embryonic stem cells) derived from foetal tissues
ES derived from blastocysts
NSC from foetal and adult CNS (progenitors of neuron, astrocytes and oligodendrocytes)
Stem cells from neural crest/derivative organs (progenitors of neurons, glia and melanocytes)
Adult stem cells ubiquitously occurring in adult tissues
HSC of bone marrow
HSC (from umbilical cord blood)
MSC of bone marrow
Stem cells from organs capable of repair and regeneration (epidermis, gut, liver, etc.)
Cancer stem cells

Based on Shakhova and Sommer (2010), Zipori (2009) and Sherbet (2013).

process of mesenchyme to epithelial transition may be viewed as potentially valuable approaches to inducing differentiation of CSCs.

Developmental signalling systems such as Notch and Hedgehog as well as Akt/mTOR are closely linked with both stem cell biology and EMT activation. Notch signalling forms a major pathway in normal development, differentiation, morphogenesis and growth. Abnormal development often follows deregulation of Notch signalling. Notch signalling can interact and enter into mutual regulation with other developmental proteins such as the Wnt proteins. The Hedgehog signalling system is another key participant in embryonic development and differentiation. It is a highly conserved signalling pathway associated with the transduction of signals relating to cell proliferation, embryonic development and pattern formation. Of prime importance is that Hedgehog signalling and growth factor pathways meet developmental systems. The mammalian target of rapamycin (mTOR) pathway has earned much importance with the demonstration that it can integrate and facilitate crosstalk between growth factor signalling pathways. The activation of PI3K/Akt also features in mTOR signalling since it leads to the phosphorylation of mTOR, which then phosphorylates the downstream targets p70S6K and 4EBP leading to cell proliferation (see Sherbet, 2013).

Recently, Shrivastava et al. (2015) have described an interesting series of experiments. They employed head and neck squamous cell carcinoma (HNSCC) cells OSC19, Cal27 and JHU29. When these cells were maintained on substratum with low cell adhesion support and in a serum-free environment, they formed the so-called oralspheres. The oralspheres displayed greater tumorigenicity than corresponding parental cells and contained large CSC subpopulations. Notch signalling correlated with CSC levels in the oralspheres. Increased Notch expression correlated with the CSC markers CD133 and Nanog. The tumours formed from the CSCs derived from the oral-spheres were more aggressive and showed enhanced expression of VEGFR1 and greater vascularisation. Earlier, Cao et al. (2011) had isolated CSCs from human hepatoma cell lines using the tumour sphere-forming strategy. The CSC isolates were identified by the overexpression of the markers, Oct3/4, OV6, epithelial cell adhesion molecule (EPCAM), CD133 and CD44. They analysed the downstream signalling and reported CSL (CBF1/RBP-Jk, Suppresser of Hairless, Lag-1)-independent Notch signalling seemed to operate concurrently with the overexpression of the Notch regulator DTX1 (deltex 1), and the histone acetyltransferase transcriptional co-activator Ep300 with which DTX1 physically interacts. This occurred in the tumour spheres rather than in corresponding controls. Exploring this situation a step beyond, one might in fact suggest an interaction with or interference by the Wnt pathway. Notch and Wnt are known to collaborate in stem cell maintenance. Notch/Wnt signalling can involve the regulatory gene Kremen 2. The latter has high affinity for and regulates Dkk2-mediated inhibition of Wnt signalling and DTX4. The DTX1 and DTX4 possess the conserved Notch-interacting domain. Although the tumour sphere studies have provided some positive results, a word of caution is not out of place. Equating sphere formation as a characteristic feature of stem cells capable of self-renewal and possessing high tumorigenic ability is not a universally accepted view. Tumour spheres do not invariably contain higher CSC subpopulations.

The pro-angiogenic signalling by Notch has been investigated in much detail. Notch signalling is another interacting pathway that has been implicated in VEGF function and induction of angiogenesis. Overexpression of the Notch ligand Jagged2 is said to be associated with the induction of VEGF. Equally, VEGF is able to induce the expression of Notch1 and the Notch ligand Delta4 in human arterial endothelial cells. In breast cancer the CD44(+)/CD24(−/low) tumour initiating or stem cell subpopulation decreases upon Notch inhibition (So JY et al., 2015).

Salinomycin has been viewed as a putative CSC inhibitor. It inhibits cell proliferation. The inhibition of proliferation has been linked with the loss of CSCs in many tumour types. Also the in vivo tumour growth in murine models has mirrored downregulated expression of genes associated with the CSC phenotype (Gupta et al., 2009). Targeting of CSCs with salinomycin downregulates Hedgehog signalling (Lu Y et al., 2015). Zuo M et al. (2015) used vismodegib and rapamycin to suppress Hedgehog and mTOR pathways and showed that this led to a synergistic inhibition of the CSC subpopulation of biliary tract cancer. The mTOR pathway integrates PI3K/Akt and NF-κB signalling. These are also known to be suppressed by salinomycin. An interesting development is achieving specific delivery of salinomycin to CSC. Yao HJ et al. (2014) have constructed a delivery vehicle of chitosan-coated single wall carbon nanotubes loaded with salinomycin complexed with hyaluronic acid. Hyaluronic acid enables the complex to home in on gastric cancer CSC carrying the cell surface CD44 receptor. CD44 is a major CSC marker and is one of an array of stem cell markers that include CD20, CD24, CD34, CD44, CD90, CD117, CD133, aldehyde dehydrogenase (ALDH), nestin, the integrin β1, Sox2, ESA and EPCAM. Although CD44*v*6 isoform has been identified closely with tumour progression and metastasis, most studies with CSC have employed antibodies that recognise many other isoforms as well. Whether the expression of different isoforms displays any cell-type specificity is yet uncertain. But the expression of CD44 isoforms can be tissue-specific. CSC niches are rich in hyaluronic acid expression. The isoform CD44s, which is the standard form, does not contain variable exons and its binding to the ECM is mainly via hyaluronic acid. CSCs of breast cancer identified by the ALDH1 express CD44s most conspicuously. However, the expression of the different isoforms has shown subtype-specific expression, which could be related to the operative signalling system (Olsson et al., 2011). One cannot exclude the consideration of the CD44 isoforms in relation to studies of therapeutically targeting CSCs.

TISSUE TROPISM OF STEM CELLS

Stem cells show marked tissue-specific tropism. The molecular basis of this tropism whether it is instigated by chemoattractants or chemokinetic factors or by a combination of both has not been established. But advantage has been taken of this homing propensity to make targeted delivery of cytotoxic drugs and antibodies to tumours. The flipside of this would be the possibility that stem cells tend to be resistant to chemotherapy, might activate EMT, induce angiogenesis and promote invasion and metastasis. The signalling systems driving these events and the identification of key effectors would determine to a large extent the success in dealing with the controlling influences of stem cells.

Tissue tropism has been valuable in therapeutic targeting of CNS lesions. Neural stem cells (NSC) have a prominent propensity of brain tropism. This feature has been suggested as a potential path to managing HER2+ breast cancers metastatic to the brain. Targeted delivery and activation of prodrugs inhibitory of growth have been regarded a viable approach to treating brain metastases (Patil and Sherbet, 2015). NSCs have been successfully delivered with anti-HER2 antibodies to inhibit tumour growth (Frank et al., 2009).

COMBINATION OF CHEMOTHERAPY AND STEM CELL THERAPY

The central postulate for providing stem cell therapy may be summarised as directed to employing low doses of drugs followed by stem cell therapy, to provide stem cell support following high-dose drug therapy or under conditions when thermotherapy on its own has little chance of providing a cure. The benefits of high-dose chemotherapy followed by transplantation of autologous haematopoietic stem cell (HSC) are not beyond debate at present and contribute little to the management of breast cancer patients. This was an overall assessment made some time ago by Vogl and Stadtmauer (2006). However, there are reports of improved PFS, but not overall survival, of patients with high-risk disease as well as those with metastatic breast cancer (Berry et al., 2011; Lotz et al., 2005; Selle et al., 2015). But as Selle et al. (2015) have argued that a compelling case can be made for continuing with high-dose chemotherapy for managing specific subgroups patients with TNBCs or with low HER2 expression.

ROLE OF TRANSCRIPTION FACTORS IN CELL LINEAGE AND MAINTENANCE

Transcription factors regulate gene expression and unsurprisingly many transcription factors are closely linked with regulating the expression of genes controlling cell proliferation, invasion and angiogenesis. Unsurprising also are the suggestions that therapeutic inhibition of transcription factors overexpressed in tumours might be a worthy option to explore to control tumour growth and spread. Much attention has been directed to the Sp1 family transcription factors. These are undeniably connected with the aggressive behaviour of cancers so much so that their expression could be clinically relevant as a molecular marker of aggressive tumours and suggestive as a potential therapeutic target. Sp1 also regulates the biological processes of cell proliferation, apoptosis, cell differentiation and immune responses, and hormonal and growth factor signalling. However, an integral function of the Sp1 transcription factors is constitutively activating housekeeping genes for cell maintenance. Equally, one ought to recognise that there are indications that Sp1 expression diminishes in parallel with neuronal differentiation of mesenchymal stem cells (MSCs) (see section of miRNAs below). Another transcription factor gene family noted for active association with normal development, proliferation, apoptosis and differentiation and ageing is the human forkhead-box (FOX) family. FOX genes regulate the Hedgehog pathway and are also overexpressed in many human cancers.

Notwithstanding the many caveats, much work has been done on transcription factors that appear to be capable of driving-specific cellular functions and features. The Ets family members for example are expressed in neural crest cells, endothelial cells and in association with EMT. Ets genes are also associated with tissue remodelling, regulation of cellular adhesion phenomena and also MMP/TIMPs (matrix metalloproteinase/tissue inhibitor of metalloproteinase). These transcription factors have also been found to be determinants of cell differentiation and so linked with cell lineage and maintenance. Ets genes participate in the delineation of HSCs and their maintenance and renewal.

Neurogenins (NGNs) are a family of bHLH (basic helix loop helix) transcription factors, of which three members have been identified. They are closely associated with cell identity, survival and maintenance. The NGNs display a complex and unique pattern of distribution in the developing brain. NGN-1 is found in embryonic neural tissues and promotes neural differentiation and inhibits glial differentiation. NGN-2 is proneural; it is required for the development of midbrain dopaminergic neurons (Kele et al., 2006). NGN-2 might have potential implication for stem cell-mediated therapies in neurodegenerative diseases. NGN-3 is associated with the formation of pancreatic islet beta cells and in dendritic growth and formation of synapses. The NGNs inhibit neuronal stem cells from differentiating into glial cells by sequestering transcription factors required for glial differentiation and promote neural differentiation by functioning as a transcriptional promoter (Sun et al., 2001). The NGN-2 gene has been implicated in early mouse spinal neurogenesis in association with and possibly induced by Sonic Hedgehog (Shh). Shh is involved with the determination of the pattern of the differentiation of neuronal cell types. The process could involve NGN-2. NeuroD is another bHLH transcription factor-regulating neurogenesis (see Sherbet, 2011a). Its function is also dependent upon Shh.

NGN-2 has been described as being able to inhibit the growth of gliomas and induce them to differentiate into neuron-like cells in culture and in the brains of murine hosts. This effect occurs in conjunction with the transcription regulator Sox11. Upon injection into the tumour NGN + Sox11 suppressed tumour growth and prolonged survival times of the host animals (Su Z et al., 2014). However, the practicality of using NGN in the clinical context requires the development of methods of delivering NGNs to the targets. Deng B et al. (2013) have produced a fusion protein TAT (transactivator of transcription domain) and LBD (a laminin-binding domain) to NGN-2. The fusion protein not only promoted neurite extension but could successfully penetrate the blood brain barrier. Another interesting finding is that NGN-1-expressing MSCs display enhanced tropism to the CNS (Choi CI et al., 2013). In this context it would be worth noting that the ECM components of gliomas, especially laminin and tenascin, might be important factors in the directed migration of neuronal and neural crest cells (Franco and Muller, 2011).

miRNAs IN NEUROGENESIS

As stated in another location, miRNAs are non-coding RNAs, which show close association with many biological functions, normal as well as aberrant.

Two important components in the biogenesis and function of miRNAs are Drosha and Dicer. The primary miRNA transcripts are processed by the so-called microprocessor complex formed of an RNase III Drosha (the catalytic subunit) and the protein DGCR8 (DiGeorge syndrome critical region 8) (the Pasha protein of Drosophila, the subunit that recognises the substrate) into pre-miRNAs. The latter are translocated to the cytoplasm and are further processed by Dicer (see Sherbet, 2013 for references).

miRNA function has been implicated in the proliferation of neural progenitor cells as well as in neuron maintenance and function. Both Dicer and DGCR8 are key players in the participation of miRNAs in the development and morphogenesis of the CNS. Drosha seems able to negatively regulate the expression of NGN-2 and NeuroD1 and neurogenesis in this way. This has been attributed to molecular similarities of NGN-2 mRNA and primary miRNA leading to the association of NGN-2 with the microprocessor in neural progenitors (Knuckles et al., 2012). On the other hand, miRNAs might be directly involved in the regulation of neurogenesis. Ristori et al. (2015) have advocated a direct interaction between Dicer and miRNA-107, which determines Dicer levels and in turn this leads to the regulation of miRNA-9 levels required for neurogenesis. A direct role has been ascribed to other miRNAs as well, e.g., miRNA-30c (Chao CC et al., 2015), miRNA-8/miRNA-200 family (Trumbach and Prakash, 2015). Direct involvement might take other routes as that taken by miRNA-15b, which is said to suppress neural progenitor cell proliferation by repressing TET3-mediated promotion of cyclin D1 and cell proliferation (Lv XH et al., 2014). Other pathways have also been postulated for miRNA function in neurogenesis. Among them are repression of SIRT1-mediated epigenetic regulation of gene expression by miRNA-34a (Hu B et al., 2014), TGF-β/Smad signalling for miRNA-376c (Liu JL et al., 2014), and the targeting Musashi1, a marker of CNS stem cells, by miRNA-23a and miRNA-125b (Gioia et al., 2014). Mondanizadeh et al. (2015) have demonstrated that miRNA-124 suppresses Sp1 expression and influences neuronal differentiation of MSCs. miRNAs seem to be able to influence neuronal migration as well. Three miRNAs of the miR379-410 cluster appeared to suppress N-cadherin expression and in parallel promoted neuronal migration and NSC differentiation (Rago et al., 2014). Neuronal migration can and does involve many ECM components; among them are laminin, integrins, N-CAM and reelin. Indeed, reelin, which regulates neurogenesis and neuronal migration (Pujadas et al. 2010), is also affected by miRNAs (Evangelisti et al., 2009).

miRNAs are ubiquitously occurring non-coding RNAs participating in multiple cellular function. It has also been the general experience that they do not display tissue specificity to a remarkable degree and furthermore they do enter into interaction and mutual regulation. Often several miRNAs can be linked with the manifestation of a normal and abnormal phenotypic feature. The activation of EMT involves many miRNA species. The reverse process of mesenchymal epithelial transition is also induced by some miRNAs and it is remarkable that some miRNAs can activate EMT, but they can also work in the opposite direction in conjunction with other miRNAs. Neurodegenerative processes are another instance of involvement of many miRNAs in the generation of the seemingly similar cellular abnormality. So attribution of specific functions can lead to erroneous conclusions if a global view of miRNA expression is not taken into account. Given the inordinate numbers of identified miRNAs and mindful of their interaction and mutual regulation of signalling, defining functional specificities would be an arduous undertaking. Any application of miRNA technology in the clinical setting would be presumptuous and premature at present.

CHAPTER 14

Inhibitor of DNA-Binding Proteins in Angiogenesis

A group of basic helix loop helix (bHLH) proteins known as inhibitors of DNA-binding proteins (IDs) are worthy of discussion here. They are dominant negative bHLH transcription factors. ID bHLH proteins possess no DNA-binding ability and function by heterodimerising with and regulating the activity of other bHLH transcription factors. As transcription factors, IDs, regulate the outcome of many signalling systems operating in cell proliferation, differentiation and determination of cell lineage. The motivation to discuss them here is their association with the regulation of angiogenesis. As shown in Table 14.1, whilst IDs 1–3 appear to be able to promote angiogenesis, ID4 appears to inhibit angiogenesis since its expression relates inversely with the expression of VEGF. It might suppress tumour growth in this way or by suppressing the growth and angiogenesis promoting effects of other IDs. It could possibly also promote the expression of suppressor genes such as BRCA1, and amend the stem cell maintenance programme. Furthermore, the loss of expression of ID4 may indicate poor prognosis. So ID4 has rightly earned the epithet of a tumour suppressor gene. With the exceptionally good correlation with the promotion of angiogenesis or its suppression, the ID family would be ideal candidates with potential therapeutic merit. Their involvement in stem cell renewal and expansion adds a further valuable dimension to our understanding of the biology of cancer development and progression.

The IDs 1–3 seem to promote the maintenance and expansion of cancer stem cells (CSCs). ID1 has been reported to increase breast cancer CSC in an MMTV-ID1 transgenic model as well as in breast cancer cell lines (Shin DH et al., 2015). They may transduce signalling by many pathways. This may be mediated by Wnt-myc signalling, but the Akt pathway has also been implicated. Indeed, Perry et al. (2011) had shown that both Wnt and PI3K/Akt signalling may be required to operate simultaneously in the expansion of HSCs. The proliferative signalling in neural stem cells seems to be subject to p53 intervention. Liu HJ et al. (2013) found that ID1 is upregulated in absence of p53 and that p53 suppresses ID1 activity. ID2 is also regulated by p53

Molecular Approach to Cancer Management. DOI: http://dx.doi.org/10.1016/B978-0-12-812896-1.00014-3

Table 14.1 Inhibitors of DNA-Binding bHLH Proteins and Their Biological Properties

ID1 (bHLHb24)	EGR (early growth response) transcription factor → ID1 cell proliferation; inhibits NF-κB and apoptosis; CSC maintenance; endothelial cell migration; angiogenesis; ↑EGFR; ↑VEGF; ↑MMPs
ID2 (bHLHb26)	EGR2 → ID2; inhibits RANKL/NF-κB → inhibits apoptosis; CSC maintenance; angiogenesis; ↑EGFR; VEGF?
ID3 (bHLHb25)	CSC maintenance; angiogenesis; ↑EGFR; ↑VEGF
ID4 (bHLHb27)	Tumour and growth suppression; stem cell programme; Cdc42 → ID4↓; ID4↓ → BRCA1↓; angiogenesis? ↓VEGF? ID4↓ → Poor prognosis

This table is based on Human Gene Nomenclature Committee, Sherbet (2013) and the references cited in the text.

and the inhibition of neural progenitor cells by ID is said to be a result of a direct binding of p53 to conserved site in the ID2 promoter (Paolella et al., 2011). Also Yes-associated protein (YAP) of the Hippo pathway may be a negative regulator of differentiation of mesenchymal stem cells and probably IDs 1–3 trigger this. One would recall here that YAP is said to co-ordinate the crosstalk between Hippo and Wnt. This co-ordination of signalling is compatible with the suggested activation of Wnt by ID1.

There are fundamental functional differences between IDs 1–3 and ID4. But paradoxically, the postulated tumour suppressor ID4 has been claimed to be able to inhibit the differentiation of stem cells and indeed promote differentiated cells to switch to a stem cell phenotype. The counter argument has also been adduced that ID4 whilst promoting stem cell maintenance and survival also promotes their differentiation and the time frame of the differentiation process (Patel et al., 2015), a view compatible with the postulated suppressor status. The overriding difference seems to lie in that IDs 1–3 inhibit the differentiation of the CSC pool. Also of much significance is that ID1 can activate epithelial mesenchymal transition (EMT) (Teo WS et al., 2014), a process known to lead to the generation of cells with stem cell-like features.

It is fairly obvious from the description of the phenotypic features of promotion of cell proliferation, endothelial migration and angiogenesis, and of CSC evolution and maintenance of the IDs 1–3 on the one hand and of the virtually diametrically opposite effects of ID4 on the other, are outcomes of the same signalling routes excepting for the nature of the regulation. Patel et al. (2015) have argued that the differences might have occurred due to the marked structural organisation of the proteins. They postulate that the functional differences arise from the markedly highly degree of molecular organisation undergone by ID4 in the C-terminus of the molecule giving greater access to interaction with other proteins at the relevant functional domains. The IDs 1–3 as a group display a different expression pattern from ID4, but there is no obvious histogenetic correlation with the distribution.

Given the emphasis on the ability of ID proteins to promote or inhibit angiogenesis, it is inevitable that the discussion should also focus on the usefulness and potential as therapeutic targets. It is noteworthy that the promotion of angiogenesis by ID1, ID2 and ID3 seems to occur more often than not in parallel with the upregulation of angiogenic growth factors suggesting a surrogate but ample provision and opportunity of suppressing them.

The marked effects on cell proliferation can also be seen as possible modes of approach to control of tumour growth. Some efforts have been made to suppress ID genes that promote tumour growth and spread. Many pathways of the regulation of IDs that operate changes in the growth and behaviour of tumours have been suggested as possible targets, especially the regulation of apoptosis signalling involving NF-κB. The postulated regulatory loop consisting of ER and ID4, BRCA1 and certain miRNAs also holds much yet undefined promise. These approaches are constrained by a lack of development of agents that can inhibit the IDs 1–3 that are counterproductive in terms of tumour growth and spread, or the development of means to activate the supposed suppressor ID4. ID4 is said to be inactivated by hypermethylation in some tumours but equally the opposite of this has also been documented. The induction of ID4 re-expression by targeted demethylation is possible. However, it cannot be seen or regarded as a practicable proposition at present. It is undeniable that targeted demethylation could offer a powerful means of regulating the inappropriate expression of genes or induction of re-expression by the reverse process. Whether this approach will work in the natural genetic environment is an open question (Sherbet, 2013). With these important caveats floating around the postulated functions of IDs, it is hardly surprising that they have aroused little clinical interest.

CHAPTER 15

Small Molecule Inhibitors of Angiogenesis and Cell Proliferation

The therapeutic potential of small molecule drugs as tumour inhibitors has been accorded much significance and there has been adequate recognition of the practicalities and the advantages inherent in the use of small molecule-based therapy. The development of small molecule drugs has focused on specific facets of the molecular environment that sustains and promotes tumour growth and spread. The inhibition of growth factor function by inhibiting receptor tyrosine kinases (RTKs) has been discussed with due weight and at length in another location (pp. 1-22). The growth inhibition by RTK inhibitors is amalgamated by their ability to control tumour invasion. Furthermore, there has been considerable emphasis on the intrinsic differential susceptibilities and weaknesses of primary and secondary tumour foci to the induction of apoptosis, the activation of epithelial mesenchyme transition (EMT) and the development of CSCs and resistance to apoptosis. The special reference here is on the means to the inhibition of angiogenesis.

INHIBITION OF ANGIOGENIC GROWTH FACTOR RTKs

The development of small molecule inhibitors (<600 Da) of RTKs has been viewed as a viable means of inhibiting angiogenesis. However, of overriding importance would be defining and achieving specific targeting of RTKs to inhibit angiogenesis, without interfering with the function of essential growth factors. The augmentation of inhibitory outcome may accrue from the deployment of inhibitors of cell proliferation together with inhibitors of angiogenesis. The rationale for this is that the loss of control of tumour growth can also promote angiogenesis and switch the tumours on to the vascular phase of growth. It is known that the activation of PI3K/Akt pathway can route signal transduction into PDK1/PKC (phosphoinositide-dependent kinase 1/protein kinase C) or mammalian target of rapamycin (mTOR) and lead to HIF-1α protein expression. The latter is induced by hypoxia and mediates VEGF expression.

Molecular Approach to Cancer Management. DOI: http://dx.doi.org/10.1016/B978-0-12-812896-1.00015-5

Many RTK inhibitors have been developed and have been approved or are awaiting approval for clinical use. Sunitinib inhibits VEGFR2 and PDGFR-B. It is known to suppress the PDGF RTK encoded by c-Kit and the Fms-related tyrosine kinase 3 FLT3 and its paralogue FGFR3. Dovitinib inhibits FGFR3 and suppresses cell proliferation. Other small molecular inhibitors of VEGFRs are lenvatinib, tivozanib, vatalanib and cediranib. Crenolanib also inhibits the HGF receptor c-met and platelet-derived growth factor receptors (PDGFRs) (Hojjat-Farsangi, 2014). Inhibition of c-met has the dual advantage of inhibiting cell proliferation as well as invasion. Cabozantinib inhibits c-met and VGFRs 1, 2 and 3 and it might turn out to be a potent inhibitor of tumour progression. It is undergoing clinical trials in patients with many forms of cancer (see http://www.cancer.gov/about-cancer/treatment/clinical-trials).

It is needless to reiterate that RTK inhibitors, which control cell proliferation by suppressing epidermal growth factor receptor (EGFR) family receptor kinases, also figure prominently in cancer treatment regimes. There is no appreciable clinical interest in taking advantage of the potential of inhibiting mTOR signalling in combination with VEGFR inhibitors. The mTOR system integrates EGFR, VEGF, IGFR, TNFR and signalling. HIF-1 inhibitors exhibit marked anti-cancer activity and many inhibitors have been identified and some are clinically evaluated. Incorporating mTOR inhibitors with inhibitors of RTK would be invaluable in combination therapy.

ALLOSTERIC INHIBITORS OF ANGIOGENESIS

In the horizon are seen novel application of established theories relating to molecular reorganisation in enterprises such as developing allosteric drugs to inhibit angiogenesis. Allosteric modulation of signalling systems was shown to be a practical proposition some while ago. Signal transduction involving cell membrane and nuclear receptors were recognised as targets of allosteric modulation. An allosteric mechanism is one wherein the binding of a ligand to a site distinct from the canonical one produces a conformational change in the receptor leading to an altered signal transduction output. The altered output could result from, among other things, the emergence of new distant active sites in a subunit or upon receptor active dimerisation or alterations in the primary active site, opening up possible interaction with ligands non-canonical to the receptor. Furthermore, allosteric effects might impinge upon the function of the natural ligand by altering the affinity of binding to the active site. If the receptor is confined to a given conformational state, the transmitted signal would be in an unaltered canonical active or inactive state, as the case may be. There is much recognition that the allosteric mode of function offers the advantages of new and more appropriate specific targets for new small molecule inhibitor drugs. Equally, allosteric perturbation of signalling can modulate the phenotypic output and lead to pathogenesis (see Nussinov and Tsai, 2013; Laskowski et al., 2009).

The inhibitors that are investigated extensively and currently employed in mTOR inhibition (see Fig. 1.3) are an important example of the allosteric mode of action. The mTOR signalling pathway is frequently upregulated in cancers. Besides, it co-ordinates several pathways of growth factor signal transduction thus providing ample scope for taking advantage of allosteric modulation of the outputs. Rapamycin and its analogues, temsirolimus and everolimus, inhibit signalling by an allosteric mode of action (Jhanwar-Uniyal et al., 2015). The activation upstream of RTKs by growth factors initiates PI3K/Akt/mTOR signalling leading to the deregulation of cell proliferation. The site of action of the non-competitive allosteric inhibitors is at a distance from the ATP-catalytic binding site that regulates PI3K/Akt-mediated inhibition. The allosteric rapamycin and everolimus inhibitors inhibit cell proliferation but they are not highly effective inducers of apoptosis. Both selective inhibition of PI3K and mTORC1 produce similar effects on the phosphorylation of the downstream mTOR effectors. However, everolimus seems to be the main inhibitor of proliferation, whilst the PI3K inhibitor is the major inducer of apoptosis. Therefore, combining a selective ATP-competitive inhibitor of PI3K with an allosteric inhibitor of mTOR would suppress cell proliferation more effectively (Badura et al., 2013) bearing in mind that loss of PTEN would significantly affect mTOR signalling.

The differential effectiveness of the selective PI3K and the allosteric mTOR inhibitors has been explained on other grounds. The rapamycin homologues inhibit mTORC1, but upregulate mTORC2 as a feedback response and confer resistance to the allosteric inhibitors. This resistance can be overcome by agents that inhibit both mTORCs 1 and 2. The mTOR kinase inhibitor CC-223 does exactly this and has led to a total mTOR blockade and achieved suppression of proliferation far superior to that achieved by rapamycin alone (Mortensen et al., 2015). CC-223 has shown some promise at the clinical stage too. Its toxicity was tolerable with some anti-tumour response (Shih KC et al., 2012). Currently, clinical trials testing is safety and efficacy when administered with erlotinib or other agents in patients with advanced non-small cell lung cancer (NSCLC). Combinations of CC-223 with other therapeutic agents are also being tested clinically in patients with advanced solid tumours, non-Hodgkin lymphoma, multiple myeloma and diffuse large B cell lymphoma. AZD2014 is another potent inhibitor of both mTORCs, which is being evaluated in several clinical trials (https://clinicaltrials.gov). This inhibitor is said to be more potent than rapamycin.

As discussed in another location, mTOR signalling can integrate EGFR, VEGF, IGFR, TNFR and oestrogen receptor (ER) signalling in combination therapy. So highly valuable it would be to assess the effects of combining EGFR and ER inhibitors with allosteric and dual mTORC1 and mTORC2 in pre-clinical studies. That might provide the impetus to initiate investigation at the clinical levels. Tumour cell lines that are resistant EGFR inhibitors show high mTOR and PDE4D (phosphodiesterase 4D) levels.

Many PDEs have been associated with the promotion of tumour cell proliferation and invasion. Inhibitors of PDE suppress tumour growth. The involvement of growth factors in PDE function is exemplified by the demonstration that the suppression of PDE4D suppressed cell proliferation and this was reversed by EGF (Xu T et al., 2014). The expression of many PDEs has been seen in breast cancers. Notably, PDE8 expression was seen in several breast cancer cell lines and breast tumour tissues. In the triple negative breast cancer (TNBC) cell line, MDA-MB-231 inhibition of PDE8 reduced cell migration but did not affect cell proliferation (Dong HL et al., 2015). The MDA-MB-231 cells are triple negative but they do express EGFR and would respond to EGFR activation by enhanced cell migration and proliferation. It is difficult to visualise a situation in which cell motility and proliferation could be uncoupled in the TNBC cell lines. The MDA-MB-231 cells may also harbour mutant p53. So, one has to be cautious in interpreting the effects of PDE8 inhibitors in relation to tumour progression.

BIM (BCL2L11) is a pro-apoptotic protein that mediates apoptosis triggered by EGFR inhibitors. Karachaliou et al. (2015) were able to show that combining EGFR inhibitors with mTOR adequately dealt with EGFR-resistant NSCLC and could be adequate therapy for EGFR-mutant NSCLC patients with high pre-treatment levels of BIM and mTOR. Activation of the EGFR/Ras/MEK signalling simulates cell proliferation and survival. So it is also helpful to know that the development of the resistant phenotype might be prevented by EGFR and MEK inhibition (Tricker et al., 2015). The synergy between EGFR and mTOR inhibitors is most valuable in ER-negative tumours that express EGFR. EGFR expression is upregulated in many tumours that are ER negative. TNBCs can show enhanced EGFR expression and the synergy can benefit this group of breast cancer patients, for this combination has been found to suppress tumour cell proliferation in vitro (Madden et al., 2014). AZD2014 inhibits both mTORC1 and mTORC2. The inhibition of mTORC2 has been reported to prevent the feedback activation of AKT signalling (Liao H et al., 2015). Possibly, AZD2014 inhibitor might offer a way to overcome the resistance to EGFR inhibitors. This is a distinct possibility since it is highly effective in ER-positive breast cancer cell lines that display acquired resistance to hormonal manipulation (Guichard et al., 2015).

SSR128129E (SSR) is a small molecule modulator of RTK function. It binds to an extracellular site of the FGFR that is distinct from the site to which the natural ligand binds and alters FGFR signalling in an allosteric manner, i.e., produces a conformational change in EGFRgenerating potent inhibition of FGFR signal transduction and possibly also alters the affinity of binding by the natural ligand for the receptor and effectively reduces the magnitude of the signal transduced by the natural ligand (Bono et al., 2013; Herbert et al., 2013).

It ought to be borne in mind here that FGFR is closely related to VEGFR and PDGFR and indeed binding of PDGF and VEGF to PDGFR can activate the latter. PDGF and FGF can upregulate each other's receptors and modulate the response of the non-canonical ligand (Shen J et al., 2009). At the moment, we have no information whether the allosteric effects might impinge upon the function of other ligands signalling angiogenesis.

VASCULAR-DISRUPTING AGENTS IN ANTI-ANGIOGENESIS

The anti-angiogenesis strategy has included the use of inhibitors of tubulin polymerisation. Among small inhibitors of angiogenesis and cell proliferation are the vascular-disrupting agents. Of the several vascular-disrupting agents, combretastatin and its analogues have received much attention. Combretastatin is a naturally occurring small stilbinoid derived from the African Bushwillow *Combretum caffrum*. The vascular-disrupting agents reduce blood supply and suppress tumour growth by inducing apoptosis and necrosis. They suppress cell migration and have been also attributed with the ability to suppress cell proliferation by cell cycle arrest in the G2/M phase (Wang ZW et al., 2016). Besides, the biological properties noted earlier, in CAM assays combretastatin inhibited angiogenesis. In vivo, xenografts of MCF7 tumours displayed reduced tumour-associated microvascular density upon treatment. Together with these effects, reduced VEGF expression and VEGFR activation have been seen (Su M et al., 2016).

There are indications that combretastatin might suppress metastasis but these need further substantiation. In murine hosts with hepatic metastases, combining combretastatin with sunitinib has prolonged host cell survival as compared with their effect as single agents. The drug combination reduced the tumour burden (Nguyen L et al., 2016). However, the tumour model used would not allow one to infer what the effects of the drug combination were on metastatic spread. With xenograft implantation, one can see whether the time to metastasis was prolonged, how extensive was the metastatic spread and whether that related to the tumour-associated microvasculature. Here,

Nguyen L et al. (2016) injected colon cancer cells intrasplenically and allowed them to metastasise to the liver. Splenectomy was performed as usual, but there is no information about the formation of tumours at the injection site or whether the vascularisation associated with them had shown any changes. This would have been of interest in the context of their finding that tumour cells, which survived the treatment, appeared to have undergone EMT.

The progress in the use of combretastatin and derivative needs to go apace with the studies on their binding to tubulin monomers and the problems linked with the solubility and delivery of the compounds. Much of the work with these drugs is at the in vitro or the pre-clinical stage. Combretastatin has been designated as an orphan drug by FDA and the EU. Some clinical trials are being carried out with combretastatin and related compounds. The outcome of the clinical studies is uncertain at present, but many trials are still in operation. The vascular-disrupting agents do not appear at this time to offer an added advantage in terms of growth control and induction of apoptosis over the conventional microtubule disruptors such as vinblastine and taxols.

CHAPTER 16

Suramin and Polysulphonated Naphthylureas as Angiogenesis Inhibitors

Suramin is an anti-parasitic and a potentially anti-neoplastic drug. Its anti-cancer effects stem from its ability to competitively inhibit protein tyrosine phosphatases by binding to their active sites. Suramain increases tyrosine phosphorylation of many signalling proteins and inhibits cell proliferation. It markedly inhibits the signalling by many growth factors by interfering with ligand/receptor binding and influences the transduction of growth factor signals along a variety of pathways. Inhibition of VEGF is believed to be a means by which suramin suppresses angiogenesis. Polysulphonated naphthylureas including suramin have been shown to inhibit bFGF- and platelet-derived growth factor (PDGF)-mediated endothelial cell proliferation and angiogenesis in vitro. Most of the studies on the inhibition of angiogenesis have been carried out in vitro using for instance Matrigel assays. Apparently, some of the findings might be artifactual because it has been suggested that suramin itself might be able to degrade Matrigel. However, Lopez et al. (2011) used animal tumour models to demonstrate that a combination of suramin and bevacizumab does result in the inhibition of angiogenesis to a greater extent than suramin or bevacizumab alone. Suramin is able to effectively block NF-κB, an essential downstream element in angiogenic signalling; especially it suppresses the expression of VEGF. Suramin has been shown to target Wnt signalling in triple negative breast cancer cells in vitro and in mouse tumour models (Koval et al., 2016) with implications for possible interference with cell motility.

Singla et al. (2014) have published an interesting study where they treated MDA-MB-231 breast cancer cells with plaxitaxel and suramin. The treatment reduced cell viability and in vitro invasion. But significantly, when the treatment regime began on day 1 of intra-arterial inoculation, a marked inhibition of metastasis to the bone was noticed. There was no reduction in metastasis but some inhibition of the growth of the metastatic deposits if the treatment was stared on day 7. This suggests that the treatment targeted circulating tumour cells more effectively than the metastatic deposits. The reduction in metastatic deposition in the bone was more marked with

Molecular Approach to Cancer Management. DOI: http://dx.doi.org/10.1016/B978-0-12-812896-1.00016-7

the combination than as single agents. Metastasis to the bone is a common feature of many tumours including breast cancer. There is no complete understanding of the mechanisms involved in the interaction of tumour cells with tissues of metastatic sites. Suramin can exert a wide-ranging array of cell membrane-related effects that can alter the degree and pattern of metastatic spread. So more focused research is required into the signalling systems that dictate specificities of the location of metastatic sites.

In this context, it may be useful to recall that osteopontin was identified as a metastasis-associated protein. It is an intermediary in promoting cell proliferation and invasion with the potential onward progression of tumours. Osteopontin co-ordinates the signalling pathways involving extracellular matrix (ECM) components, matrix metalloproteinases, S100A4, Wnt/β-catenin and NF-κB in generating the invasive and metastasising phenotype (see Sherbet, 2013). Rudland et al. (2002) reported over a decade ago that the expression of osteopontin correlated with poor survival of breast cancer patients. Suramin seems to suppress the expression of osteopontin in nasopharyngeal carcinoma cells (Jiang S et al., 2012). Suramin could affect metastasis by impinging upon the function of ECM or the invasive function activated by some of the signalling pathways.

It is needless to say that one is dealing with postulates here and so more substantive work needs to be carried out. So clinical testing of suramin is still far behind any expected schedule. Many clinical trials are in progress to assess the efficacy of suramin plus conventional therapeutic agents in patients with colorectal cancer, adrenocortical carcinoma, carcinoma of the breast cancer and prostate cancer. Some improvement in overall response has been noted in some studies. But no significant findings have been reported.

CHAPTER 17

The Anti-Cancer Potential of Flavonoids

Several phytochemicals, including carotenoids, flavonoids and polyphenols, are potent anti-oxidants. Many possess anti-inflammatory properties and have also displayed tumour inhibitory activity. Here the focus is placed on the anti-cancer potential of flavonoids, carotenoids and selenoproteins in cancer control. Ideally curcumin, the polyphenolic active ingredient of turmeric (*Curcula longa*) possessing multiple biological and medicinal properties, should have been discussed in this and the following section. Curcumin significantly inhibits NF-κB, STAT3 signalling and IGF-1-induced cell proliferation. The involvement of other signalling systems has also been suggested. In fact, resveratrol (3,4′,5-trihydroxystilbene), a polyphenolic phytoalexin and curcumin, alone or in combination seem to downregulate the activation of epidermal growth factor receptor (EGFR) and insulin-like growth factor receptor (IGFR) signalling. Curcumin has been shown to induce apoptosis in vitro by concurrent inhibition of the activations of AKT/mTOR and RAF/MEK/ERK pathways. Both resveratrol and curcumin can inhibit COX-2 and angiogenesis. Resveratrol also inhibits HIF-1-mediated angiogenic signalling. Some evidence has been adduced that curcumin suppresses in vitro invasion and suppresses metastases from tumour models. The drawbacks of poor solubility and bioavailability have prompted a search of analogues of curcumin. UBS109 is one such compound, which seems to suppress NF-κB signalling. It has been shown to inhibit the growth of xenografted HNSCC (head and neck squamous cell carcinoma) cells. Many clinical trials are underway evaluating the efficacy and the bioavailability of curcumin, which is lipophilic and poorly absorbed upon enteral administration. Much work is also being carried out to develop efficient delivery of curcumin. The emphasis placed on curcumin vindicates its perception as a potential suppressor of metastasis (see pp. 38-39, 208; Fig. 3.1 legend on p. 36 for a detailed discussion and relevant references).

Flavonoids are naturally occurring polyphenolic plant products and have had much focus on them on account of their diverse biological effects. They inhibit cell proliferation, induce apoptosis and suppress angiogenesis by

Molecular Approach to Cancer Management. DOI: http://dx.doi.org/10.1016/B978-0-12-812896-1.00017-9

interference with growth factor signalling and are anti-inflammatory. Equally important in terms of their potential as anti-cancer agents is the demonstrated ability of many flavonoids to suppress drug resistance and enhance chemosensitisation of cancer cells. Many naturally occurring polyphenols as well as their derivatives have been studied for potential use as anti-cancer agents, for effective inhibition of angiogenesis can quite effectively control tumour growth and secondary spread.

Among significant thespians in the anti-cancer scenario are the flavonoids, quercetin, myricetin and rutin, the isoflavone, genistein and the flavones, apigenin and luteolin. Here the discussion is focused on the anti-cancer action of quercetin and the flavonoid complex known as silymarin and its derivatives.

QUERCETIN INHIBITS ANGIOGENESIS AND CELL MIGRATION IN VITRO

Quercetin, the anti-oxidant flavonoid, has been tested using a carcinogen-induced murine melanoma model and it has been claimed that dietary administration of quercetin delayed the onset of carcinogenesis and inhibited IGF-1-induced cell proliferation (Jung M et al., 2013). Of interest is the report that quercetin inhibits vascular endothelial growth factor (VEGF) and therefore it would be worthwhile looking at its effects on tumour-associated angiogenesis. Many flavonoids including quercetin and myricetin have been described to be able to inhibit the synthesis and secretion of VEGF by human retinal pigment epithelial cells (Chen R et al., 2014). Quercetin suppresses VEGFR2 activation and inhibits downstream signalling via the Akt/mTOR pathway in human umbilical vein endothelial cells (HUVEC) cells. In vivo there was a marked reduction in tumour growth (Pratheeshkumar et al., 2012), which the authors have attributed to the inhibition of angiogenesis. In vitro, VEGF-induced migration of endothelial cell and tubule formation were described to have been inhibited. But the in vivo experiments are less convincing. They found a small number of endothelial markers CD31+ and CD34+ cells in the quercetin-treated group as compared with the control group. Also angiogenesis was inhibited in CAM (chorioallantoic membrane) assays. Unfortunately, no attempt was made to check the microvascular density or the effects of the drug on the incidence of distant metastases. Similar phenotypic effects are probably produced by quercetin and related flavonoids by influencing signal transduction via the NF-κB and MAPK pathways. One has to emphasise the proviso that these are mainly in vitro findings or evaluations using in vivo tumour models.

Quercetin is employed in the treatment of many human pathological conditions and many clinical trials are in progress dealing with its use in chronic obstructive pulmonary disease, and to test possible improvement of vascular function and blood pressure. Quercetin is also being studied for potential chemopreventive properties in prostate and colon cancers. However, its use in preventing progression of pre-cancerous conditions or its value in conditions of genetic susceptibility to develop cancer has received very little attention.

THE MAJOR SIGNALLING PATHWAYS INFLUENCED BY FLAVONOIDS AND THEIR DERIVATIVES

The major pathways influenced by flavonoids and their derivatives are shown in Fig. 17.1; they are the conventional PI3K/Akt, NF-κB, cIAP (cellular inhibitor of apoptosis protein) and p53 in the inhibition of cell proliferation and induction of apoptosis and the VEGF/VEGFR and HIF being the angiogenetic pathways that are inhibited (Lin Y et al., 2008; Ravishankar et al., 2015). Both methoxyquercetin and luteolin (3′,4′,5,7-tetrahydroxyflavone) effectively suppressed VEGF-induced cell motility. The effects were accompanied by the inhibition of VEGFR2 phosphorylation and significantly methoxyquercetin showed the highest affinity for VEGFR. Although the authors have gone on to demonstrate inhibition of growth of MCF7 cells, this study has depended on in vitro scratch wound healing and migration of HUVEC cells (Ravishankar et al., 2015). Endothelial cell migration is a part of the

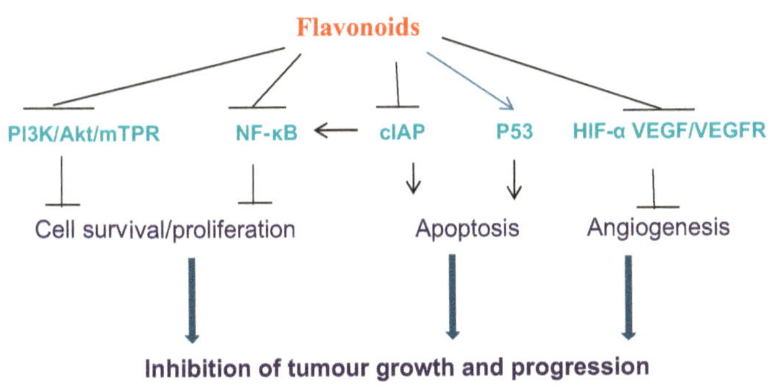

FIGURE 17.1

The potential pathways with which flavones interfere to generate their effects of tumour growth inhibition and suppression of progression. The flavonoids can induce these phenotypic effects via AMPK activation. This is not shown here, but see p. 41; Fig.1.2 on p. 9 and Table 20.1 on p. 176. Albeit the signalling by silymarin and its derivatives overlaps that by the other flavonoids discussed earlier, these have been summarised in Table 17.1 to draw attention to the specifics of the signalling cascades and their outcome. See references in the text. cIAP: cellular inhibitor of apoptosis protein.

angiogenic process and also a feature of tubule formation assay for angiogenesis. Their work lacks definitive assays for angiogenesis, e.g., tubule formation or in vivo studies of their effects on microvasculature of tumours. Important it is that they have focused more on synthesising derivative flavonoids than on assessing their biological effects. Other flavones being investigated are acacetin (5,7-dihydroxy-4′-methoxyflavone), which has been attributed with the ability to inhibit STAT phosphorylation and also VEGF, eNOS (endothelial nitric oxide synthase), iNOS (inducible nitric oxide synthase), matrix metalloproteinase (MMP)-2 and basic fibroblast growth factor (bFGF), all known pro-angiogenic agents (Bhat et al., 2013).

The isoflavone genistein (4′,5,7-trihydroxyisoflavone) possesses demonstrable oestrogenic effects, binds to oestrogen receptor (ER) and activates ER responsive genes. However, it does not invariably promote cell proliferation and may indeed inhibit the process in some cell lines. In fact, it inhibits tumour cell proliferation in general and suppresses the proliferation of endothelial cells. The oestrogenic activity seems to be due to the structural similarity of genistein to 17-β-oestradiol. It binds both ERα and ERβ and the induction of proliferation is inhibited by anti-oestrogens. The oestrogenic effects would depend upon whether ERα or ERβ was involved. The outcome of signalling depends upon a balance of the function of the two receptor isoforms, which have markedly different biological functions. ERα is pro-proliferation whilst ERβ is inhibitory of cell proliferation. Also it is imperative to know the status of progesterone receptor (PR) expression, which has profound effects on the biology of ER function.

In the context of cancer progression, it is important to acknowledge that genistein is highly inhibitory of angiogenesis. Besides, in addition to the pathways noted earlier, genistein may induce apoptosis by interfering with Bcl-2 family gene signalling. The inhibitory effects on migration could be a consequence targeting the Wnt/β-catenin signalling pathway (Spagnuolo et al., 2015). Although numerous publications mention metastatic spread of tumour among the processes affected flavonoids, there is very little substantive evidence that they inhibit tumour metastasis. Nevertheless, one has to acknowledge the report by Xiao X (2015) of the inhibition of metastatic spread of xenografted human colorectal cancers upon oral administration of genistein. Genistein downregulated MMP-2 and VEGFR3 (FLT4) providing obvious links to metastasis inhibition. Furthermore, genistein has been shown to inhibit epithelial mesenchymal transition (EMT), which plays a critical role in the promotion of metastatic spread of tumours. EMT can be blocked by the suppression of forkhead box M1 (Fox M1) transcription factor and genistein is able to downregulate that and inhibit cell proliferation, cell motility and promote apoptosis (Tian TT et al., 2014).

Another interesting prospect is that some pathways associated with the generation and self-renewal of cancer stem cells (CSCs), such as PI3K/AKT/mTOR, Wnt and Hedgehog signalling, are inhibited by genistein and other flavonoids. Notch expression has also been implicated in CSCs, again a target of genistein-mediated inhibition.

An invaluable contribution to the inhibition of cell proliferation and induction of apoptosis and to the suppression of CSCs is made by AMP-activated protein kinase (AMPK). AMPK upregulates p53 expression and the expression of apoptosis inducing family genes. Besides this, AMPK downregulates MAPK/p38/ERK and PI3K/Akt signalling. This leads to an inclusive suppression of cell proliferation and induction of apoptosis. Its ability to suppress CSC generation and propagation occurs by the downregulation of mTOR and NF-κB (see Table 17.1). Quercetin action could bring about these outcomes since it can activate AMPK. The LKB1 kinase is implicated upstream of AMPK function. Quercetin does induce apoptosis by signalling along the LKB1/AMPK axis, but possibly can work independently of LKB1. As stated earlier, flavonoids and their derivatives inhibit the angiogenic signalling via VEGF/VEGFR and HIF. In fact, quercetin can also downregulate HIF-1 prompted by AMPK activation (Kim HS et al., 2012). This is compatible with the inhibition of angiogenesis.

The perceived benefits of the intake of certain phytochemicals, especially polyphenols and their mode of action, have been reviewed recently (Thomas et al., 2015). They have highlighted the demonstrable and wide-ranging

Table 17.1 The Signalling Systems Modulated by Silymarin and Its Derivatives and the Resulting Phenotypic Effects

Targeted Signal	Phenotypic Effect
HIF1/VEGF ↓	Radiation resistance ↓; → EMT ↓
	Angiogenesis ↓
Zeb1 ↓ → E-cadherin ↑	EMT ↓
Cyclin B1/Cdk1/cyclin A2, surviving ↓	Cell proliferation ↓ apoptosis ↑
Wnt/β-catenin ↓	Motility, invasion ↓
mTOR/PI3K/Akt ↓ → STAT3 ↓	Cell proliferation, tumour growth ↓
NF-κB ↓	Cell survival ↓ apoptosis ↑
AMPK ↑ → PTEN ↑ → PI3K/Akt ↓	Apoptosis ↑
Gli1/Hh → PI3K/Akt/mTOR ↓	Apoptosis ↑
Fox M1 ↓ → PI3K/Akt/mTOR ↓	Apoptosis ↑
ERβ ↑ ERα ↓	Cell proliferation ↓

References as cited in the text; ↑ indicates of gene expression or activation of signalling pathway; ↓ downregulation of gene expression or suppression of pathway and → indicates a follow-on effect on gene expression or a signalling system.

modes of signalling and the considerable evidence concerning the effects of polyphenols currently available on tumour inhibition and associated inflammatory effects. A legitimate query would be what are the clinical prospects of polyphenols? There is little clinical interest in polyphenols and phytochemicals as a class and it is recognised that this is attributable to a lack of clinical trials to assess the benefits to human subjects. But understandably, difficulties arise from the findings that certain polyphenols might promote angiogenesis and tumour growth and progression.

HOW EFFECTIVE IS SILYMARIN AS AN ANTI-CANCER AGENT?

Silymarin is a polyphenol, a mixture of several flavonoids, isolated from *Silybum marianum* (milk thistle). The major constituent of silymarin is silibinin, with its isomers isosilybin, dihydrosilybin, silydianin and silychristin as minor components (Wagner et al., 1968). It was recognised many years ago as a potent anti-oxidant, and an inhibitor of cell proliferation and angiogenesis. Hence, this phytochemical has attracted much attention in recent years as a potential anti-cancer agent. The biological effects it exerts arise from its ability to modulate many signalling systems, which includes the inhibition of growth factor and cell survival signalling. It has a cell cycle regulatory ability and the ability to activate apoptosis pathways. The induction of apoptosis is the best studied and most convincing and persuasive of the effects of silymarin and isomers.

Indeed quite a multifaceted composite of effects has been formatted for silibinin, with suggestions that it can inhibit cell migration and invasion, suppress stem cell development and inhibit EMT activation, either as a single agent or in combination with other phytochemicals (Table 17.1). It is needless to reiterate the need for stringent criteria to be applied in defining and identifying CSCs. Nevertheless, some interesting research has surfaced. One would recall that VEGF expression has been associated with radiation resistance. Gupta et al. (2002) had shown some time ago that VEGF+/+ xenografts were most resistant than VEGF−/− ones to ionising radiation. Furthermore, endothelial cells, which survived radiation, showed increased VEGF expression. Compatible with this is the report by Nambiar et al. (2015) that silibinin suppressed VEGF expression of endothelial cells and rendered them radiosensitive. These authors have been able to show that ionising radiation also enhanced the expression of iNOS and MMP-2. It is obvious as the authors point out that invasive ability and vascularity is enhanced in the cells that survive irradiation. The radiation resistance seemed to extend to the activation of EMT as indicated by the upregulation of uPA, vimentin and N-cadherin in prostate carcinoma cells. The expression of all these angiogenic and EMT features was subverted by silibinin. Reading from these findings, one could suppose that silibinin should suppress EMT, stem cell development and endothelial cell proliferation and angiogenesis.

Signalling Pathways Modulated by Silymarin

Some significant biological outcomes of silymarin action, and indeed of other flavonoids discussed earlier, relate to cell motility and proliferation and these occur via established signalling systems. The most important attribute of silymarin is its perceived inhibition of EMT activation, since its trail follows the acquisition of cell migration, the promotion cell proliferation and the generation of CSCs. The effect on EMT has been convincingly demonstrated recently. Singh et al. (2016) reported that in vitro silymarin inhibits cell migration and reverses EMT as indicated by reduction of Zeb1 and upregulated E-cadherin expression in NSCLC cells. Concomitantly, a reduction occurred in histone deacetylase (HDAC) expression. Also the HDAC inhibitor trichostatin A (TSA) mimicked the effects (Singh et al., 2016). However, EMT is activated by many ligands. Several growth factors and tumour promoters such as MTA1 activate EMT. Also signalling systems such as EGFR, Hh and Wnt have also been implicated in EMT. Tumour suppressor proteins like LKB1 suppress EMT activation (see Sherbet, 2013). So it is hardly surprising that the expression of HDAC might be involved in the suppression of EMT by silymarin. Notwithstanding these reservations, the demonstration that it can and does suppress EMT is in practical terms does not become less attractive or less significant. It would be appropriate to mention here that TSA and silibinin, a component of silymarin, do synergistically inhibit the proliferation of pancreatic cancer cells. In fact, silibinin produced marked reduction in the expression of cell cycle regulatory proteins, cyclin B1/Cdk1/cyclin A2 and the IAP family protein called survivin (Feng W et al., 2015).

Silymarin has been shown to inhibit Wnt signalling by the downregulation of β-catenin/transcription factor (TCF) (Eo HJ et al., 2016). The β-catenin/p300-mediated increase of TCF expression is an early event of canonical Wnt signalling. This could have repercussions on adhesion-related features, e.g., cell motility and invasion. The proliferation status of cells is also liable to be influenced by this. The Wnt/β-catenin signalling is known to affect cell proliferation. The PTEN/PI3K/Akt signalling is involved in the dynamics of β-catenin accumulation in the nucleus (Persad et al., 2001) and activation of its target genes, which are numerically massive.

Unsurprisingly, the transcription factor STAT3 has come into the picture. Pre-clinical studies have shown that silibinin suppresses STAT3 activation and tumour development and progression. The STAT transcription factors are constitutively activated in many tumour cell lines. They are involved in signal transduction by growth factors, mTOR/Akt axis and in cell proliferation, regulation of apoptosis and in angiogenic signalling. Consistent with this, silibinin seems to inhibit cell proliferation and survival signalling. Both silibinin and 2,3-dehydrosilibinin inhibited in vitro and in vivo growth of basal cell carcinomas. This was accompanied by the suppression of STAT3, NF-κB and AP1 (Tilley et al., 2016). The synergy described by Montgomery et al. (2016) between silymarin and curcumin may reflect the involvement of STAT3 and NF-κB. As noted in another location, curcumin, the active ingredient of turmeric, possesses multiple biological and medicinal properties. It markedly inhibits NF-κB as well as STAT3 (Kim et al., 2012). There is further confirmation that silibinin quite demonstrably suppresses mTOR/Akt to inhibit cell proliferation and induce apoptosis (Feng N et al., 2016).

The activation of AMPK by silibinin also fits in with the general concept of involvement of mTOR. Li J et al. (2016) found that the inhibitory effects of cell proliferation and the promotion of apoptosis in vitro as well as suppression of growth of oesophageal squamous cell carcinomas as xenografts were mediated by the activation of AMPK. Some of the conclusions would inevitably attract some queries. The metastasis assay was performed by tail vein injection and assessing the localisation of the tumour cells in the lungs. This is by no proper definition a reliable parameter indicating metastatic ability. The authors also implanted the tumour cells subcutaneously, but in these experiments the incidence of spontaneous metastasis was not checked. The suppression of AMPK activation abrogated the inhibitory influence of silibinin. Metformin activates AMPK and inhibits mTOR signalling. It would be worthy of note in this context that silibinin synergistically suppresses cell proliferation and enhances apoptosis via upregulation of PTEN and activation of AMPK (Liou WS et al., 2015; Tsai CC et al., 2015). So in so far as AMPK is concerned that the findings of Li et al. (2016) stand properly corroborated.

The mTOR pathway has been postulated to provide a link of silibinin effects to the suppression of Gli1 transcription factor of the Hedgehog system and inducing apoptosis by downregulating Bcl-2 (Ma ZK et al., 2015). Gli1 is an effector of the Hh pathway in both the canonical and the non-canonical route, which can involve PI3K/Akt/mTOR and also MAPK systems (see p. 61 and Fig. 6.2 on p. 58). Thus, the effectiveness of silibinin might lie in its access to and modulation of mTOR-mediated and the integrated signalling of PTEN/PI3K/Akt and growth factor RTK systems, including the EMT phenomenon. Additional evidence has emerged that silibinin can suppress EMT. Zhang MJ (2015) was able to demonstrate that silibinin suppressed cell proliferation and induced apoptosis by downregulating Fox M1 by suppressing this integrated signalling axis. As noted in the context of plumbagin (p. 93) suppression of the transcription factor Fox M1 inhibits cell proliferation. EMT can be blocked by suppressing Fox M1 and the isoflavone genistein is able downregulate Fox M1 and inhibit cell proliferation, cell motility and promote apoptosis. In fact genistein, as stated earlier, can inhibit EMT activation and the generation of CSCs by suppressing PI3K/AKT/mTOR, WNT and Hedgehog signalling.

ER-Mediated Effects of Silymarin

Silymarin possesses oestrogenic properties and has been described as an effective inhibitor of osteoporosis. Deficiency of oestrogen leads to osteoporosis. It has been postulated that the protective effect against osteoporosis afforded by silymarin derives from its ability to modulate ERα-mediated signalling, possibly by recourse to the non-canonical route. Oestrogens may function independently of ER and in non-canonical fashion to suppress the production of osteoclastogenic cytokines. In contrast, silymarin seems to inhibit tumour cell proliferation by the canonical genomic route by upregulating the expression of the proliferation inhibitory ERβ. Silymarin inhibited the growth of MCF7 breast cancer cells also by upregulating ERβ,. The inhibition of cell proliferation and induction of caspase-mediated apoptosis were abrogated by silencing ERβ (Zheng N et al., 2016). In testosterone-induced experimental benign prostatic hyperplasia, the expression of ERβ is suppressed and ERα is upregulated and these alterations in expression are negated by silymarin (Atawia et al., 2013). Silymarin suppresses the proliferation of ER− cell lines also, but here the effect is through the suppression of NF-κB survival signalling (Yousefi et al., 2014).

Principi et al. (2013) examined the effects of combined dietary administration on the expression of ERs in colonic mucosa from patients who had previously undergone endoscopic excision of polyps. The change in individual levels of ERβ expression was not impressive, but there was a marked increase in the ERβ/ERα ratio, in comparison with the ratios in control mucosal samples, which showed only a minor increase. The increase of ERβ was paralleled by enhanced apoptosis and reduced cell proliferation. This may suggest that both are altered by the enteric administration of the phyto-oestrogens. Whether this increase in ERβ might benefit patients in terms of reduced recurrence of polyps is something to be ascertained. Of some interest would be to explore further this susceptibility of patients who had a history of polyposis to display enhanced expression of ERβ in response to the phyto-oestrogens. The colonic mucosa can possibly respond differentially, if there were a history of APC (adenomatous polyposis coli) gene mutations. It is well known that APC is involved with cell adhesion via β-catenin/Wnt signalling.

Perspective of Clinical Potential of Silymarin and Derivatives

To use a cliché, last but not least is the attribution to silymarin and related compounds the ability to overcome drug resistance, a feature that would greatly enhance the potential value of these polyphenols in the clinical context. There has been little clinical interest despite their efficacy in suppressing tumour cell proliferation, induction of apoptosis and the inhibition of EMT and, the yet not too well established, generation of CSC. There could be uncertainty with regard to the safety profile and the bioavailability upon administration. There might be some uncertainty also concerning the tissue distribution of the drug. Some in vitro studies have shown that silymarin can exert marked inhibitory effects at very low concentrations when combined with conventional therapeutic agents. The pursuit of such investigations might help to build crucially important safety profile.

DO CAROTENOIDS HAVE A PREVENTIVE OR CURATIVE ROLE IN CANCER?

Many carotenoids of plant and microbial origin have been often attributed with anti-oxidant, anti-cancer and anti-inflammatory properties. Here in the context of the potential ascriptions of phytochemicals in combating human disease, it might be appropriate to briefly refer to some carotenoids, which have been the subject of preliminary studies. As a point of departure, one should emphasise the features relevant in cancer incidence, growth and progression. The carotenoids are anti-inflammatory. They possess the ability to protect cells from oxidative damage. The anti-oxidant faculty has inevitable immunological implications. Furthermore, given that genetic instability is the driving force of cancer progression, it is interesting to note that circulating lycopene levels may correlate inversely with genetic instability. In high-grade prostate cancer, higher levels of lycopene have correlated with lower genomic changes (Nordstrom et al., 2016). Also valuable are the suggestions that carotenoids might be able to overcome drug resistance by selectively targeting P-glycoprotein, the MDR1 gene product, which is an ATP-binding cassette transporter involved in the regulation of the uptake and extrusion of drugs (Teng YN et al., 2016). It is needless to stress that these attributions would require further evaluation.

It has been claimed rather prematurely that some carotenoids have a preventive action against cancer. For, the opposite view has also been expressed that there is no association between carotenoids and tumour incidence or mortality. Nonetheless, a large case controlled study has concluded that dietary supplementation of carotenoids offers tangible risk reduction in head and neck cancer. Intake of β-carotene, lycopene, and lutein with zeaxanthin has been cited as conferring protection against these tumours (Leoncini et al., 2016). Bakker et al. (2016) have stated that high plasma levels of β-carotene and α-carotene were associated with reduced risk of ER− breast cancers. There was no obvious link noticeable in ER+ tumours. But an inverse relationship between plasma α-carotene and ER+ but not ER− breast cancer was observed by Wang Y et al. (2015). However, one could state without equivocation that these findings have to be viewed in the perspective of an important caveat that one has to differentiate between ERα and ERβ, since ERα promotes cell proliferation but ERβ inhibits it. Possibly, an inverse relationship to risk might subsist for α- and β-carotenes, lycopene and lutein/zeaxanthin irrespective of ER/PR status (Yan B et al., 2016). However, there are no correlative studies of circulating carotenoid levels with disease progression whether as an association with tumour grade or clinical stage or even in pre-clinical animal tumour models to sustain any firm conclusions. To be conclusive, the studies ought to follow the due process of subtyping the ER receptors together with PR expression status. PR expression is an important prognostic marker. Caronongan III et al. (2016) have emphasised the discernible distinction between PR and ER, with PR displaying greater correlation than ER with disease progression and prognosis.

Some carotenoids have been reported to suppress cell proliferation. This applies to plant products as well as bacterial carotenoids. Astaxanthin, the aquatic carotenoid from marine food, has been reported to suppress cell cycle progression with concomitant reduction of ERK expression and upregulation of the CDK inhibitor $p27^{kip1}$ (Kim JH et al., 2016). Fucoxanthin, another aquatic carotenoid, has been found to inhibit the cell cycle traverse and induce apoptosis (Rengarajan et al., 2013). Microbial carotenoids are also known to inhibit cell proliferation (Abbes et al., 2013; Shindo and Misawa, 2014). An interesting development is the employment of microbial hosts to produce or engineered to produce biologically active carotenoids. The PPARγ (peroxisome proliferator-activated receptor-γ nuclear receptor) signalling has been implicated in the generation of anti-inflammatory and allied responses by lycopene and lutein (Zhao WE et al., 2016). These carotenoids are said to suppress pro-inflammatory cytokines by the induction of PPARγ. Aside from this, one should note that PPAR/RXR (retinoid X receptors) heterodimers may suppress NF-κB. PPARs can interact with and inhibit NF-κB. This can happen possibly also by the agency of the suppressor ARF (alternative reading frame) transcription factor. This could be significant given the important role played by NF-κB signalling in cancer development and progression as discussed at various locations. ARF ($p14^{ARF}$) and p16

($p16^{INK4A}$) encoded by CDKN2A/INK4A locus are tumour suppressors. There is some divergence of view concerning genetic and epigenetic changes in the genes and their correlation with tumour growth and metastasis. Many of these data concerning the carotenoids are preliminary investigations and need further scrutiny. So, do carotenoids have a preventive or curative role in cancer? The answer presently is a tentative negative.

CHAPTER 18

Selenoproteins in Cancer Control

Selenium is an important element that participates in thyroid hormone synthesis, metabolism and function. It provides protection from oxidative stress resulting from reactive oxygen species and reactive nitrogen species and genetic damage. Selenium also regulates the immune system influencing both innate and adaptive responses. A large part of tissue selenium is found in metabolically active selenoproteins. Many selenoproteins have been identified and characterised, albeit not functionally. Selenocysteine P is rich in selenocysteine, with one selenocysteine residue at the N-terminus and nine at the C-terminus, which probably includes the active site, and a similar number of cysteine residues. Selenocysteine K, W and N have one selenocysteine residue at the active site. Functionally, the glutathione peroxidase enzymes GPx1, GPx2, GPx3 and GPx4 are regarded as important selenoproteins. The three selenocysteine-containing iodothyronine deiodinases form a family of three selenoproteins involved in thyroid hormone synthesis, metabolism and function. Deficiency of selenium and genetic changes in selenoprotein coding genes are known to lead to many forms of human disease, including cancer.

There is much documentation of the effects of selenium administration on the development of cancer. The potential routes of selenium signalling have been investigated (Fig. 18.1). Sometime ago, Shah et al. (2005) reported that methylseleninic acid (MSA) inhibited ERα proliferative signalling in ER+ breast cancer cell lines. Selenium is said to exert anti-proliferative effects via the canonical apoptosis signalling pathways. Selenocysteine, which resembles cysteine in structure but with selenium replacing the sulphur atom, is incorporated into many selenoproteins. Selenocysteine induces apoptosis by caspase mediation or by TRAIL/death receptor pathway (Chen T and Wong, 2008). The suppression of PI3K/Akt signalling has also been adduced. Tarrado-Castellarnau et al. (2015) have further implicated the intervention of FOXO3 in this process. MSA induced nuclear translocation of FOXO3 concomitantly with the induction of apoptosis. The transcription factor FOXO3 is known to respond to oxidative stress by forming a complex with the

Molecular Approach to Cancer Management. DOI: http://dx.doi.org/10.1016/B978-0-12-812896-1.00018-0

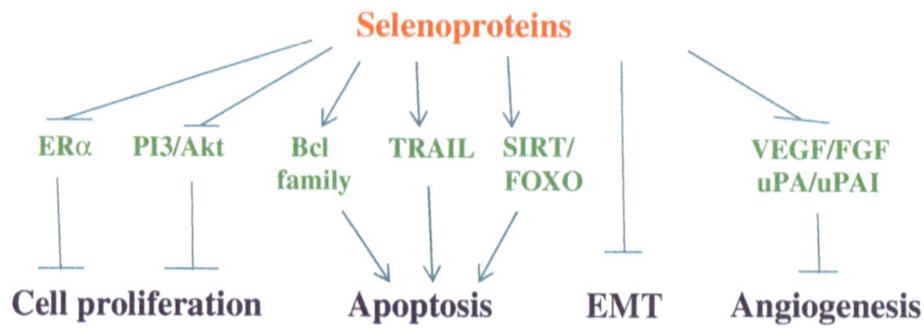

FIGURE 18.1

The signalling systems which might be activated in selenoprotein-mediated inhibition of cell proliferation and promotion of apoptosis and the postulated pathways leading to the inhibition of EMT activation and angiogenesis.

deacetylase SIRT1 of which FOXO3 is a direct target. Consistent with this, certain selenoprotein genes are upregulated in consort with genes signalling the induction of apoptosis (Zhao H et al., 2015). Unsurprisingly, the Nrf2/Keap1 pathway, which is known to regulate anti-oxidants preventing oxidative damage, has also been invoked.

Of interest in the physiology of selenium function besides selenomethionine and selenocysteine is the selenium-binding protein 1 (SBP1), which is regarded as a tumour suppressor since it is expressed at lower levels in neoplastic tissues as compared with corresponding normal tissues. Reduced SBP1 expression has been correlated with poor prognosis and there are also suggestions of correlations with angiogenic signalling. Of much significance is that SBP1 expression might be inversely related to the expression of the genes associated with EMT activation (Ying Q et al., 2015).

Yan L and DeMars (2012) reported that dietary supplementation with MSA led to reduced metastatic dissemination of experimental tumours. This occurred in parallel with decreases in uPA and uPAI (uPA inhibitor) levels as well as in VEGF, FGF and PDGF-B. This implicates the suppression of angiogenesis in the reduction in metastatic spread. Sadly, neither tumour size nor the microvascular density measurements were made in this study. One would have expected marked inhibition of tumour growth if MSA had suppressed angiogenesis.

One should recall here the selenoprotein thioredoxin reductase (TRXR), which catalyses the NADPH-dependent reduction of TRX. TRXR and TRX levels are elevated in sera of cancer patients (see p. 103). Ethaselen is a specific selenium-containing inhibitor of TRXR. It is believed to possibly inhibit lung cancer cell growth and induce apoptosis. Ethaselen exerted marked inhibitory effects on the growth of xenografted A549 cells (Tan Q et al.,

2010). It is being tested for the control of TRXR in advanced NSCLC and to check its effects on disease activity (NCT02166242).

There is little tangible activity at the clinical trials level with selenium compounds, although some trials aimed at investigating the effects on tumour growth after resection, tumour recurrence have been described. Also, some studies have taken place on selenium compounds as potential aids for cancer prevention. None have definitive and definable results. In historical perspective in the only definitive double-blind, randomized, placebo-controlled cancer prevention trial would one note reduced cancer mortality and incidence upon dietary supplementation with 200 μg of selenium per day (Clark et al., 1996). In prostate cancer where preventive effects of selenium have been mostly tested, its efficacy has been disputed (Algotar et al., 2013). Similarly, no benefits have accrued by patients with resected stage I NSCLC from selenium supplementation (Karp et al., 2013). Many studies not only have not endorsed selenium supplementation, but also have emphasised the potential risks that might be linked with it. Selenium at the levels administered in many of the clinical studies is regarded as safe. Nonetheless, it is important to keep in mind the potential of toxicity of the mineral at high doses, e.g., exceeding 500 μg per day.

CHAPTER 19

Control of Tumour Growth and Angiogenesis by Thalidomide and Its Analogues

Thalidomide was launched nearly five decades ago as a drug to deal with respiratory infections and administered to pregnant women for the relief of morning sickness. It was withdrawn from clinical use upon the discovery of its teratogenic effects. The teratogenic properties of thalidomide result from its binding to a protein called cereblon, which is found in embryonic as well as adult tissues. Cereblon is required for normal morphogenesis. Binding to thalidomide leads to a functional suppression of cereblon and this results in abnormal morphogenesis. Suppression of cereblon simulates the teratogenic effects exerted by thalidomide and a form of cereblon that does not bind thalidomide has shown reduced teratogenic effects (Ito et al., 2010).

THE THERAPEUTIC POTENTIAL OF THALIDOMIDES

Recent years have seen much focus on the immunomodulatory and anti-inflammatory properties of thalidomide. Together with the elucidation of its ability to suppress cell proliferation and angiogenesis, thalidomide has emerged as a drug with potential use in the treatment of many forms of cancer and autoimmune conditions. Furthermore, thalidomide analogues have been synthesised to combat toxicity and improve efficacy.

The thalidomides (thalidomide and its analogues lenalidomide and pomalidomide) are anti-inflammatory and immune modulatory drugs. They have been used in the treatment of multiple myeloma, pancreatic, prostate and lung cancers and also in autoimmune conditions such as graft-versus-host disease, Waldenstrom's macroglobulinaemia, and experimental autoimmune encephalomyelitis (EAE), an animal model of multiple sclerosis (MS). The growth inhibitory and immunomodulatory properties together with anti-angiogenesis potential have suggested their use in the treatment of MS (Sherbet, 2015a). The molecular mechanism by which these drugs generate the phenotypic effects and the signalling systems which they modify and

Molecular Approach to Cancer Management. DOI: http://dx.doi.org/10.1016/B978-0-12-812896-1.00019-2

moderate have been identified. Given the potential of the thalidomides in cancer treatment, the designing of adjuvant therapies to enhance their effectiveness has been advocated (Sherbet, 2015b).

THALIDOMIDES SUPPRESS ANGIOGENESIS

The rationale that suggests the potential of thalidomides in cancer treatment is that it can inhibit cell proliferation, promote apoptosis and hence could control tumour growth. By virtue of its ability to inhibit angiogenesis, it could function as an anti-metastasis agent (Table 19.1, Fig. 19.1). Many chemokines produced by tumours can promote tumour growth, induce angiogenesis and also assist with the evasion of immune surveillance. Therefore, it is of considerable interest that thalidomides suppress these chemokines and combat the immunological dysfunction associated with tumours. The ability to restore endogenous immune function has indeed been attributed to the thalidomides.

Some while ago, thalidomide was shown to inhibit VEGF- and bFGF-induced angiogenesis in corneal angiogenesis assays (D'Amato et al., 1994; Kenyon et al., 1997). Lu L et al. (2009) showed further that lenalidomide inhibited VEGF-induced P13K/Akt signalling and suppressed the pro-angiogenic HIF-1. In vitro, it inhibited tubule formation by endothelial cells. In vivo, there was much reduction in lung colonisation of B16-10 murine melanoma. Thalidomide and the analogues lenalidomide and pomalidomide inhibited the in vitro migratory behaviour of colorectal carcinoma cells. These drugs also suppressed the formation of metastatic nodules in vivo murine hosts (Liu WM et al., 2009).

Table 19.1 Salient Biological Features Influenced by Thalidomides

Biological Feature	Effector Targets
Angiogenesis ↓	VEGF, bFGF
Invasion and metastasis ↓	Cell adhesion signalling
Cell proliferation ↓	Cell cycle regulators
Apoptosis ↑	Bcl-2
Tumour growth ↓	
Immune resistance of tumours ↓	Immune checkpoint proteins
Immunomodulation	CD4+/CD8+ T cells
Immune suppression; evasion of immune surveillance ↓	Chemokines, ILs, TGF-β, VEGF

bFGF, basic fibroblast growth factor; IL, interleukin; TGF-β, transforming growth factor-β; VEGF, vascular endothelial growth factor.
From Sherbet (2015b) with permission from Anti-Cancer Research.

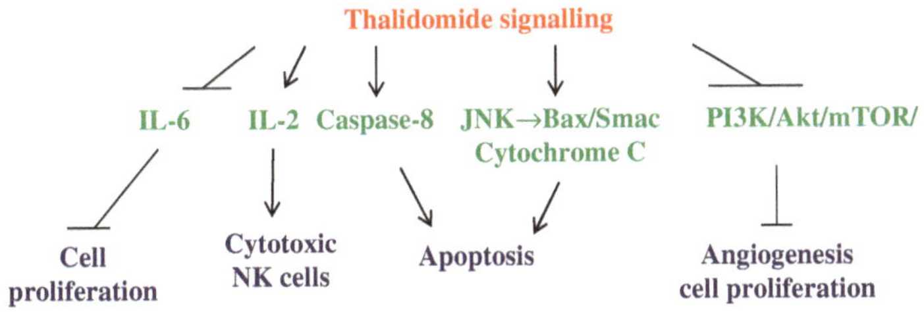

FIGURE 19.1

Pathways of thalidomide signalling to control cell proliferation and induce apoptosis and inhibition of angiogenesis in myelomas and other tumours types. Other cytokines suppressed by thalidomide and analogues include IL-8 and TNF-α. Some of the angiogenic pathways are integrated in their function by mTOR. Smac is a mitochondrial protein that promotes the release of cytochrome C leading to activation of caspase-mediated apoptosis. Regulation of Bax by JNK (Jun N-terminal kinase) is an essential element in this apoptotic signalling. This figure is based on Andersen (2005), Sherbet (2013, 2015b) and references discussed in the text.

Angiogenesis is an integral process in the pathogenesis and progression of inflammatory and autoimmune diseases. MS is a demyelinating disease of the central nervous system. Angiogenesis is a consistent feature of demyelinating plaques of MS. Many inducers of angiogenesis are expressed in these plaques and have been closely allied in MS as well as in the animal model of MS viz. EAE. This has led to the suggestion that inhibition of angiogenesis by suppressing these effectors or inhibiting the elements of angiogenic signalling pathways might provide a viable way to target therapy to manage MS (Sherbet, 2015a).

EFFECTS OF THALIDOMIDES ON CELL ADHESION-RELATED FEATURES AND INVASION

Bortezomib, a proteasome inhibitor, induces cell cycle arrest and apoptosis. It is used in the treatment of myeloma. Combination therapy of bortezomib with other therapeutic agents has produced valuable information in preclinical evaluations. Both angiogenesis inhibition and promotion of apoptosis are enhanced by combination of the thalidomides with bortezomib. Medinger et al. (2015) found that treatment of plasma cell myeloma patients with the thalidomides in combination with bortezomib enhanced clinical responses, which were consistent with suppression of angiogenesis as indicated by the levels of angiogenic markers. The responses are probably amplified by bortezomib, which promotes apoptosis by phosphorylating and cleaving Bcl-2 (Ling YG et al., 2002).

The potential of anti-metastatic effect is heightened by the inhibition of invasion. Both lenalidomide and pomalidomide have been reported to inhibit invasion in vitro by colorectal carcinoma cells and metastases in vivo (Liu WM, 2009). These effects seem to be mediated by alterations in cell adhesion signalling (Liu WM et al., 2010) as well as changes in immune responses. Liu WM et al. (2010) have implicated a mechanistic membrane-associated alteration, for they noted changes in Notch/Wnt signalling and the regulatory gene Kremen 2. The latter regulates Dkk2-mediated inhibition of Wnt signalling and DTX4 (Deltex 4, E3 ubiquitin ligase), which negatively regulates Notch. They seem to occur as a consequence of treatment in vitro with the thalidomides. The Wnt-Frizzled receptor complex can activate the canonical β-catenin pathway. Also Notch affects the function of cadherins and regulates intercellular adhesion. However, it should be noted here that Notch and Wnt proteins can exert opposing or co-operative effects in different systems. But overall, Notch would inevitably modulate cell motility or invasive behaviour, cell proliferation and apoptosis. Furthermore, one should recognise that these thalidomides alter VEGF expression and influence cell proliferation via Notch1/Delta4 or the PI3K/Akt pathways (Lu L et al., 2009; Sherbet, 2011a).

THALIDOMIDES INHIBIT CELL PROLIFERATION AND PROMOTE APOPTOSIS

The thalidomides suppress cell proliferation by interfering with cell cycle regulatory components. Fecteau et al. (2014) showed that lenalidomide supressed chronic lymphocytic leukaemia (CLL) cells in vitro by targeting cereblon. Lenalidomide-mediated inactivation of cereblon reduces the induction of p21. Cereblon is a component of the ubiquitin–E3 ligase Cul4–Rbx1–DDB1 complex and known to be directly targeted by thalidomides (Ito et al., 2010). This is said to lead to the recruitment of zinc finger transcription factors to the ubiquitin–E3 complex, their ubiquitination and degradation suppressing cell proliferation and cell viability.

NF-κB is another pathway implicated in thalidomide action. Keifer et al. (2001) demonstrated this over a decade ago. Thalidomide inhibited IKK and the NF-κB target genes IL-8, TRAF1 and c-IAP2 (see p.94). Indeed, both thalidomide and lenalidomide block NF-κB activation. Liu WM et al. (2004) noted the inhibition of NF-κB together with marked increase in Bax/Bcl-2 ratio and that the effects on the apoptosis family genes were more marked than NF-κB inhibition.

The mTOR signalling pathway is associated with several cellular processes such as cell proliferation, growth, apoptosis, angiogenesis, cell motility and invasion (see Figs 1.1 and 1.3). It could facilitate crosstalk between VEGF, PI3K/Akt and NF-κB in angiogenesis as alluded to earlier. The integration of these signalling systems by mTOR has led to the suggestion that mTOR inhibitors could be beneficially combined with the thalidomide. This has been vindicated by the synergy seen in the effects of everolimus and lenalidomide in a phase I clinical trial involving refractory multiple myeloma patients. The combined therapy correlated with the downregulation of mTOR signalling (Yee AJ et al., 2014). Temsirolimus has also been tested in combination with lenalidomide in another phase I trial in involving patients with advanced forms of cancer where some response was observed with many tumour types (Ganesan et al., 2013). However, the latter study involved only a small number of patients with each tumour type. Ganesan et al. (2013) presented the median overall survival and progression free survival (PFS) of all evaluable patients. They saw no response in HNSCC, NSCLC and endometrial carcinoma. This study is too preliminary in nature and there is a need to look at larger number of patients with specific tumour types where clinical response had been noted.

It would be worthy of note here that plumbagin, a quinoid extracted from the roots of the *Plumbago zeylanica*, has marked anti-tumour properties, which have been attributed to its ability to suppress the NF-κB/AKT/mTOR/STAT3 signalling axis (see pp. 94-95). Plumbagin reportedly accentuated the induction of apoptosis by thalidomide, apparently by STAT3 suppression and activation of the JNK apoptosis route (Sandur et al., 2010). So there is much justification for using STAT3 inhibitors to reduce the effective dosage of thalidomide administration. Adoption of a combination approach could further reduce the potential unsavoury side effects of thalidomide.

IMMUNOMODULATION BY THALIDOMIDES

Cancer development and progression occur as a consequence of the loss of surveillance attributable to a progressive suppression of the immune system. Tumours produce immune suppressants such as ILs, TGF-β and VEGF. Immune tolerance of tumours also results from the impairment of the differentiation and maturation of antigen-presenting dendritic cells and the consequent interference with the functional interaction with T- and B- lymphocytes and NK cells (Kim R, 2006; Yang L and Carbone, 2004).

Strategies designed to stimulate the immune system have been evolving over the past several years. The development and deployment of immune modulators aimed at immune checkpoints to re-activate endogenous immune responses have received much attention. Immune resistance by tumours seems to flow from tumours being able to adopt and disrupt the immune inhibitory checkpoint pathways, especially aimed against T cells that are specific for tumour antigens. Immune checkpoint proteins negatively or positively regulate T-cell response.

The interaction between the receptor and ligand leads to the inhibition of T-cell activation and cytokine production. Modulation of T-cell activation pathways has taken the form of using antibodies against T-cell receptors or ligands. CTLA4 (cytotoxic T-lymphocyte-associated antigen 4) is a checkpoint protein that suppresses immune response. PD1 (programmed cell death protein 1) and its ligands are essential for the evasion of immune surveillance. These checkpoint proteins downregulate T-cell immune responses. Hence, anti-CTLA4 and PD1 and its ligand PDL1 are being evaluated. Recently, Gorgun et al. (2015) have shown that lenalidomide accentuates the immune effects of PD1/PDL1 blockade in multiple myeloma. The heightened effects are mediated by cereblon, which is a component of one of the postulated signalling systems engaged by immune checkpoint inhibitors discussed in a later section (see Fig. 26.1).

The thalidomides can combat the immune resistance of cancers, both haematological malignancies and solid tumours. De Keersmaecker et al. (2014) examined the response of CD4+ and CD8+ cells from multiple myeloma patients to lenalidomide and pomalidomide. Both drugs increased proliferation of and cytokine production by CD4+ and CD8+ T cells, enhanced the lytic capacity of cytotoxic T lymphocytes and reduced the suppressive effects of Treg (CD4+ regulatory T cells) on CD8+ responses. Lenalidomide promoted the proliferation of CD8+ cells, but then it also enhanced a population of myeloid cells, which were CD1+/CD15+. These cells were capable of suppressing the proliferation of both CD8+ and CD4+. This had led to the postulate that lenalidomide might be promoting both activating and inhibitory components as a means of regulating the immune system (Busch et al., 2014). One should recall that target-specific CD8 cells can be generated to inhibit angiogenesis. DNA vaccines targeting VEGFR2 of the tumour vasculature have been shown to inhibit tumour angiogenesis and both new and established metastatic deposits (Xiang R et al., 2008). Jellbauer et al. (2012) could induce CD8+ cells by immunising animals with a recombinant Salmonella strain carrying a CD8 epitope from VEGFR2. In the B16-F10 melanoma tumour model, the immunised animals showed induction of VEGFR2-specific CD8+ population, which would have targeted the VEGFR2 expressing tumour vascular endothelium and reduced metastatic spread into the lungs and reduced tumour growth. One can cite many instances of specific expression of growth factors or their receptors in tumours, which can be targeted in this fashion (reviewed by Sherbet, 2015b).

CLINICAL EVALUATION OF THALIDOMIDE AND DERIVATIVES

The clinical outcome in a lenalidomide trial of metastatic renal cell carcinoma conducted in 2004 was not very encouraging, with complete response in 3%, partial response in 8% and stable disease in 21% of the patients recruited. Secondary endpoints of tumour progression, response duration and PFS were unremarkable (Amato et al., 2008). Comparable with this was stable disease response in 57% of patients obtained by Patel et al. (2008). Vestermark et al. (2008) looked at the response in melanoma patients with brain metastases. No response was noticed in brain metastases and 3 out of 35 patients showed partial response to extracraneal metastases.

Combination of thalidomide and derivative with standard chemotherapy might be warranted. The efficacy of thalidomides as single agents or in combination with other drugs has been appraised in different forms of cancer. In a phase I clinical trial, the effects of lenalidomide are being evaluated in patients with high-grade gliomas. Combination treatment of CLL with lenalidomide and dexamethasone is also being clinically evaluated; so is combination with temsirolimus in patients with Hodgkin's and non-Hodgkin's lymphoma. The thalidomides could be beneficial in multiple myeloma and other B-cell malignancies. However, the efficacy of treatment of solid tumours is uncertain. Response of some forms of tumour has been positive either with thalidomide as a single agent or in combination with conventional chemotherapy. Response can vary among tumour types with some not showing any response at all. Notwithstanding the perceived potential benefits, the side effects of therapy of thalidomide and derivatives need to be emphasised. They do exert teratogenic effects in animal models, but, being effective at lower doses, the analogues show comparatively manageable and reduced toxicity.

There is case to be made for designing new analogues of thalidomide bearing in mind certain important pharmacological aspects. Pharmacokinetics and toxicity vary in enantiomers of the so-called chiral drugs (Wienkers and Padbury, 2012). Thalidomide as a chiral drug and does display such differences with regard to its R and S enantiomers. The R isomer is not believed to be teratogenic but the S enantiomer is. This difference cannot be explored because the drug undergoes racemisation in vivo. The chirally stable thalidomide derivative alpha-fluorothalidomide was cytotoxic, but alpha-fluoro-4-aminothalidomide was not cytotoxic and was >800-fold more effective than thalidomide as an inhibitor of the pro-inflammatory cytokine TNF-α (Man et al., 2003; Lee et al., 2011). So, chiral stability and toxicity are both important considerations in the development of thalidomide analogues.

CHAPTER 20

Metformin and Its Anti-Tumour Attributes

Metformin, which is prescribed for the treatment of type 2 diabetes, has attracted much attention as a possible adjuvant aid together with conventional therapy for the treatment of several forms of cancer. In fact, patients with some forms of cancer and on metformin medication for type 2 diabetes have been found to have benefited in terms of improved prognosis. Chaiteerakij et al. (2016) have cautioned about possible bias creeping into the analyses of survival data. There are indications that metformin may reduce cancer incidence (Thakkar et al., 2013; Gandini et al., 2014; Wu L et al., 2015) but the degree of risk reduction is subject to debate.

Metformin possesses demonstrable anti-tumour properties, which seem to flow from its ability to modulate cell proliferation and cell survival signalling pathways. It can interact directly or indirectly with several signalling systems including p53, BRCA, Wnt/β-catenin, PI3K/Akt, MAPK/38-ERK, NF-κB and mTOR (Sherbet, 2013). Signal transductions by metformin along these routes create some major phenotypic effects, which would markedly impinge upon the processes of tumour progression.

POSTULATED INHIBITION OF CSCs BY METFORMIN

A salient feature of the operation of metformin is the concept that it can inhibit cancer stem cells (CSCs). Admittedly, this is not a new thought. So there is much enduring interest in assessing the outcome of administering metformin on cancer progression and of disease free survival. Metformin has been postulated to inhibit many modes of signalling leading to CSC generation and propagation. It has been shown to inhibit the COX-2/PGE2 (prostaglandin E2)/STAT3 route to signal the suppression of CSC in vitro and in vivo models of bladder cancer (Liu QL et al., 2016). In the MMTV-ErbB2 mammary tumour model, metformin downregulated HER2 and EGFR and also IGF-1R, Akt, mTOR, STAT3 and mTOR signalling (Zhu P et al., 2014). In MCF7 cells also metformin inhibits growth factor/HER2/Akt signalling

Molecular Approach to Cancer Management. DOI: http://dx.doi.org/10.1016/B978-0-12-812896-1.00020-9

(Kim J et al., 2016). The observation that induced expression of HER2 sensitises the cells to the action metformin (Zhu P et al., 2014) could be of particular interest in the context of triple negative breast cancers.

One ought to take account of the possibility that COX-2/PGE2/STAT3 signalling promotes tumour progression upon activation by toll-like receptor 4 (TLR4) (Lin A et al., 2015). Metformin is able to suppress TLR-mediated signalling (Soraya et al., 2012) and suppress COX-2 signalling in this indirect manner. Equally, therefore the suppression of CSCs could have occurred by the inhibition of the TLR/NF-κB/MAPK pathway (see pp. 233-235; Fig. 26.4). Metformin could inhibit cell proliferation and promote apoptosis, possibly by either the activation of the interferon regulatory factors route and/or in parallel by inducing pro-inflammatory cytokine production. Unsurprisingly, Zhang RR et al. (2015) have postulated that metformin suppressed the activation of epithelial mesenchymal transition (EMT) and in this way suppressed CSCs. But a useful nugget of information is that EMT suppression occurs at low concentrations of metformin.

At the present time, there is no consensus about the ability of metformin to target CSCs. This might arise from the criteria and markers used for identifying CSCs since the markers might vary according to tissue type.

METFORMIN MEDIATED ACTIVATION OF AMPK

AMP-activated protein kinase (AMPK) is a major target of activation by metformin and subserves signalling to important phenotypic effects (Table 20.1). Notable is the inhibition of EMT and the CSCs. This provides the rationale for the postulate that metformin might turn out to be a valuable therapeutic agent in its own right and additionally by activating another

Table 20.1 Phenotypic Outcome of the Activation of AMPK by Metformin

Molecular Target of Activated AMPK	Phenotypic Effect
Cyclins, cdks ↑	Cell cycle arrest
mTOR ↓	Apoptosis
[1]p53 ↑	Cell proliferation ↓
MAPK/p38/ERK ↓	Cell proliferation ↓
PTEN → PI3K/Akt ↓	Apoptosis
[2]mTOR ↓	CSCs ↓
NF-κB ↓	CSCs ↓

Based on [1]Cai XB et al. (2015); He GF et al. (2014); [2]Chen X et al. (2015); Sherbet (2013).

effector providing the same phenotypic outcome. The tumour suppressor potential of metformin may be largely attributable to its being able to target CSCs. An important mode seems to be the inhibition of the PI3K/Akt/mTOR pathway to lead to the induction of apoptosis as well as the suppression of CSCs. It is needless to add that NF-κB downregulation could be also a means by which metformin/AMPK suppresses CSCs. NF-κB is known to be associated with the propagation of CSCs and the downregulation of its transcription would be expected to suppress CSC expansion.

CLINICAL APPRAISAL OF METFORMIN

Numerous trials are underway assessing the safety and clinical benefits to patients with many different types of tumour. The results of most of the studies are awaited. The general trend has been to view the status of AMPKs as a secondary outcome to establish that metformin is working. As noted earlier, metformin/AMPK signalling leads to mTOR inhibition. The tumour suppressor LKB1 has been implicated in this flow of information downstream. LKB1, a serine/threonine kinase, directly targets AMPKs. It activates a majority of the identified AMPKs. LKB1 is associated with cell cycle regulation, microtubule dynamics, determination of cell polarity and differentiation. Homozygous deletions or loss of heterozygosity and epigenetic suppression of its expression have been encountered in many tumours. These events have been linked with tumour invasion and metastasis. With this background, it would be important to include LKB1 in the signal transduction along the metformin/AMPK/mTOR route.

It would be worthwhile emphasising here that more studies are needed to explore other agents equally capable of activating AMPK or its upstream functionary LKB1. AICAR (5-aminoimidazole-4-carboxamide 1-D-ribonucleoside), quercetin and resveratrol easily come to mind as potent activators of AMPK. Combination therapy with anti-angiogenic agents would need to be investigated. It is unclear at present if metformin affects angiogenesis but there is indirect and somewhat circumstantial evidence that it could. Metformin and resveratrol reduced HIF-1 expression upon oral administration to mice with experimentally induced hypoxia (Li XL et al., 2016). Besides this, resveratrol induces apoptosis and suppresses cell survival by modulating the p53/p21waf/Bax, PI3k/Akt and Notch signalling systems (Cecchinato et al., 2007). Quercetin also exerts its suppressive effect on cell migration via activation of AMPK and possibly by suppressing the mTOR system downstream. Luteolin and epigallocatechin gallate also activate AMPK.

These findings may lend weight to the argument that combinations of this kind could be beneficially tested in pre-clinical tumour models.

CHAPTER 21

Statins in Cancer Biology

The pharmacology of statins has been the subject of intense study on account of its use in the treatment of many pathological conditions. Statins were developed in the wake of the vast body of evidence linking blood cholesterol with atherosclerosis and coronary heart disease. The treatment of dyslipidaemia, a condition characterised by abnormal levels of lipids or lipoproteins in the blood, has mainly relied on statins. Other modes of treatment include bile-acid-binding resins such as cholestyramine and colestipol, nicotinic acids and fibric acid derivatives.

PHARMACOLOGICAL ACTION OF STATINS

Statins inhibit HMG-CoA reductase and inhibit cholesterol synthesis. This occurs within the mevalonate pathway as shown in Fig. 21.1. Bisphosphonates are also able to lower blood cholesterol levels. It has been appreciated that statins affect the biology of the cell in more ways than by interfering with the mevalonate pathway. Statins also activate the apoptotic signalling pathway and in this way seem able to regulate tumour growth. Changes in intercellular adhesion may be brought about by statins, which will impact cancer cell invasion and potentially also metastasis.

STATIN-INDUCED APOPTOSIS SIGNALLING

Statins and bisphosphonates are involved in Hippo signalling. Hence, the discussion here is centred round the role of statins in cancer management based on anti-proliferative and apoptosis promotion. Statins and bisphosphonates both lift the mevalonate-mediated inhibition of Lats, thus allowing it to phosphorylate and restrain the transcription activity of YAP/TAZ (see Fig. 7.2). This is consistent with the inhibition of cell proliferation and the induction of apoptosis by statins. Apoptosis signalling activated by simvastatin includes the conventional pathways of caspase mediation with

Molecular Approach to Cancer Management. DOI: http://dx.doi.org/10.1016/B978-0-12-812896-1.00021-0

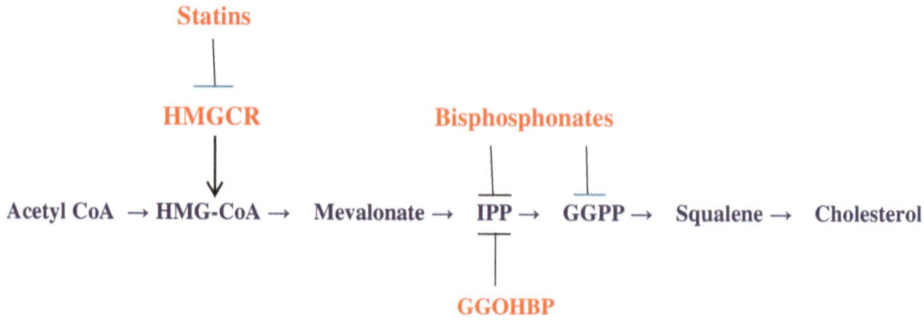

FIGURE 21.1

The points of action of statins and bisphosphonates in the mevalonate pathway. See also Fig. 7.3, which shows statins and bisphosphonate act within the mevalonate pathway and influence Hippo signalling. IPP, isopentenyl pyrophosphate; other abbreviation as in Fig. 7.3.

the downregulation of anti-apoptosis Bcl2 and upregulation of the pro-apoptosis Bax protein (Lee J et al., 2016).

Simvastatin markedly induces apoptosis and inhibits cell proliferation by inhibiting both PI3K/Akt/mTOR and MAPK/ERK (mitogen-activated protein kinase/extracellular signal-regulated kinase) pathways. The inhibition of PI3K/Akt signalling has been attributed to the upregulation of PTEN, the well-established regulator of this pathway. Indeed, some evidence has come forth that simvastatin activates PTEN, suppresses Akt phosphorylation and suppresses PI3K/Akt/mTOR. Simvastatin significantly inhibited MAPK/ERK pathway (Wang TT et al., 2016; Stine et al., 2016). Lee HY et al. (2016) noted that the downregulation of this pathway occurred in parallel with the upregulated expression of pro-apoptosis BIM (BCL2 like 11) protein of the Bcl2 family. In addition to the changes in the latter, a reduction in the expression of MMPs has been reported in statin treated MDA-MB-231 cells. This occurred together with the inhibition of NF-κB signalling (Shen YY et al., 2015). These events may be linked. For it is known that NF-κB is associated with the activation of epithelial mesenchymal transition (EMT) and with the upregulation of MMP expression. This perception of inactivation of EMT provides supplementary evidence for the total efficacy of statins in controlling tumorigenesis and tumour growth (also see another aspect discussed later).

The Ras/Raf/MAPK signalling pathway is activated by many external stimuli, such as growth factors, mitogens, inflammatory cytokines, apoptosis-inducing factors and others. External stimuli can differentially engage MAPK signalling. Growth factors/receptor tyrosine kinase (RTK) signalling activates Raf1 to engage the MAPK/ERK1/ERK2 route to lead to cell survival and proliferation. An alternative Raf1 route of signalling activates kinases such as

ASK1 (apoptosis signal regulating kinase 1) and MST2 (Ste20 family Ser/Thr kinase 3, STK3). This route of signalling seems to be adopted in the event of exposure to stress factors, inflammatory cytokines and the deprivation of growth factors. Activation of the ASK1 route to apoptosis occurs via p38/MAPK. Both these routes are involved in the induction of apoptosis by statins. Pitavastatin has been shown to enhance hydrogen peroxide-induced apoptosis of human vascular smooth muscle cells. The enhancement of apoptosis occurred as a consequence of activation of JNK and p38 MAPK but not ERK. Statin-induced apoptosis was blocked by mevalonate, farnesyl pyrophosphate or geranylgeranyl pyrophosphate (Tsujimoto et al., 2006; Wang TT et al., 2016).

The involvement of certain growth factor receptors has also reported in the induction of apoptosis by simvastatin. Lee J et al. (2016) have reported that the statin suppressed the activation of ERK/Akt by IGF-1 and its receptor IGFR. It may be recalled here that the mTOR signalling pathway is closely involved in growth factor receptor function. The PI3K/Akt activation leads to the phosphorylation of mTOR, which then phosphorylates the downstream targets p70S6K and 4EBP leading in turn to cell proliferation. Aberrant PI3K/Akt/mTOR signalling has featured prominently in a number of human tumours.

STATINS AFFECT CELL ADHESION AND MIGRATION

Some preliminary work has indicated that lovastatin inhibits cell adhesion and this effect was associated with reductions in the expression of adhesion-mediating protein such as integrins and of focal adhesion kinase (FAK). Lovastatin inhibits downstream signalling by the integrin $\alpha v\beta 3$ including FAK activation. Also affected by the treatment are β-catenin and vimentin. The downregulation of β-catenin and vimentin in synchrony may be suggestive of the suppression of Wnt signalling and indeed of EMT. The tight junction protein ZO-1 is downregulated (Yang SH et al., 2016). There is a further possibly link here with statin-mediation of the inhibition of NF-κB, cell adhesion and EMT activation. For FAK can activate NF-κB, which has been shown to suppress E-cadherin expression and to be associated with the activation of EMT (Chua HL et al., 2007).

Many of these features are reminiscent of EMT and so these alterations would have serious repercussion in terms of cell migration and metastasis. From a different angle the status of statin effects and EMT, one can obtain a novel view. Warita et al. (2014) have related the state of expression of cell surface E-cadherin to the sensitivity of cells to statin. The cells were sensitive to the action of statins in the absence of E-cadherin. When it was expressed, the cells were no longer sensitive. The suggestion here is that statins can target cells in which EMT is activated and regarded as the most likely candidate cells to form secondary tumours. However, the postulate that statins target cells that have undergone EMT activation has to be tested using more EMT markers such as N-cadherin and the transcription factors such as Snail1, Snail2 (Slug), Twist and the ZEBs and even markers for cancer stem cells (CSCs), because there is an intrinsic link between CSCs and EMT activation. Jiang P et al. (2014) found that pitavastatin and fluvastatin were highly effective in inducing apoptosis in glioblastoma cell lines, which were isolated for CSC features. An assumption is implicit in this work that the cells still retained CSC features. The susceptibility to statins reported here is on cells that had formed neurospheres, but no other CSC marker had been employed. Equating the cells able to form neurospheres with CSCs has little practical justification.

DO STATINS HAVE A PLACE IN CANCER TREATMENT?

An outcome of the study of the pharmacology and signalling systems activated by statin is the provisional or putative attribution to statins of the biological abilities of immune modulation and cancer prevention. In the clinical setting, there has been no discernible beneficial outcome from the use of statins. Many clinical studies have been reported or are being carried out. The outcome in terms of patient benefit is not overwhelmingly supportive of statins as a mode of treatment. The outcome of many clinical trials is awaited. Nevertheless, one has to look at those which do promise some hope.

Qiu ZH et al. (2016) found overexpression of HMG-CoA reductase (HMGCR) in glioblastoma samples. In vitro, enhanced HMGCR expression promoted the growth and migration of U251 and U373 cells and its suppression had the opposite effect. An aspect of statin function is their ability to target the cytoskeletal system. Simvastatin has been shown to destabilise and disrupt tubulin integrity. Simvastatin induces apoptosis of normal vascular smooth muscle cells together with contractile dysfunction by the mediation in the actin dynamics of RhoA/Rac-1 GTPases (Kang S et al., 2016). This dysfunction can and is known to inhibit cell motility with obvious consequence to metastatic outcome. So these glioblastomas could be amenable to statin treatment. Simvastatin inhibited the growth and induced apoptosis of ovarian cells (Stine et al., 2016). Compatibly, there was a reduction in the growth of tumour xenografts, but the claims of the anti-metastatic effect of the statin have not been tested at all.

A convincing and most persuasive demonstration of the effects of statins on metastatic spread has been provided by Wolfe et al. (2015). They showed that treatment of triple negative breast cancer (TNBC) cells with simvastatin caused cell cycle arrest, reduced the size of the S-phase fraction, inhibited cell proliferation and invasion in vitro. Upon introduction into host animals, the cells that had been pre-treated with simvastatin showed reduced metastatic spread. This occurred in animals after extirpation of the tumours and tested later for metastasis. Metastasis-free survival time was longer in the simvastain-treated group. Marked reduction in metastasis was also seen in animals, which had been injected via the tail vein. These authors link these effects as taking place via expression of FOXO3a, the apoptosis and PI3L/Akt-related transcription factor. They noted enhanced cell migration when FOXO3a was overexpressed. Simvastatin downregulated the expression of phosphorylated FOXO3a and Akt. Downregulation of its expression occurred in parallel with shorter metastasis-free survival of breast cancers, including TNBCs. From this, the authors suggest that FOXO3a by association may be predictive of metastatic dissemination. It would have been more helpful if the authors had checked the extirpated tumours, those where the tumour-bearing animals had shown metastasis and those which had not done so. This would have constituted more direct evidence. But this does not detract from the merit of their demonstration of the ability of simvastatin to suppress metastasis.

Viewing from a different angle, Jeon et al. (2015) had noticed clinical benefits of statin administration to patients with low grade I and II PDAC (pancreatic ductal adenocarcinoma). Statin treatment was associated with enhanced survival with a 21% reduced risk of death. The beneficial effects of simvastatin on overall survival of patients with PDAC have been confirmed by Kozak et al. (2016). A small but statistically significant improvement in progression free survival (PFS), but not overall survival, has been recorded in patients with advanced NSCLC (non-small cell lung cancer) carrying Ki-Ras mutations regarded as indicating resistance to RTK inhibitors, upon treatment with statin as compared with those treated with EGFR inhibitors (Fiala et al., 2015). Clinical findings relating to the combination of simvastatin with anti-metabolites, which inhibit DNA synthesis and repair, have been reported. Combination with the topoisomerase I inhibitor irinotecan or with the pro-drug capecitabine converted to 5-FU has indicated little effect on the PFS of patients treated for metastatic colorectal cancer (Lim SH et al., 2015). Combination of statins with taxols has been studied and much evidence has accumulated that indicates the suppression of cell proliferation and angiogenesis in experimental conditions. But very little useful information is available on the effects of combined use of statins with microtubule inhibitors even in pre-clinical studies.

Some studies have focused on cancer patients taking statins and have reported benefits in patients with many different forms of cancer. Often such studies are difficult to evaluate in terms of the efficacy of statins since one has to take into account the duration and doses of administration and the stage of disease, etc. Also relevant would be the statin being administered. Some statins are regarded as mild statins and certain other more intense. There might be concomitant or follow on pathological conditions. Also age, sex, etc., are important factors to be reckoned with. It is needless to say that some studies have found no differences between statin users and non-users in regard to disease outcome. Statins do exert marked biological effects of cancer cell migration and cell proliferation and on the apoptotic loss of cells. There are indications that statins might suppress EMT. However, more pre-clinical and clinical investigations may be essential before statins can be deemed and defined as anti-tumour and anti-metastasis agents.

CHAPTER 22

Are There Gains to be Made in Exploring Anthrax Lethal Toxin (LeTx) as a Tumour and an Angiogenesis Inhibitor?

The anthrax lethal toxin (LeTx) has been the object of much enquiry on account of its ability to influence the two fundamental processes inalienably linked with cancer progression. LeTx markedly inhibits tumour growth and invasion and angiogenesis. It is an inhibitor of mitogen-activated proteins kinase kinase (MKK) and targets many members of the MKK family of signal transducers, pre-eminently associated with the biology of tumours.

LeTx is encoded by a plasmid contained in the bacterium *Bacillus anthracis*. It is a complex of three proteins, namely the PA (protective antigen), the LF (lethal factor, an MMP) and the EF (oedema factor, an adenylate cyclase). Binding of the toxin to the cells and translocation into the cells is mediated by the PA. The PA binds to specific receptors CMG2 (capillary morphogenesis gene 2) and TEM8 (tumour endothelial marker 8) via the integrin-like extracellular domain of the receptors and the toxin is internalised. Upon binding to the receptor, PA is cleaved and activated by furin-like proteases leading the LF and EF into the cells. PA is also activated by other proteinases such as PACE4, MMPs and plasminogen activators. TEM8 expression has been correlated with tumour vasculature and might be associated also with tumour stage.

The invasion suppressing function of LeTx may be a consequence of its ability to alter cytoskeletal integrity, but the suppression of angiogenesis seems to flow from its ability to inhibit MKK signalling. Biological response modifiers differentially engage mitogen-activated protein kinase (MAPK) signal transduction. Growth factor/receptor tyrosine kinase (RTK) and hormonal and neurotransmitter/G-protein coupled receptor (GPCR) signals flow via the Raf1/MKK1 (MAP2K1/MEK1) → ERK1/ERK2 (MAPK3/MAPK1) pathway to cell survival and proliferation. But Raf1 can function by activating kinases such as ASK1 (MAP3K, apoptosis signal regulating kinase 1) and STK3 (the serine threonine kinase 3, MST2). The ASK1 route involves MKK4/7 (MAP2K4/MEK4; MAP2K7/MEK7) → JNK1-3 (stress activated protein kinases

Molecular Approach to Cancer Management. DOI: http://dx.doi.org/10.1016/B978-0-12-812896-1.00022-2

SAPK1/MAPK8-10) or the MKK3/6 (MAP2K3/MEK3; MAP2K6/MEK6)→ p38MAPK (MAPK14) and leads to inflammation and apoptotic outcome. In essence, signalling along these two routes can bring about totally opposing phenotypic outcomes. This is partly the explanation for the attribution by some of tumour and progression promoting properties to MAPK signalling while others reporting a marked tumour suppressor effect (see discussion in Sherbet, 2013).

There is considerable evidence that the LeTx-mediated suppression of tumour invasion and angiogenesis ought to be read in the background of the tumour-promoting aspects of MAPK signalling, which LeTx inhibits. Much evidence has come to light, which indicates that inhibition of MAPK signalling can control tumour growth and suppresses angiogenesis. Basically, the effects of LeTx of inactivating the MKK signalling system seem to be the reason for its anti-angiogenesis effects. Furthermore, it seems able to suppress vascular endothelial growth factor (VEGF) function and reduce tumour-associated microvasculature.

Peters et al. (2014) have reported that marked inhibition of the in vivo growth of B16 murine melanomas can be achieved using MMP-, uPA- and dual MMP/uPA-activated anthrax lethal toxins. Together with growth inhibition, they reported changes in the disease activity as indicated by blood count and enzyme parameters. These latter alterations are claimed to be indicative of inhibition of disease progression. It is not a convention to use the term progression in this sense, but in fact it is accurately used to describe the advance of the disease to a more aggressive stage in terms of invasion and formation of secondary tumours. Nonetheless, it is quite clear that tumour growth can be inhibited and advantage can be taken of the tumour extracellular matrix milieu to activate LeTx. It is needless to emphasise here the potential of LeTx in therapy. Anti-cancer drugs can be conjugated to LF and the conjugates bind to PA to deliver the drugs into the cytosol of cells. Sunitinib and sorafinib inhibit VEGF receptors and other RTKs and in this way inhibit angiogenesis. Given that LF can target the microvasculature, its combination with these inhibitors has been advocated (Wein et al., 2013). The PA can also be conjugated to growth factor ligands to target receptors such as EGFR and HER2 (Bachran and Leppla, 2016). These options have been explored in vitro and in pre-clinical tumour models. It would be useful to look at the prospect of targeting PA conjugates to HER2+ tumours (McCluskey et al. 2013) and hopefully also to HER2+ breast cancer metastatic to the brain. The conjugates might provide a potential double whammy against metastatic tumour, provided that such a conjugate can cross the blood–brain barrier (BBB). It would be worth considering since the integrity of the BBB is compromised in such situations. Besides, increasing permeability of BBB is a viable option (Patil and Sherbet, 2015).

Zhuo WL et al. (2013) found that LF might induce apoptosis by inhibiting MAPK/Akt signalling. This might turn out to be counterproductive in BBB-compromised situations. Akt signalling is said to constitutively active when the EGFR family receptors are overexpressed. Deregulation of Akt signalling is said to be associated with compromised BBB. Experimentally disrupting the integrity of the BBB has led to the activation of the Akt pathway (Jalali et al., 2010).

Although optimistically one can view LeTx as a novel option in cancer therapy, much work is needed to assess safety and tolerability of the toxin, the possibility of achieving targeted delivery of drugs and antibodies does justify the current meagre research efforts in the field.

CHAPTER 23

The HMG (High Mobility Group) Proteins in Cancer Progression

The HMG (high mobility group) proteins are non-histone chromosomal proteins grouped into three families HMGA, HMGB and HMGN. HMGA is made up of two subfamilies, HMGA1 and HMGA2. HMGA2 (HMG AT-Hook 2) proteins may act as transcriptional regulators by virtue of the presence of three copies of the DNA-binding functional motif called the AT-Hook. The AT-Hook binds to the minor groove of AT-rich promoter and enhancer DNA regulatory sequences. The HMGA2 proteins subserve many biological functions, e.g., in embryonic development, the regulation of genetic transcription and in DNA repair. But owing to the unique DNA-binding motifs, they may be involved in exclusive substrate binding, induce changes in the substrates and thus modulate the phenotypic outcome of biological processes (reviewed by Reeves, 2010). The HMGs display some differences in emphasis with regard to their function, despite the identity of their role in oncogenesis. The biological actions of HMG are regulated by post-translational modifications, which may affect or be reflected in their interaction with DNA and other transcription regulators thus emphasising some differences in the signalling systems activated by them generating the differences that are noted in the resultant phenotypic outcome (Figs 23.1 and 23.2).

HMGA2 SIGNALLING IN EMT ACTIVATION, INVASION AND METASTASIS

HMGA2 is overexpressed in some forms of cancer and has been associated with the regulation of the cell cycle traverse, activation of epithelial mesenchymal transition (EMT), and cancer invasion and metastasis. Its expression has correlated with clinical stage, lymph node involvement and prognosis. Berlingieri et al. (1995) showed that inhibition of HMGA2 in normal thyroid cells using anti-sense HMGA2 cDNA suppressed their transformation by Kirsten murine sarcoma virus, providing an unambiguous link of HMGA2 with the promotion of cell transformation. It might regulate cell proliferation

Molecular Approach to Cancer Management. DOI: http://dx.doi.org/10.1016/B978-0-12-812896-1.00023-4

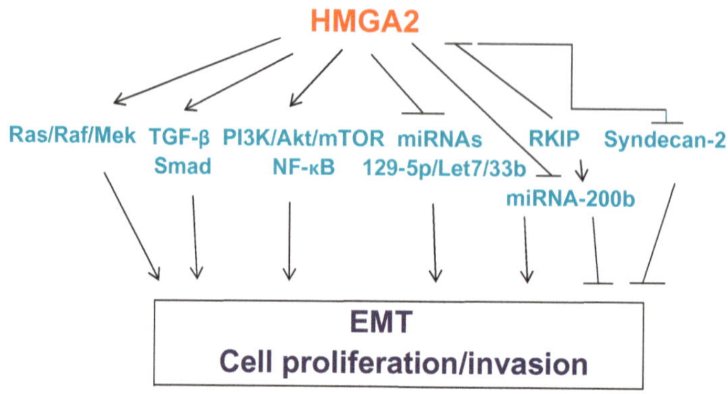

FIGURE 23.1

The putative pathways by which HMGA2 promotes EMT. HMGA2 is also involved in the promotion of angiogenesis. This is not shown here.

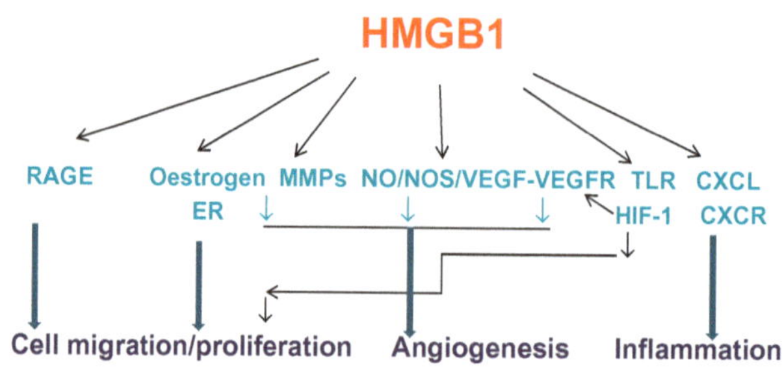

FIGURE 23.2

The pathways by which HMGB1 produces its phenotypic effects, which are suppressed by appropriate inhibitors.

by mediating the overexpression of cell cycle regulatory proteins. With cell proliferation and invasion being the phenotypic hallmarks of EMT, it is of much interest to note that downregulation of HMGA2 has resulted in the loss in vitro of cell motility and expression of EMT markers (Zhao XP et al., 2016). The signalling systems activated by HMGA2 to mediate EMT and the associated alterations in cell proliferation and invasion are presented in Fig. 23.1 and are discussed in detail later.

The EMT pathway initiated by HMGA2 is modulated by many miRNAs. In neuroendocrine tumours, miRNA-129-5p and let-7f/let-7 family members are downregulated. Transfection of miRNA-129-5p has led to the inhibition of cell proliferation. The overexpression of Let-7 miRNAs similarly suppresses cell proliferation. When Let-7 was inhibited the expression of HMGA2 increased together with other transcription factors (Dossing et al., 2015). The Lin-28b/Let-7 signalling pathway is involved in the regulation of HMGA2 expression. Lin-28B-mediated suppression of Let-7 expression and overexpression of HMGA2 protein frequently associated with tumour invasion and progression have been frequently encountered (Helland et al., 2011). This is compatible with the fact that HMGA2 activates the transcription factor Snail and to the activation of EMT.

The inhibition of HMGA2 by miRNA Let-7 was reported some while ago. In lung cancer cells, induced expression of Let-7 correlated with the downregulation of HMGA2 and reduction of cell proliferation. The effects depended upon the presence of Let-7 target sites in the 3′UTR of HMGA2 (Lee YS and Dutta, 2007). Although not reported in many tumours, the expression of the Let-7 miRNAs has indeed negatively correlated with high expression of HMGA2 in the paediatric atypical teratoid/rhabdoid tumours (Zhang KQ et al., 2014). The miRNA Let-7b seems able to suppress HMGA2. Di Fazio et al. (2012) showed that the HDAC inhibitor panobinostat upregulated Let-7b expression with parallel downregulation of HMGA2 in HepG2 cells. The downregulation of HMGA2 was replicated in Hep2 xenografts. Zhang P et al. (2015) showed that upregulation of miRNA-33b by the curcumin analogue, diphenyl difluoroketone (EF24), inhibited the initiation of EMT by HMGA2. Targeting of the miRNA generated mechanistic changes relating to cell migration, formation of stress fibres and focal adhesion assembly and the activation of Src and RhoA mediated by HMGA2. Actin polymerisation is a Src-dependent process and RhoA of the Rho family GTPases mediates stress fibre formation and actin polymerisation. Both Src tyrosine kinase and RhoA are important determinant of cell proliferation, adhesion and cell migration and are also well-established participant in cell migration.

Another mode of miRNA participation has brought the suppressor gene RKIP (Raf kinase inhibitor protein) into the picture. The miRNA-200b is induced by RKIP and it is inhibited by HMGA2. It is shown that miR-200b inhibits expression of lysyl oxidase and suppresses invasion. RKIP is also believed to function by inhibiting syndecan-2 by downregulating HMGA2, independently of miRNA involvement (Sun M et al., 2014). One has to state an important proviso in this context that Syndecan-1 and -2 both can exert contradictory effects, often dependent upon the tumour type and the localisation of the proteoglycan. The loss of their ectodomain or deletions in the cytoplasmic tail can generate different biological effects on adhesion and cell migration with consequence for cancer invasion and metastasis. Indeed, in the context of angiogenesis, one should recognise that syndecans have also been attributed with the ability to suppress endothelial cell migration and inhibit angiogenesis. Syndecan-2 shed from the cell surface by the excision of the extracellular domain inhibits angiogenesis (De Rossi et al., 2014).

Among the pathways activated by HMGA2 in the promotion of cell proliferation are the PI3K/Akt/mTOR pathway (Tan L et al., 2016). Earlier,

Yu KR et al. (2013) had shown that this was caused by the inhibition of the anti-proliferative $p16^{ink4}$ and the cell cycle regulator and tumour suppressor $p21^{waf1/cip1}$. The involvement of p53/p21 signalling might also explain why the downregulation of HMGA2 induces apoptosis. It is needless to reiterate here that the PI3K/Akt/mTOR and PI3K/Akt/NF-κB are prominent EMT signalling axes. The Ras/Raf/MEK/ERK can also lead to EMT and is probably involved in HMGA2-induced EMT activation, since downregulation of HMGA2 results in the reduction of Snail and enhanced expression of E-cadherin (Watanabe et al., 2009). Finally, transforming growth factor (TGF)-β is a well-known and powerful inducer of EMT and promoter of cell invasion. HMGA2 is involved in sustained activated EMT state maintenance by Ras/TGF-β signalling. Thuault et al. (2006) showed that HMGA2 mediated the induction of EMT by TGF-β via the canonical Smad pathway. The HMGA2 can also signal by the non-canonical PI3K/Akt/mTOR route, promote cell invasion and activate EMT.

INHIBITORS OF HMGA2 BINDING TO DNA

DNA-binding molecules non-covalently bind with DNA either by intercalation or by binding to the major or minor groove. The search for small molecules that recognise and bind to specified sequences of the minor groove of the DNA has led to the identification of some useful molecular species, which could influence genetic transcription by producing allosteric alterations in the DNA helix. These alterations could potentially disrupt the interaction of transcription factors with DNA (Chenoweth and Dervan, 2009).

HMGA proteins regulate gene expression by changing the DNA conformation by binding to AT-rich regions of the minor groove. They are described as architectural transcription factors. Besides binding to the DNA, they are able to bind to other transcription factors. Thus, although they do not possess intrinsic transcription capability, they can modulate the activity of other transcription factors by interacting with them (see Cleynen and Van de Ven, 2008). The HMG proteins can temporally regulate genetic transcription, a feature valuable in its participation in developmental processes and also in tumour progression. The latter involves and requires such temporal genetic regulation.

Given that HMGA2 targets the DNA minor groove, netropsin has been recognised as a possible candidate to prevent the generation of its phenotypic effects (Miao Y et al., 2008) by competing with HMGA2. Netropsin and the related compound distamycin bind to AT-rich sites of the minor groove of the DNA. Berenil also preferentially binds to AT-rich regions. These compounds are growth inhibitors and also exert anti-tumour effects. They exhibit differential binding affinities to DNA. Netropsin binds with maximum affinity (Wegner and Grummt, 1990). The binding is believed to induce conformational changes in the DNA and alter gene transcription patterns.

Alonso et al. (2015) have described some compounds that interfere with the interaction of HMGA2 with DNA. They confirm that notable are netropsin and the DNA intercalator and binder of the minor groove DAPI (4,6-diamidino-2-phenylindole dihydrochloride) and Hoechst 33258, which seem to be active at nanomole levels. Szerszenowicz and Drozdowska (2014) have synthesised analogues of netropsin and bis-netropsin, which inhibit in vitro cell proliferation. Alonso et al. (2015) have also found two bisintercalators (WP631 and WP762) that inhibit HMGA2.

Netropsin and distamycin as HMGA inhibitors are of some special interest. Inducible NOS2 is an active participant of angiogenesis. HMGA1 is able to bind an AT-rich tract in the NOS2 promoter and promote its expression. Netropsin suppresses NOS2 promoter activity, which requires the AT-rich HMGA1 DNA-binding site (Grant et al., 2009). One has to concede that the angiogenesis suppressor effect of netropsin has not been the subject of much investigation, but this study does underline its potential in the inhibition of angiogenesis by deactivating HMGA/NOS2 signalling. Distamycin derivatives are not only anti-angiogenic but are also markedly inhibitory of tumour growth and metastasis. These compounds do inhibit angiogenic growth factors but there is no evidence at present of the involvement of HMGA proteins in the anti-angiogenic effect or in the suppression of metastatic spread. Similarly, berenil/platinum complexes are markedly cytotoxic to and induce apoptosis of tumour cells, but it is not clear if HMGAs have role in this effect.

Currently, none of these compounds has made much headway barring isolated demonstrations of their anti-proliferative activity. An instance is the postulated involvement of cdc25 in HMGA action and its negation by netropsin. The cdks, which promote cell cycle progression, are activated by the cdc25 family phosphatases. HMGA1 is believed to target cdc25 to induce cell proliferation. Netropsin has been found to suppress cdc25 expression and inhibit in vitro invasion and growth of medulloblastoma cells (Lau KM et al., 2012). Another practical demonstration of the potential practical value of netrospin is that it competes with the Epstein–Barr virus nuclear antigen EBNA1 and leads to the loss of viral genome from Burkitt lymphoma cells. This effectively reduced the proliferation of the lymphoma cells (Chakravorty and Sugden, 2014). However, this has to be viewed in the background of the possible presence of HMGA in the system. HMGA1 was shown some while ago to be highly expressed in the lymphoid cell line CB33, and reducing its expression by transfecting anti-sense constructs into Burkitt lymphoma cells reduced transformation as indicated by the failure of these cells to form colonies even when maintained over a prolonged period and this was accompanied by reduced cell proliferation (Wood et al., 2000).

SHORT HAIRPIN RNA (SHRNA)-MEDIATED INHIBITION OF HMGA2

Other forms of suppressing HMGA2 have also been tried. Silencing of the expression HMGA2 by shRNA transfection was shown to suppress cell proliferation of and in vitro invasion by SW480 (Xu GM et al., 2012). Wei CH et al. (2013) transfected the gastric cancer cell line MKN-45 with HMGA2 shRNA. The transfectants showed enhanced apoptosis accompanied by reduced PI3K/Akt and Bcl2 signalling. The expression of HMGA2 is upregulated in AT/RT tumour tissue and could be suppressed by the use of HMGA2 shRNA. The AT/RT cell lines responded to the treatment with reduced cell proliferation attended by enhanced apoptosis. There was reduction in the growth of tumour xenografts of AT/RT tissue.

The tactical and strategic problems associated with the packaging and delivery of small RNAs such as shRNA and siRNA have been discussed in detail by Moore et al. (2010). Transfection and infection with vectors carrying the small RNA are the preferred routes. However, the practicality of stable integration and achieving specificity of delivery are unresolved at present. This applies equally to the deployment of miRNAs. The study of miRNAs has provided valuable information, probably more relevant in diagnostic and assessment of disease prognosis. Equally valuable it would be to look at their relevance to chemoresistance. But targeting miRNAs as a treatment modality seems too undefined and uncertain at the present time. Targeted delivery of small molecules is not impossible. The homing propensity of stem cells could be a valuable approach (see Patil and Sherbet, 2015). An added incentive to pursue this line of work is that HMGA protein expression correlates with stem cell features. HMGA1 expression is associated with the activation of EMT and by implication would be associated with the emergence of CSCs. However, conclusive evidence providing simultaneous or parallel expression of HMGA and of CSC markers is not available at present.

Nothing remarkable has emerged from the signalling spectrum activated by HMGA2, but there is much scope for deploying established inhibitors of the major signalling involved in conjunction with some HMGA2 inhibitors discussed here. Given the wide spectrum of cellular activities with which HMGA proteins are engaged, it is intriguing that netropsin and related natural and synthetic analogues have not found much favour with the research community.

There are plausible and logical grounds for concern. Distamycin A may be mutagenic and is said to enhance the mutagenic effects of ethidium bromine. CC-1065, also a minor groove binder, exhibits properties of an alkylating agent (Turner and Denny, 1996). There is no direct evidence that netropsin is mutagenic. The induction of frameshift mutations by netropsin was reported some time ago. It may be relevant to note that CC-1065 binds to the same site as netropsin. In fact, netropsin can displace CC-1065 bound to DNA (Chidester et al., 1981). Although there could be these obvious concerns, the use of netropsin and analogues conjugated with appropriate therapeutic agents is worth looking at in pre-clinical models. Some studies have shown that netropsin enhances the cytotoxic effects of camptothecin. As a conjugates, netropsin and analogues could be more effective in suppressing cell proliferation and tumour growth. Netropsin and distamycin A were successfully used as vectors for targeted delivery of alkylating agents (Bielawski and Bielawska, 2008). These authors demonstrated the effectiveness of such targeted alkylation in MCF7 and MDA-MB 231 breast cancer cells and how some alkylating agents affected the downstream signalling by growth factors. These are more than mere matters of scientific curiosity.

HMGB1 IN THE INDUCTION OF ANGIOGENESIS

HMGB1 in common with HMGA2 markedly influences tumour progression by promoting cell proliferation, cell migration and angiogenesis. Besides these attributes, it is involved in inflammation and a process that should not be divorced from tumorigenesis and tumour progression. Inflammatory cells play a critical role in tumorigenesis. The inflammatory microenvironment has been linked with EMT and the appearance of CSC (Fig. 23.2). Indeed, HMGA1 expression is associated with the activation of EMT and by implication would be associated with the emergence of CSCs.

Several molecular targets of HMGB1 have been identified. Prominently, some of them, e.g., NOS2 and VEGFs/VEGFRs are in the angiogenic signalling pathway. Also among the targets is oestrogen/ER which has links with cell proliferation and conceivably also with invasion. A majority of the studies of HMGB1 have confirmed its link with the induction of angiogenesis. The suppression of HMGB1 by antibodies reduced vascular density in chorio-allantoic membrane angiogenesis assays and this was accompanied by a downregulation of the growth factor signalling axis. Suppression of HMGB1 had only a minor effect on endothelial cell proliferation but it did reduce cell migration (van Beijnum et al., 2013). There is a hint here of differential functioning of HMGB1 in endothelial cell activities. Endothelial cell proliferation and migration go hand-in-hand. Many biological activities of endothelial cells are orchestrated by angiogenic agents. Cell migration and proliferation do engage different signalling pathways, but they could interact, crosstalk and mutually regulate one another. So it is difficult to visualise any uncoupling of cell proliferation and migration.

HMGB1 induces the expression of vascular endothelial growth factor (VEGF), platelet-derived growth factor (PDGF) and their receptors and matrix metalloproteinases (MMPs). The major signal transduction route seems to be receptor for advanced glycation end products (RAGE) and toll-like receptor (TLR)-4. The involvement of NF-κB is also an important consideration. Recently, RAGE- and TLR-mediated signalling has been found to differ in their phenotypical outcome. In corneal angiogenesis, Lin Q et al. (2011) were able to show the association of RAGE with TLR-4, but not with TLR-2. TLRs can generate different responses depending upon the adaptors that they engage. But TLR-4 and TLR-2 are not known to use different adaptor molecules. The situation is too complex to unravel since signalling pathways can be disengaged from one another even when the same adaptor is mediating the effects.

Anyhow, TLR-4 mediation seems to be an important requirement for HMGB1 to upregulate HIF-1 and induce angiogenesis (Park SY et al., 2015). HMGB1 has three redox-sensitive cysteines (C23, C45 and C106). Its function is dictated by the thiol/disulphide redox state of the cysteines, in cytokine-stimulating or chemotactic activity (Yang H et al., 2013). Zhu LY et al. (2015) were able to distinguish the functional forms that induce VEGF-A secretion and cell migration. They associate the disulphide form with the secretion of the angiogenic factor via TLR-4 and the all-thiol form with RAGE-mediated migration of endothelial cells. The binding of HMGB1 to the RAGE receptor activates the MAPK/ERK1/ERK2 cascade to promote both invasion and cell proliferation. So, as discussed in the context of S100A4 which is also a RAGE ligand, it would be practicable to inhibit the RAGE signalling system to thwart HMGB1-induced tumour progression.

The induction of arthritis in animal models has shown overexpression of HMGB1 together with upregulation of VEGF in areas of the synovium with inflammation and angiogenesis. Blocking these effectors reduced the severity of arthritis accompanied by the downregulation of the mediators of inflammation and angiogenesis IL-1 and IL-6 and TNF (Biscetti et al., 2016). Shakir et al. (2015) have pointed out that HMGB1 could be acting via the HIF-1α/CXC ligands/CXCR4 and CXCL12 to induce angiogenesis and lymphangiogenesis and possibly aid the aggressive behaviour of pancreatic cancer. HIF-1α is a target of HMGB1, which it activates to induce angiogenesis in rheumatoid arthritis (Park SY et al., 2015). In diabetic retina exposed to HMGB1, VEGF/VEGFR2 signalling is activated. Although CXCL12 and CXCR4 interaction is also accentuated, the interaction of HMGB1 occurs with RAGE rather than with CXCL12/CXCR4 (Abu El-Asrar et al., 2015), raising the possibility of the operation of two distinct signalling pathways in the induction of inflammation and angiogenesis. Inflammation and angiogenesis have been closely associated in many pathological conditions but the distinct modes of signalling may enable devising synergistic inhibition of both pathways.

The induction of MMPs is one of the manifestations of the initiation of angiogenesis. The upregulation of MMP-9 and the downregulation of tissue inhibitor of metalloproteinase (TIMP) by HMGB1 support the involvement of MMPs in the process. When HMGB1 is inhibited, MMP expression is reduced indicting a direct link between their expression (van Beijnum et al., 2013; Mohammad et al., 2016).

The association of HMGB1 with angiogenesis/lymphangiogenesis would be inevitably reflected in tumour dissemination. Although much emphasis is placed on haematogenous dissemination of cancer, the signalling by VEGF-A, VEGF-C and VEGF-D via VEGFRs has correlated with tumour spread by the lymphatic route. But angiogenesis and lymphangiogenesis are not greatly dissimilar. Both blood and lymphatic vessels would be practical routes to tumour extension due to the many anastomoses between them. In colon carcinoma specimens, HMGB1 levels have correlated with lymphatic microvessel density and extension of the primary lesions to the lymph nodes. The tumour tissues have also revealed the presence of VEGF-C (Li Y et al., 2015).

VIABLE APPROACHES TO HMGB1 INHIBITION

MMPs are active participants of the angiogenic process. Consistent with the induction of angiogenesis by HMGB1 is the postulate that MMPs are a downstream target of HMGB1. A sizeable body of credible evidence has been presented in support of this. Glycyrrhizin, which is extracted from the roots of the plant *Glycyrrhiza glabra* (licorice), was shown some time ago to bind to and inhibit the chemoattract and mitogenic activity HMGB1 (Mollica et al., 2007). It also reduced the migration inducing ability of HMGB1 in 3T3 fibroblast cells but it is not clear if the migration response of endothelial cell was also inhibited. Glycyrrhizin inhibits the induction of angiogenesis. In vivo, it is able to suppress tumour recurrence (Smolarczyk et al., 2012). Suppression of MMPs could be a reason for this. In cases of proliferative diabetic retinopathy, glycyrrhizin reduces the levels of MMP-9 in the vitreous fluid. Upon injection into vitreous chamber HMGB1 upregulates MMP-9 and inhibits TIMP. Also targeted inhibition of MMP-9 negated the MMP upregulating effect of HMGB1 (Mohammad et al., 2016).

An interesting snippet of information concerns the perceived anti-proliferative and potentially angiogenesis suppressing effects of riboflavin. The products of irradiation of riboflavin were shown to inhibit cell proliferation, and cytotoxic through Fas/FasL signalling. The photoproducts also downregulated VEGF and MMP together with the upregulation of TIMP (De Souza Queiroz et al., 2007). It is of much significance in the context of the present discussions to note that riboflavin reduced the expression and extracellular release of HMGB1 in an experimental model of inflammation induced by zymosan. Riboflavin seemed also able to inhibit the angiogenic iNOS and NO (Mazur-Bialy and Pochec, 2016; Mazur-Bialy et al., 2015).

Cilostazol (6-[4-(1-cyclohexyl-1*H*-tetrazol-5-yl)butoxyl]-3,4-dihydro-2-(1*H*)-quinolinone) is a quinolone derivative, which may mentioned here for its potential bearing on the function of HMGB1. Human microvascular endothelial cells displayed increased tubule formation in vitro upon exposure to HMGB1 or to medium conditioned by HMGB1-stimulated rheumatoid arthritis fibroblasts. This angiogenesis-like effect was inhibited by Cilostazol. The pro-angiogenic effect of HMGB1 seemed to result from increased expression of HIF-1α and VEGF. Also enhanced expression of NF-κB was seen. These increases were counteracted by Cilostazol. It is postulated that Cilostazol inhibited NF-κB-mediated transcription by activating the deacetylase SIRT1, leading to the suppression of HIF-1α and VEGF (Kim HY et al., 2014). This mode of inhibition of HMGB1-induced angiogenesis has been confirmed using the anti-angiogenic Emodin (6-methyl-1,3,8-trihydroxyanthraquinone derived from *Rheum emodi* the Himalayan rhubarb) (Qu et al., 2015), However, no further facts have emerged concerning either of these inhibitors. In the light of the numerous reports that Cilostazol promotes angiogenesis by upregulating many angiogenic agents, any discussion concerning this has to be held in abeyance at present. However, a further valid comment is that microvascular endothelial cells are known to differ from macrovascular endothelial cells, e.g., in the expression status of MMPs/TIMPs. This basic difference could be reflected in these studies rather than being a response to HMGB exposure.

Of the two HMG proteins discussed here, one can see the preponderance of angiogenic signalling in the operation of HMGB, whilst in comparison, EMT signalling is a prominent mode of action of HMGA2. This is quite legitimately emphasised in Figs 23.1 and 23.2. Despite these differences in emphasis perceived in their function, both seem to be ideal targets for manipulation of tumour progression.

ARE ID PROTEINS RELEVANT IN HMG PROTEIN FUNCTION?

It is interesting to explore if a link exists between HMG and ID proteins, especially since HMG-box domains occur in transcription factors, such as the

Sox family members, which are powerful inducers of pluripotent stem cells. Transfection of ID1 and ID2 into Sertoli cells increased the expression of HMGB-11 (Sox11) protein. The transfected cells showed enhanced proliferative ability (Chaudhary et al., 2005), but there is no suggestion here that this had occurred as a consequence of enhanced expression of HMGB-11. A similar link occurs in the induction of proliferation of CSC by TGF-β, where parallel changes take place in the expression of ID1 and ID3 and Sox2 and Sox4 (Anido et al., 2010). Some ID proteins and HMGB1 may be downregulated in tandem upon the activation of nuclear receptors such as ER. It is possible that their pathways of signalling might interact. Also one has to know whether ERα or ERβ is involved since they have diametrically opposite effects of cell proliferation. The IDs 1–3 themselves are active promoters of cell proliferation, angiogenesis and support CSC maintenance (see Table 14.1). Protein–protein interactions may be involved, but there is no direct evidence can be adduced for this. The specifics of the interaction of their pathways are unclear at present. However, there are some common grounds to suggest that colluding or mutually suppressing outcome from interactive signalling. The ID4 is a suppressor protein and may interact with and negate the tumour promoting property of HMGB1. The ID proteins can heterodimerise with specific bHLH proteins and prevent them from binding to E-box sequences of target genes. Most HLH proteins possess a domain with basic residues, which participates their binding to E-box sequences. Some bHLH proteins, e.g., E12/E47 and Twist, and HMG proteins such as LEF1 can recognise E-box sequences in the transcription initiation sites of target genes and regulate their transcription.

CHAPTER 24

MTAs in EMT Activation and Tumour and Metastasis Promotion

The MTA (metastasis associated) family of tumour and metastasis promoter genes identified and cloned some years ago as important activators of epithelial mesenchymal transition (EMT) and promoters of invasion and metastasis are now well established in that role (see Toh and Nicolson, 2014 for a recent review). So it is a matter of much surprise that very little, if any, note has been taken of this gene family as possibly providing viable options in clinical approaches to cancer management. Much pre-clinical work has underscored their latent value but this has not led to natural progression of effort.

THE SIGNALLING BY MTAs IN AGGRESSIVE NEOPLASTIC STATE

The MTAs exert a wide range of biological effects, which are brought by their function as transcriptional co-regulators in histone deacetylation and nucleosome remodelling. Chromatin remodelling is an essential requirement that allows transcription factors to access the DNA and regulate genetic expression. MTA1 is a component of the NuRD (nucleosome remodelling and histone deacetylase) co-repressor complex. The NURD is recruited to gene loci related to many biological events of genetic transcription-related cell proliferation, normal and abnormal development and differentiation and in oncogenic processes. So MTAs are involved in NuRD-mediated genetic expression by regulating the access of transcription factors to the genes. The most important functional domain of MTA1 is the ELM2-SANT domain, which recruits HDAC1. The ELM2 (Egl-27 and MTA1 homology 2) domain occurs N-terminal to the DNA-binding domain SANT (SM00717) and so the ELM2-SANT domain might mediate DNA binding. This domain is believed to target the MTA1–NuRD complex to genomic DNA. The MTA1–NuRD regulates many genes and their downstream signalling. Several signalling pathways are activated by MTA1 and these are shown in Fig. 24.1.

Molecular Approach to Cancer Management. DOI: http://dx.doi.org/10.1016/B978-0-12-812896-1.00024-6

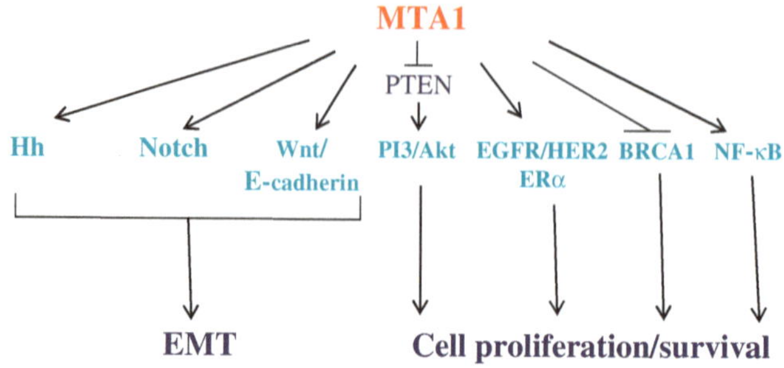

FIGURE 24.1

MTA signalling pathways leading to the activation of EMT, induction of cell proliferation and promotion of cell survival. Although shown herein as separate physiological entities, cell proliferation and survival are in fact a manifestation of EMT. Many of the cell proliferation pathways are engaged following EMT activation. Growth factors such as EGF are established activators of EMT.

The MTA family has six members and splice isoforms of which MTA1, 2 and 3 seem to be the well-studied ones. The MTA1 gene occurs as alternative splice isoforms. The MTAs are expressed in many forms of cancer. The expression of MTA1 has been associated with EMT activation, tumour cell proliferation and survival, invasion and aggressive disease. In contrast, MTA3 inhibits the transcription factor Snail and leads to an upregulated expression of E-cadherin and inhibition of EMT. MTA1 induces cancer cell invasion by regulating the expression of cell adhesion-related proteins and by influencing cytoskeletal dynamics. The signalling pathway activated by MTA1 interacts and engages in crosstalk with many signalling systems such as Wnt/E-cadherin/β-catenin, Hh, notch, cell cycle regulatory and cell proliferation pathways. It inhibits the function of some tumour suppressors. MTA1 is also involved with cell proliferation and survival signalling. The metastasis promoting ability has been attributed to the induction of the expression of angiogenic effectors.

Among major activators of pathways leading to the activation of EMT, cell proliferation and survival are the growth factors and their receptors. They are established activators of PI3K/Akt and ERK/MAPK signalling. HER2-induced cell proliferation takes the Akt/MAPK/ERK signalling route. Induction of cell proliferation is an aspect of EMT activation, and growth factor-induced EMT involves STAT3 functioning via Snail and twist mediation. E-cadherin suppresses invasion and its loss leads to the acquisition of cell motility. The transcription factors Snail, ZEB1 and ZEB2 repress its transcription and in this way induce EMT. To complete the composite structure of EMT activation, it should be recognised that NF-κB binds to the Snail promoter and induces Snail expression. Non-EGF family growth factors such as TNF-α induce EMT in a Snail or ZEB1/ZEB2-dependent fashion (see p. 4). These signalling systems have been shown to operate in the MTAs scenario. Furthermore, MTAs affect the normal functions of suppressor genes such as BRCA and p53. The promotion of proliferation by MTA1 is strengthened further by this. The downregulation of BRCA may promote cell proliferation by upregulating or downregulating the expression of transcription factors such as p53 and c-myc.

MTAs IN EGFR FAMILY SIGNALLING

The EGFR family receptors, EFGR and HER2, come under the remit of responses to MTA1 action. The receptor HER2 is overexpressed in neuroendocrine tumours of the ileum. Along with HER2, the HGF receptor c-met and MTA1 are also overexpressed, but vascular endothelial growth factor (VEGF) is not (Azzoni et al., 2011). It is not beyond the realm of possibility that HER2 might activate MTA1. The promotion of tumour progression by HER2 can involve MTA1. It was demonstrated some time ago that HER2 induces MTA1 expression, which suppresses ER/ERE (oestrogen receptor/oestrogen response element)-mediated transcription of target genes and this is reversed by the histone deacetylase (HDAC) inhibitor trichostatin A (Mazumdar et al., 2001; Ciocca et al., 2006). Oestrogen-mediated effects along this signalling axis are said to be co-regulated by MTA1 with other co-repressors, among them is an oestrogen inducible protein NRIF3. The NRIF3 has an ERE in its promoter (Mishra et al., 2003; Talukder et al., 2004). This has been proposed as being able to regulate the effects of oestrogen on tumour cells. These observations seemingly provide a firm footing for the operation of the MTA in the oestrogen/ER axis. However, as yet there is little authentication that phenotypically the events causally connect MTA1 to the function of HER2 or other EGFR family members, but that possibility cannot be excluded. In fact, confirmation of such an association, whatever might be the underlying reasons for it, is bound to be of help in the management of tumours such as breast cancer. Not only do many breast cancers express HER2 but HER2+ breast cancers have a propensity to metastasise to the brain (Patil and Sherbet, 2014). So MTA1 could provide additional means of combating the primary breast tumour and potentially also metastatic cancer in an additive or synergistic mode with humanised antibodies.

MTAs IN CANONICAL AND NON-CANONICAL ER SIGNALLING

A postulate has gained ground that MTAs might be implicated in the non-canonical signalling by oestrogen and progesterone and their receptors. The

ER/PR signalling axis has assumed much significance in the management of breast cancer patients. Besides operating by the canonical path of regulating genetic transcription by binding to EREs in responsive genes, the ERs can also function in a non-genomic fashion, which does not involve direct genetic regulation. They can influence cell proliferation by the activation of PI3K/MAPK signalling. The G-protein coupled receptor GPCR30 has been recognised as a membrane receptor of oestrogen and activation of GPCR30 leads to signalling in the non-genomic mode. Indeed, critical to the argument is that oestrogens generate a variety of effects in some systems with the activation of GPCRs. Oestradiol and other ligands activate GPCR30 and promote cell proliferation and cell invasion by driving PI3KAkt and MAPK/ERK signalling. Oestrogens can also upregulate the expression of matrix metalloproteinases (MMPs). These are prime examples of non-canonical GPCR30-mediated signalling. Other pathways such as EGFR and Notch signalling been drafted in by implication of crosstalk with the GPCR30 system. It is thought that the manipulation by MTA1 of the ER/PR signalling axis might take place by the non-genomic non-canonical route. However, it ought to be stressed that there is no direct evidence for this. An MTA1 variant has been shown to contain an ER-binding motif and this sequesters ER to the cytoplasm precluding genomic action but the variant MTA1 can initiate the activation of non-genomic mode of function (Kumar et al., 2002). Equally, recognising that MTA1 is a powerful suppressor of ER-mediated transcription, direct suppression of ER is also a conceivable outcome. So it would be expedient to consider the contrasting view that MTA1 enhances the level of ERα, which is consistent with the association of the latter with enhanced cell proliferation (Kang HJ et al., 2014). Whilst it is generally accepted that MTA1 promotes cell proliferation, it ought to be noted that ERα has been found to downregulate MTA1 and suppress cell proliferation and invasion in vitro (Deng L et al., 2015). This does not conform to the cell proliferation promotion property of MTA1. An alternative view may be that the suppression of proliferation and invasion could have been the outcome of the expression and activation of PR, which would suppress cell proliferation. Deng L et al. (2015) have suggested that the three functional ER-element half-sites, which they have identified in the MTA1 promoter, lead to decreased transcription and expression of MTA1. Equally, the ERα effect could be due to its binding to and the downregulation of PR. PR does contain ERE half site/Sp1-binding site and ER does bind directly to this site (Petz and Nadulli, 2000). Furthermore, the non-canonical mode of progesterone signalling needs to be reckoned with here. As stated earlier, progesterone can generate its biological effects via mPRs and PGRMC1s and this can occur even in absence of the conventional nuclear PRs.

MTA EXPRESSION IN CLINICAL SAMPLES REFLECTS AGGRESSIVE DISEASE

In the context of the apparent circumspect approach to the clinical utility of MTAs, it would be worthwhile to focus on some recent information of the role of MTAs in determining tumour behaviour. The sub-cellular distribution of MTA1 determines its target and governs its function. Cytoplasmic localisation might be involved in its interaction with the cytoskeletal system leading to the modulation of cell motility, whilst in the nucleus MTA1 might be concerned with the manipulation of genetic expression. MTA1 expression and its sub-cellular distribution, especially in the nucleus, have strongly correlated with state of the disease and its progression of several tumour types to the metastatic state. Nagaraj et al. (2015) have reported that MTA1 expression as judged by immunohistochemical staining was more intense in high-grade ductal breast carcinoma and correlated with clinical stage. They also noticed increases in the microvascular density with increasing grade. Compatible with this, in vitro MTA1 induced the expression VEGF and angiogenesis. This study used only 10 ductal carcinoma specimens and it is difficult to visualise how one can significantly infer any correlation of MTA expression with tumour grade/stage and microvascular density. Nonetheless, the indications of the association of MTA1 with aggressive disease are reassuring. Besides, even patients with node negative breast cancer with high MTA1 expressing primary tumours appear to carry a higher risk of recurrence (Martin et al., 2006).

The adverse effects of high MTA1 expression are quite convincingly demonstrated in a study of gastric cancer where both overall survival and disease free survival were much poorer in patients with high MTA1 as compared with patients with low MTA1 tumours. Furthermore, forced expression by transfection of MTA1 gastric cancer cells in vitro upregulated the expression of cyclin D1 and downregulated p21. In vitro invasion assays also showed enhanced invasive ability of the cells with high MTA1 levels. The study also indicates enhanced expression of MMPs (Yao Y et al., 2015). This suggests possible links with angiogenesis and progressive disease. Indeed, in nasopharyngeal carcinoma MTA1 expression correlated not only with clinical stage, but also with the presence of distant metastases. Furthermore, metastasis free survival was far lower in patients with high MTA1 expression than those with low MTA1 expression (Yuan TZ et al., 2014). Liu TB et al. (2013) had observed such a correlation in cervical cancer. MTA1 expression significantly correlated with lymph node spread, was predictive of tumour recurrence and appeared to be good indicator of overall survival and disease free survival.

Some mechanistic explanations have been forthcoming for the perceived link between the expression of the gene and tumour invasion and progression. MTA1 expression correlated with the expression of EPCAM in lung cancer cell lines. Silencing of MTA1 reduced in vitro invasion and this was reversed by forced overexpression of MTA1. The expression of both MTA1 and EPCAM in lung cancer tissue was also interrelated and positively correlated with clinical stage and metastasis to the lymph nodes (Zhou N et al., 2015). The loss of E-cadherin and alterations in the cytoskeletal dynamics and associated signalling systems would strongly impact the tumour invasive ability. The upregulation of VEGF expression and induction of angiogenesis occurring concomitantly with enhanced MTA1 would inevitably suggest how this protein might promote distant spread of primary tumours.

Of the two other MTAs which have received some attention, MTA2 appears to influence invasion in vitro and metastasis in vivo breast cancer models. The expression levels of MTA2 correlated with the expression of markers of poor prognosis (Covington et al., 2013). These findings related to ER negative breast cancer cells. However, one ought to read this together with the view that ER negative breast cancers often tend to be EGFR positive. In sharp contrast with other members of the family and in conformity with its established role, MTA3 is able to suppress EMT activation by supressing the transcription factor Snail with consequent increase of E-cadherin expression. MTA3 mRNA and protein expression were reported to be lower in tumour tissues as compared with corresponding normal tissues and also inversely related to metastatic potential (Dong HM et al., 2013). Similarly, reduced MTA3 levels have occurred with increased Snail and E-cadherin expression in choriocarcinoma cells after genistein treatment (Liu XX et al., 2011). However, some of these studies are subject to the caveat as to whether the ERα or ERβ/MTA3/Snail/Slug/EMT axis operates in the cellular environment. Whilst Liu XX et al. (2011) show that ERβ mediated the effect, but others have suggested the involvement of ERα. These contradictions can have many explanations. Conventional wisdom says that ERα is pro-proliferation whilst ERβ is inhibitory of cell proliferation. Also it would be essential to bear in mind that the ER signalling axis interacts with many other signalling systems that impinge upon the process of cell proliferation. The status of PR is an essential component of the oestrogen/ER signalling axis in that PR is regulated by ER and has a major role in determining the state of progression of tumours (Caronongan III et al. 2016). MTA3 expression has negatively correlated with tumour grade and overall survival of patients with gliomas may be a marker of good prognosis (Shan SQ et al., 2015).

There are dissenting views concerning MTAs and tumour progression. The expression of MTA1 in breast cancer samples was neither related to tumour size, grade or nodal status nor to disease free survival and overall survival of

90 patients investigated. These findings do call into question the utility of MTA1 expression in patient management. This study also reported a negative relationship between MTA1 levels and in vitro invasion of breast cancer cell lines. The inverse link to invasion was supported by direct correlation with E-cadherin and also extended to the expression of ER and PR (Tong D et al., 2007). However, it ought to be noted that in that study the distinction and grouping of the breast cancer cell lines was based on published data. The authors themselves did not measure in vitro invasion. The cell lines would have gone through numerous passages in culture, which could have affected their behaviour in vitro and in vivo. In colorectal cancer also high MTS1 expression is said to be inversely related to tumour node metastasis stage, local invasion and also metastatic spread. The inverse relationship was noticed also with respect to VEGF C and VEGFR3 (Li J et al., 2015). But in overall perception, the evidence is overwhelming that MTA1 does promote invasion and metastasis together with the identification of some of the effectors of invasion and angiogenesis. Therefore it is somewhat intriguing why so little effort is directed to at least pre-clinical studies looking for potential inhibitors of MTA1.

ARE THERE VIABLE OPTIONS FOR SUPPRESSING MTA1?

The options open to the suppression of MTA1 for suppressing tumour growth and spread ought to be considered on the sheer weight of the evidence of the biological effects exerted by MTA1 on most of the important fronts of cell invasion and metastatic progression.

The inhibition of the metastatic process by using gadolinium metallofullerenol nanoparticles, which have been shown to be capable of suppressing MMPs (Meng H et al., 2012), does seem to offer a viable option. Breast cancer cells treated with the nanoparticle inhibited invasion in vitro of breast cancer cells, and in vivo models of the treated cells displayed reduced metastatic spread. Taking the cue from this work, Pan YM et al. (2015) have shown that these nanoparticles can inhibit metastasis in pancreatic cancer. This occurred in conjunction with the downregulation of MMP-2/9 and MTA1 and HDAC1. This study also noted that the RECK protein was upregulated with increased acetylation of its promoter. One would recall that RECK is a cysteine-rich, extracellular membrane-bound glycoprotein that can downregulate MMP activity. The link with the suppression of metastasis is provided by the downregulation of HIF-1α, which is a known inducer of angiogenesis.

It might be worthwhile noting an indirect connection of MTA in the PTEN/PI3K/Akt signalling cascade. That involves resveratrol, a naturally occurring phytoalexin. We showed some time ago that it suppresses cell proliferation and induces apoptosis. Resveratrol regulates cell survival and apoptosis in three different ways. It inhibits survival signalling by Notch and its downstream effectors, induces the levels of p53 and its effectors p21waf and Bax, inhibits PI3K/Akt, activates Gsk-3β and reduces cell proliferation (Cecchinato et al., 2007). The suppressor PTEN, which inhibits PI3K/Akt, is suppressed by MTA1. Suppression of MTA1 enhances the acetylation of PTEN. Resveratrol inhibits MTA1 and promotes acetylation and reinstates inhibitory action of PTEN on PI3K/Akt (Dhar et al., 2015). Resveratrol is also capable of upregulating the expression of death receptors (Ko YC et al., 2011).

Of late, it has emerged that enhanced p53 occurs by the suppression of MTA1 by resveratrol. Resveratrol and derivative compounds pterostilbene enhanced acetylation and the expression of p53 in PC cells. In vivo, PC tumour xenografts showed reduced growth with increased apoptosis, reduced invasion and metastatic ability coupled with decreased angiogenesis. Pterostilbene suppressed MTA1 more efficiently and led to higher p53 acetylation than produced by resveratrol (Li K et al., 2013). This is a distinct possibility since resveratrol is able to inhibit HDACs and increase acetylation of its molecular targets (Venturelli et al., 2013). However, as discussed earlier, resveratrol inhibits MTA1 and interferes with PTEN/PI3K/Akt and NF-κB signalling also; so the operation of these pathways cannot be excluded. The status of p53 mutations is also an important factor. Hepatocellular carcinoma displays many genetic changes, including p53 mutations in poorly differentiated tumours. Often the incidence of mutations has correlated with disease progression. The gain of function mutants is frequently hyperacetylated. Mutations of p53 are probably less frequent but do occur in hepatoblastomas, where deregulated Wnt signalling has been seen (Oda et al., 1995).

Curcumin is an inhibitor of both NF-κB and Wnt/β-catenin signalling. It has anti-proliferation and anti-invasion properties. Lu YM et al. (2014) have shown that curcumin inhibits the proliferation of NSCLC cell lines 95D and A549 cells and their in vitro invasion. This occurs concurrently with the downregulation of MTA1 expression. They have confirmed that suppressing MTA1 using MTA1 siRNA produces the same inhibitory effects. Further downstream of MTA1, the Wnt/β-catenin pathway was also inactivated. Taken together, these results have been interpreted as suggesting that curcumin exerts its effects of inhibition of proliferation and inhibition by inactivating the MTA1/Wnt/β-catenin signal transduction cascade.

A new link has been interleaved in the MTA1/Wnt/β-catenin signalling axis. The Epstein–Barr virus-encoded latent membrane protein 2A (LMP2A) actively promotes EMT in nasopharyngeal carcinoma cells. This has been attributed to the activation of mammalian target of rapamycin (mTOR) signalling by LMP2A leading to the upregulation of MTA1 expression. MTA1 in turn activates the Wnt/β-catenin pathway to EMT (Lin Z et al., 2014). The perceptible sequel of LMP2A → mTOR strengthens MTA1 expression → Wnt/β-catenin activation → activation of EMT can potentially offer opportunities for a viable approach to the inhibition of cancer invasion and EMT with established inhibitors of mTOR and MTA1 individually and probably more effectively in combination. Wnt/β-catenin also targets MMPs, which also affect cell migration. Furthermore, Wnt signalling integrates with Hh and TGF-β in mutual regulation. This makes the Wnt signalling system too complex for easy interpretation. Quite obviously, there is a wide range of options that could be followed up to suppress or mitigate the promotion of tumour progression by MTA proteins at least in pre-clinical tumour models.

CHAPTER 25

S100A4 Has Potential Benefits as a Therapeutic Target

S100A4 is a calcium-binding protein whose expression correlates significantly with cancer metastasis and which wields a wide spectrum of biological effects. S100A4 is overexpressed in many forms of cancer and cancer-derived cell lines and also in non-neoplastic cell lines. The expression of S100A4 is regulated by methylation. The incidence of hypomethylation has correlated with tumour progression. Its expression has been linked also with pathology of Crohn's disease, rheumatoid arthritis and psoriasis, among others. Besides the association with disease processes, S100A4 is known to subserve many normal physiological functions. It regulates macrophage motility, and contributes to fibrosis and remodelling of diseased and damaged tissues.

S100A4 SIGNALLING IN CANCER BIOLOGY AND PATHOLOGY

The expression of S100A4 has closely correlated with recurrence, progression and prognosis of many forms of cancer. The growth and metastasis promoting function of the protein flows from its ability to regulate the cell cycle, cell proliferation and apoptosis, to remodel the extracellular matrix (ECM), to modulate cytoskeletal dynamics and cell motility and to induce angiogenesis. S100A4 activates and integrates several signalling systems, which generate the phenotypic expression of these features characterising cancer (Table 25.1, Figs 25.1 and 25.2).

S100A4 seems able to target cell cycle regulatory genes, modulate apoptosis signalling and signalling by growth factors and their receptors. The modulation of growth factor/receptor signal transduction has been implicated in the activation of epithelial mesenchymal transition (EMT) leading to the acquisition of invasive ability by interactive signalling with Wnt/β-catenin and NF-κB. S100A4 has been shown to upregulate the transcription factor Snail and in this way suppress E-cadherin expression, a prominent event in EMT activation.

Molecular Approach to Cancer Management. DOI: http://dx.doi.org/10.1016/B978-0-12-812896-1.00025-8

Table 25.1 S100A4 Signalling in Cancer Growth, Invasion and Progression

Cell proliferation, tumour growth
P53-Rb/stathmin/p53, p21waf, p16; P53/stathmin/microtubule dynamics/cell division; p53 and apoptosis family genes; caspases; calpain/Fas (?); *PI3K/Akt*/mTOR
Invasion, intercellular adhesion
Modulation of cytoskeletal dynamics; E-cadherin/β-catenin complex enzyme system/ECM remodelling; *PI3K/Akt/* mTOR, EMT
Tumour vascularisation
Activation of MMP/TIMP; plasmin plasminogen pathway; activation of angiogenic factors/endothelial cell proliferation; p53-mediated inhibition of endothelial cell proliferation; RAGE/VEGFA-dependent endothelial proliferation and angiogenesis
Differentiation signalling
Activation of Wnt, Notch (?); terminal epidermal differentiation; induction of differentiation-related transcription factors; activation of G proteins, PLC and DAG.

From Sherbet, G.V., Lakshmi, M.S., 2006. The modus operandi of S100A4 signalling in cancer growth, progression and prognosis. In: Sherbet, G.V. (Ed.), Molecular and Cellular Pathology of Cancer Progression and Prognosis. Research Signpost, Trivandrum, pp. 359–377.

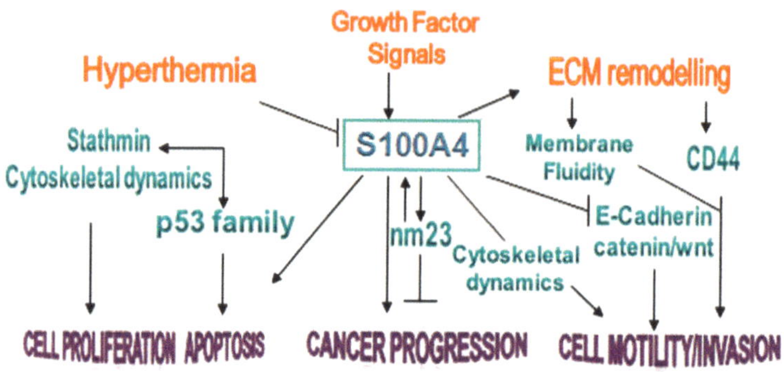

FIGURE 25.1

The pathways activated by S100A4 to transduce signals to induce cell proliferation, apoptosis, invasion and angiogenesis in tumour growth and progression. *From Sherbet, G.V., 2011b. S100A4 (S100 calcium binding protein A4). Atlas Genet. Cytogenet. Oncol. Haematol. 15, 877–886 (updated in 2013) with permission from the Atlas of Genetics and Cytogenetics in Oncology and Hematology.*

MOLECULAR APPROACH TO TARGET S100A4

S100A4 is arguably a molecular target of considerable potential possessing a wide range of biological activity that can alter and regulate the major phenotypic features of cancer and could provide suitable prospects for developing new therapeutic procedures. Some effectors of the S100A4-activated pathways might also lend themselves as foci of extensive therapeutic interest as discussed at length earlier (see Sherbet and Lakshmi,

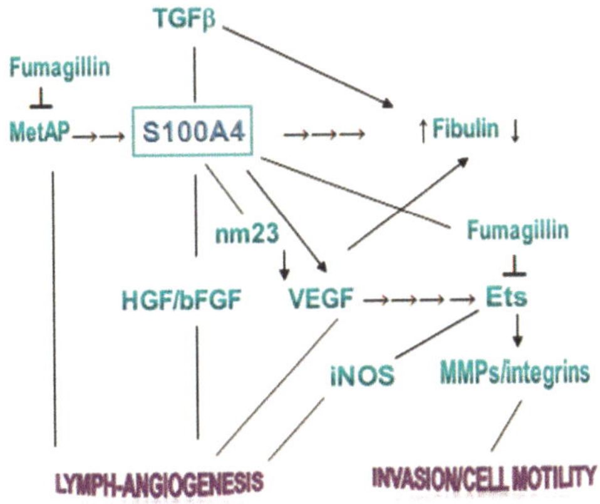

FIGURE 25.2
The modes of induction of cell motility by angiogenesis. *From Sherbet, G.V., 2011b. S100A4 (S100 calcium binding protein A4). Atlas Genet. Cytogenet. Oncol. Haematol. 15, 877–886 (updated in 2013) with permission from the Atlas of Genetics and Cytogenetics in Oncology and Hematology.*

1997, 2006; Sherbet, 2009, 2011a, 2011b, 2013). So here the discussion is restricted to the identification of the foci in the signal transduction cascades activated by S100A4 that might be clinically beneficial and amenable to therapeutic targeting.

Niclosamide Inhibits S100A4-Induced Cell Proliferation, Invasion and Angiogenesis

The anti-helminth drug niclosamide is able to suppress the expression of S100A4, inhibit cell proliferation, invasion and promote apoptosis and inhibit metastatic spread of tumour xenografts. It targets the Wnt/β-catenin pathway to suppress S100A4-mediated promotion of invasion. This is evident from its ability to reduce the expression of VCAM-1 and ICAM-1 in human umbilical vein endothelial cell (HUVEC) cells. These adhesion molecules are known to induce cell migration and activate EMT, with the participation of Wnt/β-catenin. Niclosamide also inhibits angiogenesis. In vitro angiogenesis assays using Matrigel, albeit not totally or positively persuasive, have shown that niclosamide inhibits the proliferation and migration of HUVEC cells and also suppresses tubule-like formations. In vivo, it suppresses VEGF-induced angiogenesis (Huang MC et al., 2015). It is also able to suppress HIF-1α/VEGF-mediated induction of angiogenesis and inhibit endothelial cell proliferation. The effects occur by the inhibition of MAPK and PI3K/Akt signalling (Hsu CW et al., 2016). Another mode of angiogenesis signalling that niclosamide inhibits is by access to the Akt/mTOR and the

IKK/NF-κB paths (Huang MC et al., 2015) that are liable to affect cell survival too.

Effects of Niclosamide on EMT and the CSC Phenotype

Exciting is the prospect that niclosamide might reverse EMT and inhibit the cancer stem cell (CSC) phenotype. Breast CSCs as characterised and defined by the sphere-forming assay are enriched for the expression of a panel of CSC markers. These cells possessed high tumorigenic potential compatible with the CSC character and were susceptible to apoptosis upon exposure to niclosamide (Wang YC et al., 2013). Liu JJ et al. (2016) used SKBR3 and BT474 cells resistant to lapatinib, a receptor tyrosine kinase inhibitor capable of inhibiting HER2 and EGFR signalling. These cells display higher levels of EMT and CSC markers than corresponding control cells. Upon treatment with niclosamide, these lapatinib-resistant cells lost both EMT and CSC features. These events were accompanied by the induction of apoptosis and inhibition of HER2-mediated growth and loss of invasive ability. HER2 expression could enhance invasion by modulating the expression of matrix metalloproteinases (MMPs). MMPs 2 and 9 may be related to the presence of HER2 as reported some while ago (Pellikainen et al., 2004). These findings tie in with the inhibition of MMP9 in the suppression of migration by niclosamide (Tomizawa et al., 2015).

The nexus of niclosamide with S100A4 is that it reduced S100A4 expression at the mRNA and protein levels and suppressed cell migration and metastatic spread. Treatment of colon cancer cells reduced colony formation and inhibited the metastasis to the liver of intrasplenically xenografted colon cancer cells. The suppression in metastasis corresponded with reduced S100A4 mRNA levels in the splenic tumours of the treated mice as compared with control tumours. The treatment with the drug also appeared to have a long-term effect in that the metastasis suppressor effect persisted for several days after the treatment was discontinued. The effects seemed to be structurally specific to niclosamide, for they were not replicated by the several derivative compounds. Also of interest was the finding that Wnt signalling showed a marked reduction in the niclosamide-treated cells (Sack et al., 2011).

EMT has strong associations with the function of a family of transcription factors that include Snail, Twist, Zeb and TCF3. Zeb and TCF3 are closely concerned also with Wnt signalling. However, niclosamide suppresses many other pathways, NF-κB, Notch, ROS and mTOR among them (Pan JX et al., 2012), that are actively involved with the activation of EMT and generation of CSCs, all affiliated to the operation of S100A4. This does not detract from the merits of the demonstration of the inhibition of Wnt/S100A4 as a means of inhibition of cell proliferation, invasion and metastasis by niclosamide.

Niclosamide has been found to be an effective inhibitor in pre-clinical studies using many human cancer models, as a single agent or in combination with conventional chemotherapeutic agents, but without any attempt to link the inhibitory effects with the blocking of S100A4. It is undergoing clinical trials in patients with colon cancer. In prostate cancer, it is being tested in conjunction with enzalutamide to suppress the androgens that aid the progression of prostate cancer (NCT02532114). Niclosamide is said to reduce the expression levels of androgen receptor splice variants such as AR-V7 (Liu CF et al., 2014), which is associated with of drug resistance in hormone refractory prostate cancer. But none of these trials have S100A4 as an outcome.

Sulindac Influences S100A4 Signalling

Sulindac, the non-steroidal anti-inflammatory agent, can modulate Wnt/β-catenin as well as NF-κB signalling that can have repercussion on the invasive behaviour of cancer cells. Sulindac downregulates the expression of S100A4 in vivo tumour models. The growth and metastasis of intrasplenically xenografted human colon cancer were inhibited. S100A4 levels were lower in both primary and liver metastases. In vitro, β-catenin/TCF signalling was downregulated (Stein et al., 2011). Sulindac is also regarded as a non-specific COX-2 (cyclooxygenease 2) inhibitor. COX-2 is an inducer of invasion and angiogenesis. One can visualise that sulindac can inhibit these processes by the COX-2 inhibition route. Phosphosulindac has been postulated to target breast CSC. No progress has been made with sulindac at the clinical level.

Flavonoids in the Inhibition of S100A4

The flavonoid Xanthohumol derived from the hops plant *Humulus lupulus* suppresses cell proliferation, invasion and tumour progression. This flavonoid has been shown to inhibit TNBC (triple negative breast cancer) cell lines by suppressing anti-apoptosis Akt and NF-κB survival signalling pathways. Xanthohumol has also been attributed with the ability to suppress EMT activation, which is said to occur in parallel with the inhibition of S100A4 (Viola et al., 2013).

Phenothiazines and the Inhibition of S100A4 Signalling

A class of compounds worthy of attention are phenothiazine and derivatives, which have shown some inhibitory activity against S100A4. There is ample justification for this awareness in that the phenothiazine family members have been found to inhibit signalling systems that induce cell proliferation, invasion and angiogenesis. They have also been imputed to be active against drug resistance. The phenothiazines downregulate ABCB1 [ATP-binding cassette, sub-family B (MDR/TAP) 1] gene and inhibit the expression of the transporter P-glycoprotein in drug resistant cells and render them sensitive to the cytotoxic action of phenothiazines (Spengler et al., 2011). Several derivatives of phenothiaziane have been described. Two amine derivatives inhibit cell proliferation by affecting the function of cell cycle regulatory genes and those associated with the induction of apoptosis (Latocha et al., 2015). Thioridazine suppresses the growth of tumours formed by gastric cancer cell implants in animal models. The growth inhibition resulted from the induction of apoptosis by the inhibition of caspase-dependent signalling (Mu JS et al., 2014). The PI3K/PDK1/Akt and the downstream mTOR axis are involved in cell proliferation and angiogenesis. The phenothiazines suppress cell proliferation by inhibiting the PI3K/PDK1/Akt signalling axis (Choi et al., 2008). These drugs can activate PP2A (protein phosphatase 2). Perphenazine dephosphorylates PP2A substrates (Gutierrez et al., 2014; Chien WW et al., 2015). PP2A and PTEN both negatively regulate the anti-apoptosis PI3K/Akt signalling and induce apoptosis. On the angiogenesis front, thioridazine is able to suppress the growth of xenografts of ovarian cancer. This is accompanied by reduced tumour-associated vasculature. In parallel, the PI3K/PDK1/Akt signalling is inhibited, which accounts for the growth inhibition. VGFR2 mediated activation of PI3K/Akt/mTOR and the induction of angiogenesis is also suppressed by thioridazine (Park MS et al., 2014).

S100A4 targets many proteins upon assuming an open conformation after Ca^{2+} binding. In this altered conformation, it can bind to the target proteins via specific domains of S100A4 that become accessible as a result of the conformational change. S100A4 interacts with myosin-IIA and this binding regulates its ability to promote invasion and metastasis. Phenothiazines are inhibitors of S100A4–myosin-IIA interactive function (Garrett et al., 2008). The phenothiazine TFP (trifluoperazine) binds to the hydrophobic target-binding pocket. It is postulated that sequestered and induced to oligomerise in this way the prospective S100A4–myosin-IIA interaction is prevented (Malashkevich et al., 2010). This would lead to the abrogation of the metastasis promoting activity of S100A4.

Inhibition of S100A4/RAGE Signalling Suppresses Angiogenesis

RAGE (receptor for advanced glycation end products) is a protein of the IgG superfamily. The full-length RAGE is a transmembrane protein. The extracellular region contains three IgG-like domains, one a variable V-type that binds the ligands and two constant C-type domains. The V-type domain is responsible for interaction with multiple RAGE ligands. RAGE also occurs as splice variants, which have been implicated in the regulation of the function of the full-length RAGE by competitive ligand binding or by displacing the full-length receptor from the cell membrane. Gene splicing generates proteins with altered ligand-binding domains or produces variants with deleted transmembrane domain and cytoplasmic tail. Of three known variants, RAGEv1 is a soluble receptor. This has the full extracellular domain but lacks both transmembrane and the cytoplasmic domains. The soluble variant inhibits tumour invasion and angiogenesis and hence it is strongly implicated in the suppression of metastatic spread (Kalea et al., 2010; Steranczak et al., 2013). The endogenous secretory RAGE is the cytoplasmic domain that also inhibits tumorigenesis.

Numerous ligands that bind the soluble variant have been identified, among them are AGEs (advanced glycation end products), and RAGE is known to bind to and mediate the function several S100 proteins including S100A4. Besides S100 proteins, the HMGB1 protein amphoterin and the amyloid-β peptide are also RAGE ligands. The functional significance of binding of S100A4 is gradually being elucidated (Ding Q and Keller, 2005; Leclerc et al., 2009). The induction of cell migration by S100A4 is inhibited by the inhibition of RAGE using siRNA. This also inhibited the phosphorylation of extracellular signal regulated kinase (ERK) and MMP-2 (Spiekerkoetter et al., 2009). S100A4/RAGE/VEGFA-dependent signalling is a significant signalling axis in endothelial proliferation and angiogenesis. This might potentially offer the possibility of suppressing this mode of signalling to counteract the induction of angiogenesis. The soluble extracellular domain of RAGE (sRAGE) acts as a decoy receptor and suppresses the whole length RAGE-mediated pro-inflammatory NF-κB activation by S100A4 (Chuong C et al., 2009). Dahlmann et al. (2014) have shown that S100A4—RAGE interaction activates the MAPK/ERK signalling and enhances cell motility, and these effects can be inhibited by sRAGE- and RAGE-directed antibodies.

The S100 family calcium-binding protein S100P promotes cell proliferation and survival by activating ERK and NF-κB signalling. The effects of S100P are suppressed by amphoterin (HMGB-1)-derived peptide that inhibits RAGE activation and also by anti-RAGE antibodies (Arumugam et al., 2004). Arumugam et al. (2012) have developed a small peptide based on S100P sequence that can inhibit the binding of RAGE ligands to sRAGE. The peptide inhibited the binding of S100A4 to RAGE and suppressed the activation of NF-κB signalling both in vitro and in vivo. Systemic administration of the peptide inhibited the growth of glioma and pancreatic cancer cells introduced into host animals. The pancreatic cancer cells were injected into the pancreas and Arumugam et al. (2012) found that intraperitoneally injected peptide reduced invasion and formation of metastatic deposits in the liver. Although orthotopic injection is one of the methods generally used, subcutaneous grafting can lead to the formation of lung metastases. The xenografting of resected primary tumours into immune compromised host animals would have provided more convincing proof of the effect of the RAGE antagonist peptide. The glioma cells were injected subcutaneously, but no information was available regarding metastatic spread. Given the marked association of S100P in the progression of pancreatic cancer, these findings are prime examples of future leads to therapy.

FPS-ZM1 (*N*-benzyl-4-chloro-*N*-cyclohexylbenzamide) is a specific RAGE inhibitor, which prevents the binding of amyloid-β peptide to the V-domain of RAGE and inhibits the subsequent biological outcome (Deane et al., 2012). The peptide described by Arumugam et al. (2012) can inhibit the binding of amyloid-β peptide to RAGE, so the possibility has to be checked if FPS-ZM1 is capable of inhibiting S100A4 interaction too.

A different approach has been taken by Putranto et al. (2013). Ligand binding leads to the phosphorylation of the intracellular domain of RAGE and to the recruitment of two adaptor proteins viz. Toll-interleukin 1 receptor domain-containing adaptor protein (TIRAP) and myeloid differentiation protein 88 (MyD88), which facilitate the downstream signalling (see pp. 233,234; Fig. 26.4 for TLR, toll-like receptor, signalling). Putranto et al. (2013) have devised inhibitors of the binding of RAGE to the adaptor protein TIRAP and block the intracellular signalling cascade. This mode of signal inhibition might have the advantage of being effective against any RAGE ligand.

Monoclonal Antibodies Against S100A4

The thought of employing antibodies was aired some time ago. Some monoclonal antibodies have been tested to counteract the effects of S100A4 and for their efficacy in suppressing cell migration in vitro and metastasis of tumours in vivo (Klingelhofer et al., 2012; Grum-Schwensen et al., 2015). This research group has argued that the effects are generated by the suppression of the T-cell movement to the primary tumour, with the associated reduction in angiogenesis and metastasis. Equally, the migration of S100A4 expressing stromal cells to the metastatic site, which is an important event in secondary spread, may be a factor. O'Connell et al. (2011) showed that depleting the S100A4+ stromal fibroblast population resulted in the reduction of metastases. Irrespective of the nature or mode of the blocking of S100A4, other studies have supported the inhibition of angiogenesis and metastatic spread by antibodies directed against S100A4. Hernandez et al.

(2013) have produced an anti-S100A4 monoclonal antibody capable of inhibiting endothelial cell migration, angiogenesis and also capable of inhibiting the growth of xenografts of tumours derived from S100A4 expressing tumour cell lines. This represents an extensive study showing the involvement of MMPs in the invasion phenomenon, RAGE mediation of S100A4 signalling, among others. However, crucially one would have liked to know the status of metastasis in the experimental in vivo system and whether the antibody had had any effect on that.

Targeting MetAP2 to Inhibit S100A4-Mediated Angiogenesis

MetAP2 (methionine aminopeptidase-2) is an enzyme overexpressed in many forms of cancer. It was identified as a molecular target of fumagillin and analogues, which are powerful inhibitors of endothelial cell proliferation and angiogenesis in vitro and in vivo (Ingber et al., 1990). Fumagillin and analogues bind and inhibit MetAP2. The ring epoxide group of fumagillin covalently binds to histidine 231 in the active site of the enzyme (Griffith et al., 1998). Fumagillin and its synthetic analogues inhibit MetAP2 and inhibit HUVEC cell proliferation in vitro and endothelial cell migration and angiogenesis in vivo. They inhibit tumour growth of xenografted tumours. Growth inhibition seems to be aided by the induction of apoptosis. The inhibition of angiogenesis appears to result from the downregulation of VEGFR. It has been suggested that these inhibitors specifically target endothelial cells. However, they would be expected to inhibit protein synthesis in general. Fumagillin inhibits the transcription factor Ets-1, which controls the expression of several genes implicated in tumour growth, invasion and angiogenesis (see Sherbet and Lakshmi, 2006 for references).

Fumagillin and ovalicin have been used for treating obesity. TNP-470, another analogue, which inhibits angiogenesis, had been in clinical trials for the treatment of brain and breast cancer, Kaposi sarcoma and renal cell tumours. The identification of fumagillin and analogues as potent inhibitors of MetAP2 has raised the possibility that they might be effective in the inhibition of S100A4-mediated induction of angiogenesis. S100A4 interacts in a calcium-dependent manner with a domain between monoacid residues 170 and 229 of the N-terminal half of MetAP2. The binding did not alter the enzymatic activity of MetAP2 but it was postulated that this binding could regulate its activity by altering its subcellular location (Endo et al., 2002). The interaction between S100A4 and MetAP2 has suggested a means of inhibiting the perceived angiogenic outcome. A synthetic peptide with sequence correspondence with the S100A4-binding domain of MetAP2 not only interacts with and binds to S100A4 but also inhibits angiogenesis in vitro and in vivo. Upon intratumoral injection into xenografted prostate tumour, the peptide inhibited tumour-associated vasculature and led to tumour regression (Ochiya et al., 2015).

A few clinical trials are underway to test the efficacy of Beloranib, an analogue of fumagillin and SDX-7320 (SynDevRx), which is a fumagillin derivative conjugated to the polymer poly(*N*-hydroxypropylmethacrylamide), in obesity and some forms of cancer.

Does Amlexanox Have a Role as an Inhibitor of S100A4?

Amlexanox (2-amino-7-isopropyl-5-oxo-5H-chromeno[2,3-b]pyridine-3-carboxylic acid), an inhibitor of inflammatory mediators and a phosphodiesterase inhibitor, has obvious therapeutic potential. Amlexanox also inhibits cell proliferation and migration. It inhibits PI3K/Akt/MAPK and NF-κB signalling. This could bring about its phenotypic outcome on cell proliferation and migration in vitro. The cell cycle is inhibited in G1 via the operation of the IκB kinase (IKK)-related kinases TBK1/IKK-epsilon, possibly also the Akt/MAPK pathway (Moser et al., 2016). Given that this pathway can inhibit MMPs, the inhibitory effects of amlexanox on cell migration have become more revealing of the involved mechanisms. That it can promote the depolymerisation of actin filaments is supplementary evidence for its effect on cell motility. It binds many S100 family proteins, e.g., S100A1, S100A2, S100A11, S100A12, S100A13 and S100P. Some of the interactions with S100 proteins occur in the context and involvement of angiogenic growth factors and so possibly have a bearing on and could inhibit angiogenesis. But strangely conspicuous by its absence is S100A4, which is known to markedly influence actin polymerisation dynamics.

Mutations in the calcium-binding EF hand of S100A4 do reduce its ability to bind target proteins and reduce its metastasis promoting ability (Zhang S et al., 2005). The mutant proteins are unable to dimerise and interact with myosin heavy chain IIA (Kim and Helfman, 2003). However, mutant S100A4 does bind to p53. Nonetheless, it would be of much interest to see if amlexanox binds to S100A4 and interferes with the interaction of the latter with its target proteins such as p53, RAGE and myosin, among others. The mode of function of amlexanox could be more than mere interference with molecular interaction of S100 proteins with their targets. It impedes the release of FGF-1 from its complex with p40 synaptotagmin-1 (Carreira et al., 2003). Equally, it has been shown to bind to the interface of FGF-1 interaction with S100A13 and prevent the formation of FGF-1 releasing complex (Rani et al., 2010). Irrespective of the mechanism involved, it is fairly obvious that the FGF-1 release pathway might be amenable to therapeutic manipulation.

The Inevitable Question Is Quo Vadis?

The salient signalling pathways which S100A4 activates encompass growth factor receptors in the regulation of cell proliferation and the cell division cycle and the apoptotic pathway, among others. On the metastasis front, the participation of S100A4 in cancer invasion by ECM remodelling, alteration of cell membrane fluidity, and in the modulation cell cytoskeletal functional dynamics is well established, so is its link with neovascularisation. The discussion of these attributes underscores the viability of appropriate strategy for therapeutic approach to target it. S100A4 is a normal gene, not exclusively linked with cancer but deregulated in its expression leading to the expression of the cancer phenotype.

The quest for targets for therapeutic manipulation has to fulfil several criteria. Is the postulated target a biomarker for tumour invasion, growth and metastatic progression? Is the maker widely expressed in human cancers? Do the signalling pathways of the potential target lend themselves to pharmacological manipulation? The answer to these queries is arguably yes. If so, much pre-clinical work is needed with potential inhibitors as single agents or in combination with conventional cytotoxic agents. This could lay the groundwork to pose these questions in clinical trials.

CHAPTER 26

Notable Approaches to Cancer Immunotherapy

In conventional wisdom, immunotherapy is regarded as active therapy when the immune system is stimulated, restored or reactivated to mount an immunological assault on cancer cells in contrast with procedures that involve the administration of monoclonal antibodies to target them. Several strategies have been adopted for delivering active immunotherapy in cancer treatment. The focus here is on the efficacy of inhibition of immune checkpoint protein in the control of cancer, but a brief reference has been made to small molecule drugs that appear to possess potential tumour inhibitory properties.

THE CD28 FAMILY IMMUNE CHECKPOINT PROTEINS AND LIGANDS IN IMMUNOTHERAPY

Several modes of approach have been adopted in immunotherapy, especially for targeting the development and deployment of immune modulators at immune checkpoints in order to re-activate endogenous immune responses. Immune resistance by tumours seems to flow from tumours being able to adopt certain immune checkpoint pathways especially against T-cells that are specific for tumour antigens. Immune checkpoint proteins negatively or positively regulate T-cell response (Pardoll, 2012). These proteins belong to the CD28 family, which also includes PD1 (programmed cell death protein 1 encoded by the PDCD1 gene, CD279), CTLA4 (cytotoxic T-lymphocyte antigen-4, CD152), BTLA (B and T-lymphocyte attenuator, CD272) and ICOS (inducible T-cell co-stimulator CD278) and share around 30% sequence homology (Okazaki and Honjo, 2007) (Table 26.1).

The Mechanisms of Action of Immune Checkpoint Proteins

The interaction between the receptor and its ligand leads to the inhibition of T-cell activation and cytokine production. T-cell activation involves the interaction of TCR (T-cell receptor) with MHC (major histocompatibility complex) antigens on the antigen-presenting cells and the interaction of immune

Molecular Approach to Cancer Management. DOI: http://dx.doi.org/10.1016/B978-0-12-812896-1.00026-X

Table 26.1 The CD28 Family of Receptors and Their Ligands and Their Expression Profiles

Receptor	Expression	Function	Ligand	Expression
CD28	T constitutive	↑	B7.1 (CD80)	DC, B, monocytes
CTLA4	T upon activation	↓	B7.2 (CD86)	DC, B, monocytes
ICOS	T upon activation	↑	ICOS-L (B7-H2)	DC, B, monocytes/non-lymphoid
BTLA	T and B upon activation	↓	HVEM	DC, B, monocytes/non-lymphoid
PD1	T and B upon activation	↓	PD-L1 (CD274) PD-L2 (CD273)	DC, B, monocytes/non-lymphoid

BTLA, B and T-lymphocyte attenuator; CTLA4, cytotoxic T-lymphocyte-associated antigen 4; HVEM, herpesvirus entry mediator; ICOS, inducible T-cell co-stimulator; PD1, programmed cell death protein 1 encoded by the PDCD1 gene. This table is based on Okazaki and Honjo (2007).

checkpoint proteins of the CD28 family with the appropriate ligand. This latter interaction prevents the apoptosis of the lymphocyte that can occur after TCR–MHC interaction. B-cell activation can be T-cell dependent or occur independently of T-cell intervention. In T-cell dependent activation, the initial signal is TCR–MHC interaction and co-stimulation by CD40 receptor–ligand interaction. The latter is an important event, indeed a requisite component of both T- and B-cell immune responses and humoural and cellular immunity. In T-cell independent activation, the extraneous antigen binds directly to B-cell receptor. As shown in Table 26.1, the immune response is negatively or positively regulated depending upon whether co-stimulatory and co-inhibitory molecules are engaged in the interactions.

Inhibition of Immune Checkpoint Proteins and Its Biological Outcome

Modulation of T-cell activation pathways has taken the form of using antibodies against T-cell receptors or the ligands (Pardoll, 2012). Among immune checkpoint proteins of note that are being investigated for targeted inhibition are PD1 (encoded by the PDCD1 gene) and its ligand PD-L1. PD1 is a transmembrane protein of the immunoglobulin family. It occurs in stimulated B and T-cell lines and is thought to modulate B-cell responses by recruiting the tyrosine phosphatases SHP-1 and SHIP-1. The binding of PD1 receptor by its ligand negatively regulates both T- and B-cells (Riley, 2006; Thibult et al. 2013). The negative signalling has provided a causal link with the pathogenesis of many autoimmune conditions and cancer and has led to the recognition of PD1 as a potential target in disease control.

Monoclonal Antibody-Mediated Targeting of PD1 and Its Ligands

Antibodies against PD1 and PD-L2 are being clinically evaluated. Langer (2015) has recently reviewed the efficacy of the CTLA4 inhibitor ipilimumab, and the anti-PD1 antibodies nivolumab and pembrolizumab in non-small cell lung cancer (NSCLC). Nivolumab has been reported to elicit reasonable overall survival of patient with previously treated advanced NSCLC, especially 1–3 year overall survival of 56%–27% who had been administered nivolumab at the recommended dosage of 3 mg/kg (Gettinger et al., 2015). However, objective response rate was low. The response rate following treatment of advanced melanomas is less than 40% but toxicity is described as tolerable (Ivashko and Kolesar, 2016). Combination of nivolumab and ipilimumab has resulted in greatly enhanced progression free survival (PFS) of patients with advanced melanoma as compared with nivolumab alone. The latter also seemed to be superior in outcome to ipilimumab (Wolchok, 2015). Weber et al. (2012) have defined the unique patterns of response of patients with melanoma to the administration of these antibodies. The administration is often accompanied by immune-related adverse events. It is needless to reiterate importance of the kinetics of response in the identification of patients who might benefit from the treatment and the early recognition of these adverse events, especially in the light of some reports that the responses to treatment have correlated with the adverse events (Weber et al., 2012). The adverse events could constitute an important factor in judging the overall beneficial response. Baksh and Weber (2015) have drawn attention to other immune checkpoint proteins such as BTLA, VISTA (V domain-containing Ig suppressor of T-cell activation), CD160, LAG3, TIM3 and CD244, which might possess therapeutic potential. Treatment with PD1 antibodies has met with much success in the treatment of haematological malignancies (see Armand, 2015).

Targeting of B and T-Lymphocyte Attenuator

BTLA is another immune checkpoint protein under investigation for potential use in cancer treatment. The major problem in this case seems to be that BTLA and CD160 ligands both bind herpesvirus entry mediator (HVEM), a co-stimulatory tumour-necrosis factor receptor. The interaction of HVEM with LIGHT (TNFSF14 tumour necrosis factor superfamily member 14), its endogenous ligand, induces a positive immune response, whilst the interaction of HVEM with BTLA or CD160 negatively regulates T-cell responses. Thus the outcome would depend which ligand binds to HVEM (Murphy et al., 2006; Cai G and Freeman, 2009; Crawford and Wherry, 2009).

Another relevant consideration is the possible influence of steroid hormone receptors on the expression of checkpoint proteins (Kolacinska et al., 2015). We do know that oestrogen receptor, progesterone receptor and HER2 influence tumour behaviour. However, the precise nature and significance of the relationship between the levels of checkpoint protein expression, the expression of steroid receptors and distant dissemination of the primary tumour can only be speculated at present.

The Clinical Potential of VISTA Inhibition

Attention is currently also being focused on VISTA, an immune checkpoint protein ligand with homology to PD-L1, which suppresses T-cell activation and immune responses, but not of B-cell activation (Lines et al., 2014a). Anti-VISTA antibodies promote T-cell activation. In pre-clinical studies, the inhibition of VISTA has been found to suppress tumour growth and enhance host survival, apparently by reducing the development of tumour-specific Foxp3(+)CD4(+) regulatory T-cells (Le Mercier et al., 2014; Lines et al., 2014a). Similarly, inhibition of CTLA4 suppresses Foxp3 and regulatory T-cell differentiation (Sakaguchi et al., 2009).

In the genetic background of VISTA deficiency, experimental mice show an accrual of activated T-cells together with enhanced production of inflammatory cytokines and chemokines, but these events are not accompanied by signs of autoimmune disease. Cross breeding these animals with a strain of mice that are prone to develop experimental autoimmune encephalomyelitis (EAE) does lead to enhanced incidence and intensity of EAE. This suggests the genetic condition of EAE susceptible mice might have complemented the VISTA-deficient genetic background. In other words, VISTA deficiency only lowers the threshold of T-cell activation but not totally inhibit it (Wang L et al., 2014). It could be that VISTA can bind to more than one checkpoint protein receptor. Nonetheless, VISTA is demonstrably an immune checkpoint protein ligand as shown by Liu J et al. (2015) who used VISTA-deficient, PD1-deficient and VISTA/PD1 double knockout mice. Both VISTA-deficient and PD1-deficient mice showed chronic inflammatory responses and spontaneous T-cell activation. These phenotypic effects occurred in synergy and in higher levels in the double knockout mice. PD1 and CTLA4 gene polymorphisms have been encountered in inflammatory and autoimmune conditions. Such genetic alterations, which would influence the biological outcome, have been thought to portend predisposition to disease development and do need to be reckoned with in assessing the eligibility for and overall efficacy of immune checkpoint inhibitors.

Clinical trials have emphasised the potential of combining VISTA blockage with PD1 and CTLA4 inhibitors and the likely benefits provided by combination therapy with conventional chemotherapeutic agents (reviewed by Lines et al., 2014b).

Signalling Pathways of Immune Checkpoint Proteins and Their Ligands

The mechanisms of function of PD1/PDLs are not fully understood at present. There are several interacting signalling systems that might come into the reckoning (Fig. 26.1). Gorgun et al. (2015) have shown that lenalidomide accentuates the immune effects of PD1/PD-L1 blockade in multiple

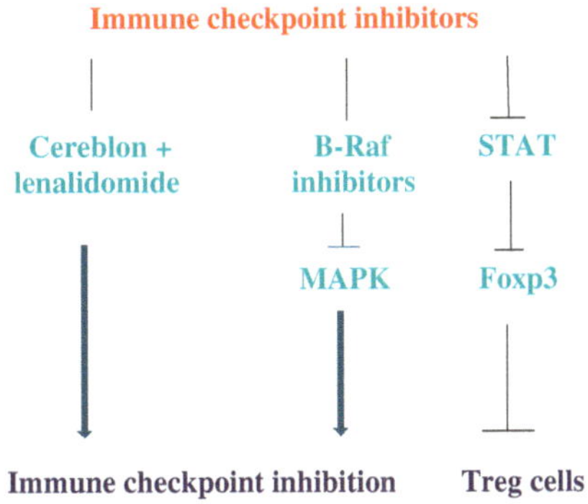

FIGURE 26.1
The postulated signalling systems engaged by immune checkpoint inhibitors.

myeloma. The heightened effects may be mediated by cereblon, which is a component of one of the pathways of action of thalidomide and its analogues (Sherbet, 2015a, 2015b). It ought to be noted, however, that only a proportion of cancer patients is believed to respond to this form of therapy (Sui et al., 2015).

B-Raf^{V600} mutations have been encountered in around 50% of melanomas. There have been some attempts to check if combination of B-Raf inhibitors with inhibitors of checkpoint proteins might provide clinical benefits. The Ras/Raf/MAPK signalling pathway is activated by many external stimuli, such as growth factors, mitogens, inflammatory cytokines, apoptosis inducing factors and others. Activation of the mitogen-activated protein kinase (MAPK) pathway is a frequent phenomenon in cancer. Ras activates the MAPK signalling cascade through its effectors C-Raf, A-Raf and B-Raf. External stimuli can differentially engage two signalling routes of MAPK. Some growth factors engage Raf to activate the route to cell survival, proliferation and differentiation, whilst stress factors, UV irradiation, deprivation of growth factors and inflammatory cytokines activate an alternative route and lead to inflammation and apoptosis.

The demonstration of the benefits of combining ipilimumab with B-Raf inhibitors in patients with melanoma metastases in the brain (see Di Giacomo and Margolin, 2015) is a good example of interaction with a major signalling system linked with tumour progression. However, Postow et al. (2015) found no differences between melanoma patients with wild-type B-Raf as compared with patients carrying B-Raf mutations in respect of response rate and PFS upon treatment with nivolumab and ipilimumab, but combination of nivolumab with ipilimumab was superior to ipilimumab monotherapy. In any case, given the complexity of the MAPK signalling system, it is difficult to relate the perceived relationship between B-Raf to the expression of immune checkpoint protein expression and the effects of their inhibitors.

Cytokines such as interleukins signal in conjunction with their receptors by activating the JAK/STAT signalling system. It was noted earlier that inhibition of VISTA suppressed tumour growth and cell survival, apparently by reducing the development of tumour-specific Foxp3(+)CD4(+) regulatory T-cells (Le Mercier et al., 2014; Lines et al., 2014a). Foxp3 is a transcription factor involved in the development and function of regulatory T-cells. The expression of Foxp3 induces CD4+ cells to differentiate into T regulatory cells. This is mediated by the activation of STAT5 signalling by IL-2 (see Villarino and Laurence, 2015). These findings are compatible with the perceived oncogenic and immunosuppressive functions of STAT3. Indeed STAT3 inhibition improves the inhibition of tumour growth by anthracycline-based chemotherapies. The additive effects are seen only in tumours developing in immunocompetent but not in immunodeficient mice (Yang H et al., 2015).

In the pathogenetic scenario of autoimmune conditions such as EAE, which mimics MS, and AIA (antigen-induced arthritis), PD1 seems to engage a different signalling system. PD1 (−/−) mice have been found to develop autoimmune conditions such as EAE. The latter condition seems to involve the activation of STAT signalling and enhanced STAT binding to the promoter of miRNA-21 and upregulation of its expression. This miRNA is said to directly target the expression of PDCD4 protein (Iliopoulos et al., 2011). One might recall here that PDCD4 subserves the cellular functions of cell cycle regulation and apoptosis. It is downregulated in tumours and so conferring on it the epithet as a tumour suppressor (see Sherbet, 2013). It is noteworthy here that EAE is dependent on a specific molecular profile and a defined genetic environment. For instance, many genes associated with susceptibility to MS are differentially regulated in EAE (Hoppmann et al., 2015). Of particular interest is the expression of caspase 1 and SMAC (second mitochondria-derived activator of caspase). The activity of IAPs (inhibitor of apoptosis proteins) is regulated by SMAC and mimics of SMAC. Reduction in SMAC expression leads to the inhibition of apoptosis and promotes tumour progression. SMAC mimics induce apoptosis together with activation of anti-tumour activity and increased infiltration of lymphocytes with reduced PD1 expression (Emeagi et al., 2012).

These considerations do add a further signalling dimension to the mode of function of immune checkpoint proteins. Inevitably, it is difficult to dissect out the various modes of signalling to isolate the specific signalling pathway activated in a given experimental setup, since the physiological outcome could be a composite of engagement of more than one signalling pathway or a consequence of crosstalk between the activated pathways. Hence, understanding the modes of signalling is crucially important in the search for immune checkpoint inhibitors before attempting to translate laboratory findings to pre-clinical and clinical studies. Many clinical trials on human malignancy are in progress. These address the efficacy and safety of combining immune checkpoint inhibitors of both receptor and ligand with conventional chemotherapeutic agents and also with newer agents such as cancer stem cell (CSC) inhibitors.

THE CD47 SIGNALLING SYSTEM AND THE EVASION OF IMMUNE SURVEILLANCE BY TUMOURS

CD47 regulates many signalling systems associated with cancer biology, notably CSC self-renewal, and tumour initiation, growth and invasion. It is an active regulator tumour growth together with thrombospondin-1 (TSP-1). Suppression of CD47 leads to tumour inhibition (Roberts et al., 2015; Soto-Pantoja et al., 2015) and to the suppression of CSCs (Lee TKW et al., 2014). By virtue of its ability to regulate NO and VEGFR signalling, it would be reasonable to expect it would influence angiogenesis and therefore metastatic spread. Here by design, the focus is on immune regulation as relevant to evasion of immune surveillance by cancer.

The expression of CD47 on cancer cells protects them from destruction by the immune system. Angiogenic and immunosuppressive responses are not totally unrelated biological phenomena and may often occur simultaneously. These systems may also regulate each other. In cancer cells not only angiogenesis is regulated by the immune system, but also some anti-angiogenic molecules may possess the property of immunosuppression (Motz and Coukos, 2011; Tartour et al., 2011).

CD47 engages in interactions with many membrane proteins such as integrins and modulate their signalling via FAK (focal adhesion kinase) and paxillin. FAK activation can have repercussion on NF-κB/E-cadherin-mediated activation of EMT. Inappropriate activation of FAK can lead to the activation of proteinases and promotion of cell migration and angiogenesis. Of interest in this context is the biological effect of interaction between CD47 and the anti-angiogenic TSP-1. TSP-1 inhibits angiogenesis by antagonising NO signalling. TSP-1 can also interfere with the binding of CD47 with VEGFR2 and prevent its phosphorylation (Kaur et al., 2014). The angiogenic pathway involving hepatocyte growth factor (HGF) and its RTK receptor c-met is also influenced by CD47 via interaction with TSP-1. This aspect of CD47 is discussed in another location. TSP-1-mediated signalling is also involved in the regulation of T-cell immunity. So here by design, the focus is on immune

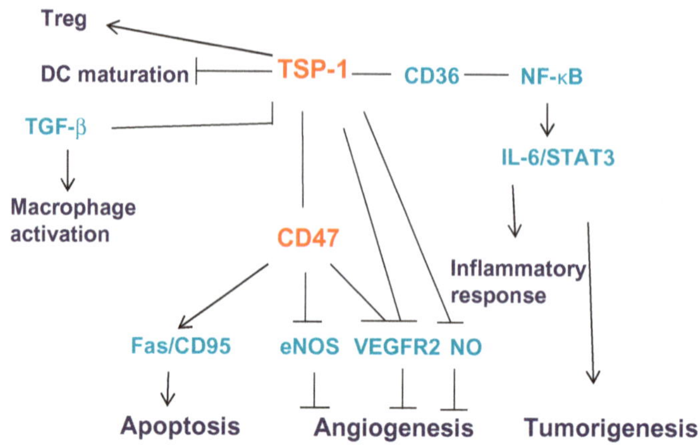

FIGURE 26.2
The modes of regulation by TSP-1/CD47 of immune response and tumour growth and dissemination via suppression of angiogenesis. This figure takes into account the perception that TSP-1 can also act as a CD47 agonist.

regulation as relevant to evasion of immune surveillance by cancer as a mode of immunotherapy (Fig. 26.2).

CD47 Interaction With Signal Regulatory Protein-α

Cancer cells evade immune surveillance with the expression of CD47 on the cell surface. CD47 and SIRP-α (signal regulatory protein-α) play a major part in the evasion of immune surveillance. CD47 serves as ligand or a counter receptor for SIRP-α. SIRP-α is one of three SIRP family proteins. These proteins are immunoglobulin family proteins possessing Ig and Ig-like ligand-binding variable V-set domain and two domains similar to the C1-set domains of IgG, T-cell receptors, MHC antigens and β_2-microglobulin (Barclay and Brown, 2006). SIRP-α is particularly highly expressed in macrophages or dendritic cells, whilst CD47 is expressed ubiquitously (Murata et al., 2014) (Fig. 26.3).

The activation of SIRP-α is known to induce apoptosis and inhibit tumour growth. The blockade of CD47 can inhibit tumour growth by inhibiting the suppressive effects of SIRP-α, promotes macrophage activity and leads to tumour inhibition (Roberts et al., 2015). CD47 suppression can also promote SIRP-α mediated effects. This is compatible with the views that processes such as inflammation associated with autoimmune conditions are mediated at least in part by the PAR (protease activated receptor)-2 pathway and most agents, which activate this pathway promote inflammation (Cottrell et al., 2003). CD47 indeed can activate this pathway. CD47 seems to provide a molecular environment for the pathogenesis of MS, for it seems

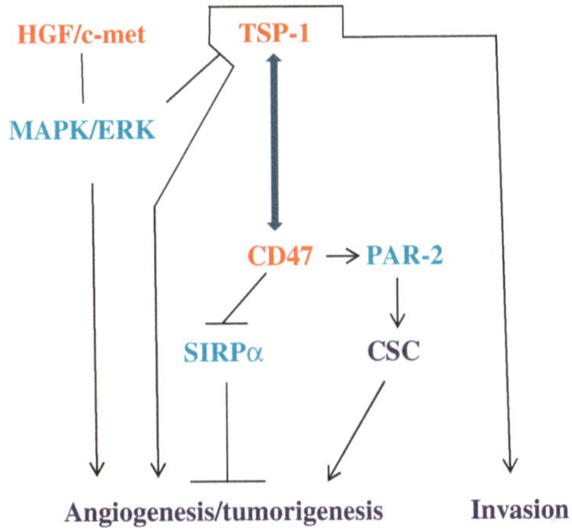

FIGURE 26.3

The effects of TSP-1 and CD47 interaction on angiogenesis and tumorigenesis. CD47 can interact with VEGFR2 and suppress angiogenic signalling. Also it should be recalled here that p53 can upregulate TSP-1 and possibly prevent angiogenesis. As discussed in another location, the TSP-1 domain-containing ADAMTS1 (a disintegrin and metalloprotease domain) protein is anti-angiogenic. The suppression of TSP by HGF/c-met/MAPK/ERK pathway also said to be able to promote invasion. Other growth factors such as EGF can also crosstalk with HGF/c-met signalling. This figure is based on references cited in the text and Sherbet (2011a). Do note that the relevant figure in Sherbet (2011a) should have shown MAPK/ERK as suppressing TSP-1.

to differentially regulate the expression of genes coupled with the risk of developing the disease (Hoppmann et al., 2015). CD47 is a significant regulator of CD4+ T cells that are important movers of EAE. CD47 promotes the secretion of cathepsins. Mice that are CD4+ T-cell deficient are not susceptible to develop EAE in the molecular environment such as the deficiency of cathepsins.

The importance of CD47 in tumour promotion is impressively supported by the finding of a link with CSCs. This seems to be result of the activation of the cathepsin S/PAR-2. Lee TKW et al. (2014) serially propagated hepatocellular carcinoma (HCC) cell shpheroids and obtained a cell population enriched for the expression CSC markers and resistance to chemotherapy. These CSCs showed enhanced CD47 expression. Supressing CD47 reduced the CSC population in the carcinoma. Thus has arisen the postulate that CD47 expressing CSCs initiate tumour development and metastasis and this directly related to poor prognosis for patients. It is suggested that linkup between the CSC phenotype and CD47 expression involves the activation of HCC secreted caspase S/PAR-2 pathway by CD47 leading to the regulation of hepatic CSC.

Cioffi et al. (2015) suggest the targeting the stem cells as a viable treatment option irrespective of the adopted pathway. Monoclonal antibodies have been effectively targeted to HCC xenografts leading to the inhibition of tumour growth as well as promotion of macrophage infiltration into the xenografts (Xiao ZY, 2015). However, targeting monoclonal antibodies to the tumour is not a workable postulate (see Patil and Sherbet, 2015).

How Does CD47 Expression Relate to Disease Prognosis?

By virtue of its ability to regulate NO synthesis, it would be reasonable to expect it would influence angiogenesis and therefore metastatic spread. TSP-1/CD47 signalling seems to suppress angiogenesis. One would expect that activation of this pathway would be prognostically favourable. CD47 acting either as a receptor for appropriate ligands or as ligand can have either agonistic or antagonistic outcome. This would be dependent upon the ambient molecular environment. So in partial compatibility with the interregulation of angiogenesis and immunosuppression discussed earlier, high levels of CD47 expression levels have been linked with poor prognosis. CD47 expression is said to be upregulated in osteosarcoma as compared with osteoblasts. High expression has correlated with reduced disease free and overall survival. Unfortunately, no clinical data relating to the patients have been provided for proper assessment of the effects on prognosis. Antibody-mediated suppression of CD47 halved invasion in vitro and metastasis of osteosarcoma cells in vivo (Xu JF et al., 2015). Yoshida et al. (2015) have reported similar findings from experiments with gastric cancer cell lines. Both these studies found the CD47+ cells to be CD44 positive and construe a link with the CSC phenotype. As stated earlier, this can occur by activation of the PAR-2-mediated signalling by CD47. Cioffi et al. (2015) have pointed out that CD133 + pancreatic CSCs occurred in the CD47+ cell population. Not unexpectedly CD133+ /CD47+ cells were more tumorigenic than CD133 − /CD47 − cells.

CD47 Synergises With Other Invasion/Metastasis Promoting Genes

CD47 has been reported to enhance tumour metastasis in synergy with inhibitor of the RTK receptor c-met of HGF. The HGF/c-met signalling is known to promote tumour invasion and angiogenesis and thus aid metastatic spread. Baccelli et al. (2014) found that luminal type breast cancer patients who were CD47 + /c-met + had poorer survival as compared with double negative patients and double positivity correlated with metastatic spread to the lymph nodes. This synergy whilst a useful feature in assessing disease state is unsurprising. HGF/c-met signalling could be activating Ras/MAPK signalling. The latter is known to inhibit TSP-1 (see Fig. 26.3). This simply underscores the importance of the genetic background in which the angiogenic and immune responses might be expected to mutually regulate one another.

Therapeutic Targeting of CD47 Signalling

Some studies have claimed not only that blocking CD47-inhibited tumour growth but have also begun to address the inevitable question whether inhibitors can be delivered effectively and tumours are targeted efficiently. Wang YH (2013) incorporated anti-CD47 siRNA into a liposome-protamine-hyaluronic acid nanoparticle and administered them systemically into tumour-bearing animals. They found marked reduction in the growth and lung colony formation by B16-F10 melanoma cells introduced by the intravenous route in response to siRNA administration. Although the authors use the term spontaneous metastasis, this assay does not measure metastatic spread, possibly only an adhesion-dependent colonisation of the lungs. One might legitimately ask how target specificity can be achieved since CD47 is a ubiquitously expressed membrane protein. The enhanced expression found in tumour targets does not ensure exclusive and specific targeting. Liposomes tagged with melanoma-associated markers would be essential in order to achieve this.

An essential part of any exercise aimed at CD47 signalling in the control of tumour growth and progression should be to determine the signalling scenario operating in the given cell type or tumour and when they might produce totally antagonistic effects. So novel strategies need to be designed and evolved to override some of the complex interactions and crosstalk between the signalling systems operating at the time.

TOLL-LIKE RECEPTOR SIGNALLING AND CANCER IMMUNOTHERAPY

Toll-like receptors (TLRs) were so named on account of their homology to the Drosophila protein Toll. TLRs are transmembrane receptors. Most of them are located in the plasma membrane but some occur in the endosome membrane. TLRs actively participate in innate immunity and in the defence against pathogens by being able to recognise patterns or motifs of extraneous macromolecules. Among motifs recognised by TLRs are lipopolysaccharide (LPS), proteoglycans, lipoproteins and macromolecules such as bacterial DNA and RNA.

TLR Signalling Pathways

The activation of TLRs by the recognition motifs leads to the operation of several signalling systems that lead to the production of pro-inflammatory cytokines interferons (IFNs), and also cytokines involved in the generation of immune responses. The internal domains of the TLRs function with adaptor proteins MyD88/TIRAP to activate MAPK transduction pathways and NF-κB by IKK or PI3K/Akt mediation. The adaptor TRIF (TIR-domain-containing adaptor protein-inducing IFN-β) is linked with the activation of the transcription factors IRFs (interferon regulatory factors). The TLR family includes 11 members and many of these are involved also in cancer biology. They may differ in function; the differential phenotypic effects are engendered by the adaptor molecule engaged (Fig. 26.4).

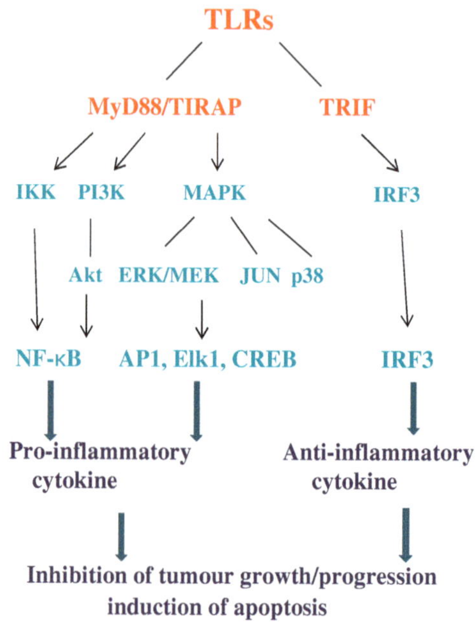

FIGURE 26.4

The pathways activated by the internal domains of TLRs, which are modulated by the adaptor proteins MyD88/TIRAP and TRIF. A MyD88 adaptor-like protein and TRAM (TRIF-related adaptor molecule) are also TIR-domain-containing adaptor proteins involved in the signalling. These are not shown in the figure. The emphasis in this figure is on the participation of TLRs in inducing innate and adaptive immunity, which can lead to tumour suppression or promote tumour growth and progression. The infiltration of tumours by immune cells can suppress or promote cancer progression depending upon the molecular microenvironment. Cytokines of immune cells and stromal cells can generate these contrasting effects. NF-κB signalling leads to the production of pro-inflammatory TNF-α and interleukins. Immune cells that infiltrate tumours produce these cytokines, which would affect tumour growth and progression. The TRIF/IRF3 pathway leads to the production of anti-inflammatory IFN-β and results in the inhibition of tumour growth. Although IRF3 signalling is shown here, TLRs can induce other anti-inflammatory cytokines quite independently of TRIF signalling. As discussed in the text, TLR signals would activate NK cells, CD8+ and negatively regulate Foxp3+ known to suppress anti-tumour immune responses. In totality, these signalling systems would inhibit tumour growth and induce apoptosis. The TLR agonists, as expected, enhance these signalling pathways. Elk1 is an Ets family transcription factor and CREB (cAMP response element-binding protein)/ATF-2 (activated transcription factor) are involved in the expression of pro-inflammatory cytokines consequent upon LTR (long terminal repeat) activation.

TLRs in the Suppression of Metastatic Spread of Cancers

TLR agonists have been attributed with the ability to suppress the invasive behaviour of tumour cells as well as being able to suppress angiogenesis. Therefore they may be projected as ideal candidates to target the process of metastatic spread. In sharp contrast is the view that TLRs can positively regulate tumour progression. This is supported by the demonstrations, discussed at length in a later section, that some TLRs may induce the propagation of sub-populations that are capable of cell renewal and survival, enhance the invasive behaviour of tumour cells and promote angiogenesis.

TLR Agonists in Cancer Control

The participation of TLRs in inducing innate and adaptive immunity has given rise to the thought that TLR agonists could be employed in cancer treatment. One can envisage two distinct approaches. In one approach, the ligands are designed to activate TLRs to achieve the stimulation of immune responses against the neoplasm. In the second approach, the ligands would selectively activate a TLR signalling axis that leads to tumour suppression by activating intratumoral factors. Both these approaches have had positive outcomes. The TLR7 ligand imiquimod activates anti-tumour immunity and induces apoptosis and autophagy of target cancer cells. Imiquimod enhances p53 expression and initiates p53-dependent apoptosis (Huang SW, 2016). Indeed, gardiquimod, also an imidazoquinoline compound and agonist of TLR7, activates MAPK signalling and several other genes, including p53 and PTEN (Wang F et al., 2016).

The TLR8 agonist VTX-2337 (USAN: motolimod) activates NK cells. Its potential practical application is suggested by its ability to sensitise NK cells from patients with HNSCC (head and neck squamous cell carcinoma). The NK cells became more responsive to stimulation by the NKG2D or Fc γRIII after VTX-2337 treatment (Dietsch et al., 2016). Dendritic cells interact with and activate NK cells, which regulate CD8+ T-cell effector function. The TLR5 agonist entolimod has been reported to suppress metastasis by activating the CD8+ cytotoxic function (Brackett et al., 2016). In that study, the authors used both experimental and spontaneous metastasis in murine tumour models and have demonstrated marked improvements in the survival of animals upon treatment with entolimod, together with a remarkable suppression of spontaneous metastases in the lungs. As these authors have themselves pointed out, of the several TLR agonists identified, only imiquimod has reached the stage of clinical evaluation. Some have led to the stimulation of metastatic progression. Seen in this light, the work of Brackett et al. (2016) appears highly worthy of follow-up studies.

Systemic administration of synthetic TLR4 agonist, glucopyranosyl lipid-A (GLA-SE), reduced the development of metastases of mammary adenocarcinoma and colon carcinoma xenografts. Matzner et al. (2016) ascribe this reduction of metastases to enhanced NK cell activity. Commendable though this work is, one ought to point out that the authors have relied mostly on experimental metastasis assays, which involved the injection of tumour cells intravenously and their retention in the lungs is assessed. They have claimed that the degree of lung retention would reflect the number of metastases that would have developed over a subsequent period. However, in this method the lungs are the first encountered seeding vascular substratum from where tumour cells can be carried to form metastases in the liver. The spleen to liver metastasis assay performed involved the injection of cells into the spleen and checking for hepatic metastases. Neither is this an appropriate assay for spontaneous metastasis. Controversially, they have argued that administration of the agonist in the perioperative period reduced cancer metastasis. It is historically well established that upon induction of neovascularisation huge numbers of cells are released from the primary tumour and some would inevitably intravasate into the new vasculature and would seed at distant metastatic loci. So a relative late perioperative window is not a most suitable window for preventing metastases. Strikingly, one can hardly see the evidence here that supports this claim.

Ando et al. (2015) have used the TLR agonist LPS with the NK cell ligand alpha-galactosylceramide and have achieved enhanced metastasis inhibitory effects in experimental tumour models. The reduction in metastasis was concomitant with enhanced CD8 + cells and the increase in the expression of CXCL9 and CXCL10 in the mediastinal lymph nodes. Equally, this can also occur with the inhibition of angiogenic iNOS, which LPS is capable of, as another research group has already shown (Ito et al., 2015). Some TLRs can induce iNOS expression, so this might indicate a co-ordinated signalling TLR and LPS via iNOS downregulation and the activation of anti-tumour immune responses.

The possibility of eliciting anti-tumour responses has been considered with alacrity also with the second path of approach. The stimulation intratumoral production of IFN-β has been shown to be possible by peritumoral administration of the TLR3 agonist poly (A:U). This effect is said to be mediated by IRF3 (Nocera et al., 2016). Poly (I:C) (poly inosine-poly cytidylic acid) also stimulates IFN-β and activates NK cell function and inhibits lung metastases of murine hosts carrying B16-F10 melanomas (Guillerey et al., 2015). The activation of NK cells and also CD8+ cells is also obvious from the fact that the TLR5 ligand flagellin stimulates IFN-γ and controls the lung deposition of B16-F10 cells introduced intravenously into host mice (de Melo et al., 2015). The use of assays for metastasis by intravenous injection is always subject to the reservation that they do not reflect spontaneous metastasis and that the lung nodule formation may be a reflection of adhesion-dependent retention of the tumour cells in the lungs.

Clinical Trials With Imiquimod

Several trials are underway assessing the effects of this agonist on breast cancer recurrence and metastasis. Other forms of tumours investigated are NSCLC, gliomas, basal cell carcinoma, prostate cancer and CIN (cervical intraepithelial neoplasm). There has been sharp focus on the treatment of basal cell carcinoma (BCC), a lowly metastatic skin tumour. Among the modes of the treatment of BCC are radiotherapy, 5-flurouracil and photodynamic therapy, and immune modulators such as TLR agonists. Both the latter forms of treatment are suitable for treating superficial BCC.

Some positive findings have been reported in sustained clearance of superficial BCC at 5-year follow-up in 80% of patients treated with 5% imiquimod cream; these patients had been followed up after they showed initial clearance after 12-week treatment (Quirk et al., 2010). Actinic keratosis lesions also responded with complete or partial clearance of 30% and 48% for imiquimod at 2.5%, and 35% and 59% for imiquimod at 3.75%, respectively. Placebo effects in the two groups were at 6% and 22% (Swanson et al., 2010). Local skin reaction, e.g., erythema, occurred in some patients. Other studies have shown similar erythema with both placebo and imiquimod cream. Imiquimod application has produced beneficial effects albeit only in 2 out of 10 patients with skin metastases of breast cancer. The response was partial but it was accompanied by regression of the lesion and lymphocytic infiltration and production of cytokines indicating that the imiquimod has elicited immunological responses (Adams et al., 2012). Nonetheless, how the efficacy and safety profile of imiquimod compare with other modes of treatment is debatable.

Photodynamic therapy employs aminolevulinic acid or its ester methyl aminolevulinate. The administration of these prodrugs leads to the formation and accumulation of protoporphyrin IX. Upon photoactivation or activation by ultrasound, protoporphyrin IX generates singlet oxygen and other free radicals, which damage cells and induce apoptosis and autophagy (Wachowska et al., 2011). Both these methods of activation have led to tumour regression. Like imiquimod, aminolevulinic acid is quite effective in suppressing superficial BCC and attempts to employ both these agents have seen much success. Also being tested is combination of imiquimod with radiotherapy or conventional chemotherapy. The potential and the feasibility of imiquimod treatment in low-risk squamous cell carcinomas, invasive squamous cell carcinoma and cutaneous metastases of malignant melanoma have been explored. Some of these have been discussed in preceding sections.

Among other human tumours under the imiquimod compass are gynaecological tumours. Complete clearance of cervical and vaginal intraepithelial neoplasia has been described in a small number of cases as an encouraging outcome (De Witte et al., 2015). Rook et al. (2015) reported complete regression of the disease in 2 out of 12 patients and partial regression in 9 out of 12 patients with early-stage IA–IIA cutaneous T-cell lymphoma following topical treatment with 0. 03% and 0.06% resiquimod, another imidazoquinoline compound. The agonist produced high responses at both concentrations. Complete responses occurred in the 0.06% group. Responses also appeared more rapidly among patients in the higher dosage group. It is unsurprising but valuable to note that untreated lesions also seemed to regress, which suggests the induction of a systemic immune response upon resiquimod treatment. Photodynamic therapy was found to systemically stimulate the immune system and upon topical application potentially stimulate anti-tumour immune responses (Reginato et al., 2014). The comparative merits of imiquimod and photodynamic therapy in terms of clinical benefits and cost effectiveness of the two modes of treatment have been investigated by many. However, these studies have singularly failed to address the crucial question of whether the immune system is systemically influenced by these treatments or what form the immune modulations might have taken. This is essential from the viewpoint of not only combating the growth of the primary lesion but also suppressing the seeding of the primary tumour at distant sites and form metastatic lesions.

Equally important is to devise agonists that can be administered orally and stimulate innate immune responses and curb tumour growth and spread. Oral or intratracheal administration of SM-276001, a TLR7 agonist, reduced tumour growth and suppressed metastatic deposition in the lungs (Koga-Yamakawa et al., 2013). Inevitably, these experiments had to employ experimental metastasis systems, but the feasibility of drug administration by non-topical routes is the most salient feature of these studies. The administration of TLR agonists carried in liposomes is another option that has received some attention. Fox et al. (2014) have incorporated imiquimod and GLA into liposomes taking advantage of the differential solubility of the two agonists. The two agonists generated synergistic effects and could potentially accentuate the beneficial outcome.

Despite apparent success, there are important provisions to formulate with reference to the targeting the nanoparticles carrying the drug, targeting of the nanoparticles to the site of action, release and control of the delivery of the incorporated drugs and the potential immune responses elicited by the introduction of nanoparticles.

CpG-ODNs as TLR Agonists and Tumour Suppressers

CpG-ODNs (CpG oligodeoxynucleotides) are short synthetic single-stranded DNA molecules containing CpG motifs. They stimulate cells bearing TLR9 to activate innate immune responses by the production of pro-inflammatory cytokines and Th1 the helper T-cells. Several CpG-ODNs are efficient inhibitors of tumour growth. In an orthotopic diffuse malignant peritoneal mesothelioma xenograft model, CpG-ODN1826 administration has produced marked reductions in tumour growth both in early and late stages of tumour development (De Cesare et al., 2016). A similar outcome has been recorded with orthotopic HCC model in which the CpG-ODN YW002 suppressed the growth of HCC xenografts and prolonged the survival of host animals. These effects occurred together with marked anti-tumour immune responses (Jia HJ et al., 2016). Aside from their ability to suppress tumour growth, CpG-ODNs may render the tumours radiosensitive. This would be of potential benefit in patient management.

The CpG-ODNs have been delivered efficiently into the lungs of murine hosts with Lewis lung carcinoma xenografts using the non-immunogenic biodegradable polymer polyketal (poly(1,4-phenyleneacetone dimethylene ketal)) nanoparticles described by Hefferman and Murthy (2005) as carriers. This has resulted in tumour regression associated with the induction of anti-tumour responses (Sato et al., 2015). CpG-ODN 1826 enhanced radiosensitivity of the human lung cancer cell line A549 in a rat model. Not only that, simultaneous administration of CpG-ODN 1826 and radiotherapy is said to have reduced the production of VEGF-C (Yan W et al., 2015). Jeanbart et al. (2014) have postulated that targeting the delivery of CpG-ODNs to sentinel nodes might elicit greater anti-tumour response. However, it ought to be recognised that if the sentinel node contains tumour cells, it is more likely than not that the downstream nodes will also contain tumour cells. It is not conceivable that nanoparticles conjugated with tumour antigens and the adjuvant delivered to sentinel nodes would be restricted to the sentinel node alone and would not drain into the non-sentinel lymph node network. This might neutralise the postulated concept of targeting the sentinel node, but inhibitory effect of the agonist would be unaffected. Another mode of administering CpG-ODN as an aerosol has been described to actively induce anti-tumour immunity and suppress tumour metastasis in murine tumour models (Sfondrini et al., 2013).

A few clinical trials are underway to assess the effect of MGN1703, a structurally modified CpG-ODN and a highly efficient immunomodulator (Schmidt et al., 2015). MGN1703 is being tested on advanced colorectal cancer and SCLC (small cell lung cancer). A preliminary study has shown that MGN1703 is safe and well-tolerated (Weihrauch et al., 2015). In a series of metastatic colon carcinoma patients administered with 60 mg of MGN1703, an improvement in PFS was noted. Also there was 65% overall survival over a 17-month period (Schmoll et al., 2014).

TLRs Can Promote Tumour Growth and Progression

The emphasis here has been by design on the potentialities of TLRs and their agonists as a mode of immunotherapy. However, one should not lose sight of the many claims that TLR signalling might promote tumour growth and spread. That TLRs can positively regulate tumour progression is supported by the demonstration that some TLRs may induce the propagation of subpopulations that are capable of cell renewal and survival, enhance the invasive behaviour of tumour cells and promote angiogenesis. All these features are characteristics of metastatic progression. Much evidence has recently emerged that supports this view.

In gastric cancers and in normal stem cells, TLR2/MyD88 maintains the expression of stem cell features (Echizen et al., 2016). Conversely, bone marrow stem cells downregulate the TLR3/MAPK and NF-κB signalling axes (Wang JC et al., 2016). The MAPK and NF-κB signal transduction may be disengaged from one another albeit the pathways are mediated by the same adaptor molecules. For example, the TLR4 agonist LPS can influence MAPK/JNK and NF-κB signalling differentially. In the context of the dissemination of the primary tumour, it would be relevant to note that the TLR4 agonist LPS increased invasion in vitro of HCC cells together with the upregulation of MMPs, but that experimental setup also noted the upregulation of the cytokines 1L-6 and TNFα, which would promote apoptosis. LPS markedly upregulated the expression of TLR4 on the surface of HCC cells and seemed to activate the MAPK/JNK signalling cascade, but did not affect NF-κB (Dong YQ et al., 2015).

TLR9 signalling induces the expression of stem cell markers transducing its signals by the induction of NF-κB/RelA and STAT3 (Moreira et al., 2015). TLR9 activation and its perceived link with NF-κB have implication for angiogenesis given that NF-κB is a major effector of angiogenesis and that TLR9 activation can upregulate VEGF. TLR9 has been reported to promote both tumour growth and angiogenesis. Tumours induced by mutated Ki-Ras showed higher tumour growth in TLR9+/+ as compared with TLR9−/− background. The TLR9+/+ animals also showed poorer survival. Furthermore, these tumours produced VEGF and had higher tumour-associated vascularity. The TLR9 was expressed by the mononuclear cells infiltrating the tumour suggestive of a link with tumour progression (Belmont et al., 2014). High levels of TLR7 in tumour cells of oral squamous cell carcinoma correlated with poor prognosis, but high expression in stromal fibroblasts seems to relate to good prognosis. The high expressers were also characterised by low number of CD3+/CD4+ lymphocytes and but more FoxP3+ infiltration. Compatible with their ability to suppress anti-tumour immune responses, lower levels of FoxP3+ infiltration seemed to accord superior survival time (Ni YH et al., 2015).

Much support can be found for TLR-mediated promotion of progression. Some TLRs, including TLR4, are associated with local recurrence and metastatic spread of tumours. Compatibly, TLR4 seems to take part in the promotion of angiogenesis/lymphangiogenesis by HMGB1 as indicated by the induction of VEGF-C and in vitro endothelial cell proliferation and tubule formation in a TLR4-dependent manner (Han LH et al., 2016). TLR4+ HCC cells are not only invasive in vitro but also express stem cell markers. The concurrent expression of TLR4 and stem cell markers correlated with microvascular invasion and high TLR expression was associated with tumour recurrence and poor survival (Liu WT et al., 2015). LPS stimulation of TLR4 increases adhesion to fibronectin and to hepatic sinusoidal endothelium. These effects are accompanied by phosphorylation of p38 (Rousseau et al., 2013). Quite obviously TLR activation here promotes adhesion by the conventional route adopted in cellular adhesion receptors in the metastatic cascade, wherein integrins mediate cell adhesion by binding to the ECM components via the p38 MAPK system. Invasion is also liable to be enhanced by upregulation of MMPs upon TLR activation, as shown in the case of TLR9 some time ago (Merrell et al., 2006). Activation of TLRs 1 and 2 has led to the promotion of cell proliferation, which might have resulted from the upregulation of the expression of the anti-apoptosis protein Bcl-xL (Cottalorda et al., 2006), which would be expected to promote tumour growth.

A new dimension can be added to the TLR signalling network. TLR4 stimulation by LPS has led to enhanced cell proliferation of HNSCC cells but also increased their migratory ability. These effects occurred together with increased cytokine production. Interestingly, pre-treatment of cells with rapamycin eliminated these effects. This paralleled the inhibition of NF-κB signalling (Ren G et al., 2014). The mTOR signalling pathway integrates signalling systems cell proliferation, growth, apoptosis, angiogenesis, cell motility and invasion. The PI3K/Akt/mTOR/NF-κB signalling axis actively supports tumour progression by inducing cell proliferation and angiogenesis (see Epilogue Table 1). Inhibiting this pathway effectively suppresses angiogenesis and many inhibitors that suppress angiogenesis and invasion have been identified. Rapamycin and its analogues, temsirolimus and everolimus, inhibit signalling by an allosteric mode of action. The engagement of the mTOR signalling axis upon TLR activation thus provides another avenue of approach to inhibit tumour growth and progression.

TLRs Agonists and Inhibitors in Pathology: A Post-Script

Genetic alterations in TLRs would also have negative or positive effects on tumour growth and progression. Loss of function mutations or deletions of TLR can suppress the normally exerted anti-tumour effects of TLRs. Polymorphisms of LTRs have been frequently reported. The molecular mechanisms by which polymorphisms might affect TLR signalling and function are largely undefined at present. Polymorphisms have been reported in many TLRs and this would modulate and modify cellular immune responses by altering the expression of cytokines and lead to vulnerability to diseases (Misch and Hawn, 2008). TLR polymorphisms have been associated with susceptibility to allergic and autoimmune diseases and also with some forms of cancer. Fibroblasts carrying a TLR3 Leu412Phe SNP (single nucleotide polymorphism) seemed to promote progression of idiopathic pulmonary fibrosis and poorer prognosis for the patients (O'Dwyer et al., 2013). TLR4 SNPs have been associated with atherosclerosis, but it is unclear whether pathogenesis of this disease, which is attributed to innate immune responses generated by TLRs, has a causal link with modulation of TLR function by the SNPs. SNPs in TLR4 have been linked with the progression of rheumatoid arthritis (Davis et al., 2015). Recently, Zidi et al. (2016) have suggested that some polymorphisms in TLR2, TLR3, TLR4 and TLR9 may be associated with the progression of cervical cancer. The signalling outcome of TLR activation can also be modulated by SNPs in the adaptor proteins, which they engage. Indeed, signalling by the TLRs would be affected differently depending upon whether the TLR or the adaptor molecule harbours the SNP. Klimosch et al. (2013) identified an SNP in the TLR5 gene of colon carcinoma patients that was linked with enhanced survival, but an SNP in the adaptor MYD88 was associated with reduced survival.

In summary, the contrast of the findings relating to the function of TLRs in tumour development and progression is stark and striking. This makes it imperative that one considers the potential factors and the molecular and genetic environment that could create the vicissitudes of function in order to devise appropriate strategies to promote and accentuate the suppresser effects and neutralise any plausible activation of systems that might promote tumour progression. Some salient features are easily identifiable, such as for instance the possibility that TLRs can engage different adaptors, which could activate the different signalling routes. Equally, one ought to recognise that a nominated adaptor protein can differentially activate alternative signalling systems, the reasons for which are not lucid enough at present. Also genetic alterations can and do affect the signalling systems and change phenotypic outcome from tumour suppression to tumour progression.

THE THERAPEUTIC POTENTIAL OF SMALL MOLECULE DRUGS AS TUMOUR INHIBITORS

Cyclic di-GMP in Tumour Growth Control

Among small molecule drugs that appear to be capable of controlling tumour growth, *cyclic* diguanosine monophosphate or cyclic di-GMP (c-di-GMP) has attracted much attention. The immune-stimulatory properties of c-di-GMP were recognised some time ago (Karaolis et al., 2007; Yan and Chen, 2010). The reported inhibition of tumour growth by c-di-GMP seems to be a consequence of its ability to activate NK cells. Although the means to deliver the drug in a targeted fashion are yet to be evolved, the nucleotide can be loaded into liposome and delivered efficiently into the cytoplasm of tumours. Nakamura T et al. (2015) found that c-di-GMP targeted to B16-F10 melanomas in this way led to the production of type I IFN and activation of NK cells. However, the purported anti-tumour effect is not convincing. The melanoma cells were injected into the tail vein. The introduction of liposomes containing c-di-GMP is described as having reduced tumours in the lungs. This does not indicate tumour inhibition by any criteria. It shows reduced tumour cell localisation in the lungs, which could be merely an adhesion-dependent effect.

Indoleamine-2,3-Dioxygenase (IDO) Inhibitors Overcome Evasion of Immune Surveillance

Indoleamine-2,3-dioxygenase (IDO) is a rate-limiting enzyme involved in tryptophan catabolism by the kynurenine pathway. The importance of IDO is underlined by the demonstration that tryptophan breakdown is an essential feature of immune tolerance. IDO is overexpressed in tumour cells and expressed in an inducible manner in antigen-presenting cells and this enables tumours to evade immune surveillance (Moffett and Namboodiri, 2003). Hence, inhibition of IDO has been advocated for cancer therapy. Nakamura et al. (2015) were able to demonstrate that the IDO inhibitor 1-methyl-d-tryptophan (d-1MT), as a single agent or when combined with cyclophosphamide, inhibited the proliferation of A20 BALB/c B-cell lymphoma cells in vitro and inhibited the growth of the lymphoma in vivo. Thaker et al. (2013)

noted that metabolites of IDO promoted cell proliferation and tumorigenesis; they recorded tumour inhibition by the inhibition of IDO. However, Takamatsu et al. (2015) do not subscribe to that view. They noticed no colon cancer suppression in spite of the detection of immunomodulatory activity. Besides, mucosal invasion seemed higher in IDO deficient mice.

Another suggested route for accentuating the effects of IDO inhibitors is combination with of agonists of TLRs that exert anti-tumour effects. Ito et al. (2015) have argued that this is counteracted by many factors including IDO itself. They have claimed that imiquimod suppressed tumour progression and promoted survival in IDO (−/−) deficient mice more markedly than in the wild-type counterparts based on the presence of IDO mRNA in the lymph nodes. No effort was made to check the lymph nodes for tumour cell or the lung for the distal spread. A further suggestion is to engage MSC (mesenchymal stem cells). The latter are immune-suppressive and this involves IDO activity since blocking IDO negates the effects of MSC (Ciccocioppo et al., 2015). Although much information is on record about the biochemical action of IDO, most of the work using IDO inhibition is at a preliminary stage. Nonetheless, the prominent IDO inhibitors d-1-methyl-tryptophan and INCB24360 are being tested in clinical trials in patients with advanced melanoma, ovarian and fallopian tube cancers, primary peritoneal cancer in remission, advanced solid tumours and also myelodysplastic syndromes.

The Epilogue

I began this work on the premise that molecular approaches based on the identification of genetic determinants and the operation of their signalling pathways are worthy of research focus because they provide opportunities of devising targeted treatment of cancer. I want to avoid hyperbolic assertions, but do observe that several targets for molecular intervention have been recognised, which relate to the regulation of cell cycle progression, cell proliferation, and tumour growth and invasion and metastasis. So these genetic determinants and their downstream signalling that activate epithelial mesenchymal transition (EMT) accompanied by the generation and perpetuation of cancer stem cells (CSCs) could be accessible and targeted and designed for therapy to suppress invasion, angiogenesis and metastasis. I also recognise that this is easier said than done. For, admittedly, the molecular approach is not a novel approach but we see new portals. What portals have we opened? This epilogue provides a precis of the salient features in that perspective with pointers to prospective progression for evolving new ideas and novel anticancer agents.

It ought to be recognised at the outset that no hard and fast distinction or differentiation can be made of signalling systems activating cell proliferation and the induction of angiogenesis. Indeed loss of growth control can allow angiogenesis to occur. In other words, the link-up of the loss of control of tumour growth with a switch to the vascular phase of growth may turn out to be an important event in tumour progression. Similarly, EMT activation and the appearance of CSCs are closely allied with cell proliferation and survival signalling. This is precisely why one finds much overlap between the discussions of cell proliferation signalling, EMT activation, the appearance of the CSC phenotype and the induction of angiogenesis.

Much credence is given here to the signalling systems activated by growth factors to promote tumour growth, invasion and metastasis. These systems are integrated by mammalian target of rapamycin (mTOR). The mTOR signalling cascade is deregulated in many tumours. This signalling system is prominently active in the regulation of cell proliferation and survival as well as in angiogenesis. The HER2/mTOR axis may be a valuable route to patient management, notwithstanding the perceived resistance to mTOR inhibition. Besides this, the pre-eminence of this signalling system is emphasised by the apparent integration of epidermal growth factor receptor (EGFR), vascular endothelial growth factor (VEGF), IGF receptor (IGFR), tumour necrosis factor receptor (TNFR) and oestrogen receptor/progesterone receptor (ER/PR). The mTOR system seems to achieve this by interacting with and modulating signal transduction by these growth factors and their receptors along the PI3K/Akt/NF-κB axis. On account of its being able to influence manifold signalling systems, mTOR inhibitors are seen as viable therapeutic tools on their own or in combination therapy (Fig. 1.2 and Epilogue Table 1).

I have placed much prominence on the part played by mTOR and receptor tyrosine kinase (RTK) inhibitors together with dual inhibitors of mTOR/PI3K in regulating angiogenesis apart from the exerting marked effects on tumour growth, both of which are unquestionably major elements in tumour progression. Hence much attention has been directed to target them for manipulation by therapeutic deployment of the inhibitors. For instance, suppressing the systems linked with EGFR family receptors is currently a proven beneficial mode of treatment in HER2+ primary breast cancers and central nervous system metastases. Conjugates of cytotoxic drugs with HER2 antibodies can be efficiently targeted to cancer cells overexpressing HER2 and are markedly cytotoxic and inhibit angiogenesis. The tropism of neural stem cells can be availed to target therapy to brain lesions. Neural stem cells can be genetically engineered to generate anti-cancer prodrugs and targeted and activated upon delivery.

Epilogue Table 1 An Overview of the Regulators of the mTOR Signalling in Cancer Initiation, Development and Progression

Positive regulators of mTOR
EGFR; IGFR IRS; VEGFR; TGF-β/endoglin
ER/PR
MTA; S100A4
Negative regulators of mTOR
AMPK; plumbagin; metformin
Hh/Smo inhibitors
Allosteric inhibitors of mTOR and RTKs
Dual mTOR/PI3K inhibitors
Drug laden neural stem cells
Signal transducing pathway
PI3K/Akt/NF-κB
Phenotypic outcome
EMT; CSCs; cell proliferation; survival; angiogenesis

This is an experimental but a novel approach to suppress brain metastases. It is needless to reiterate that the HER2/mTOR could provide a valuable route to patient management despite the occasional development of resistance to inhibitors of signalling. The IGF/IGFR/IRS signals interact with ER/PR and also operate the PI3K/Akt, the mitogen-activated protein kinase (MAPK) and the mTOR pathways to modulate the expression of apoptosis family genes. This actively raises the possibility that the crosstalk between these signalling systems might be the reason why the IGF/IGFR/IRS system has often been ascribed a role in the development of drug and radiation resistance of tumours.

A whole corpus of growth factors seems to come within the compass of mTOR (Fig. 1.2). Many selective RTK inhibitors have been identified for potential use in cancer treatment. Also available are inhibitors of specific signalling pathways. Appropriately, considerable attention has been devoted to the development of small molecule RTK inhibitors and some of them have been approved for clinical use. Several allosteric inhibitors of angiogenesis are known. Among them are inhibitors of the mTOR signalling pathway. RTK inhibitors suppress growth factor-mediated activation of PI3K/Akt/mTOR. Selective PI3K inhibitors may function differently from allosteric mTOR inhibitors. The mTOR kinase inhibitors can block mTOR and also suppress proliferation. The mTOR pathway interacts with growth factor receptor and ER signalling. So mTOR inhibitors can overcome the resistance to EGFR inhibition, possibly by suppressing Akt activation. There is considerable synergy between EGFR and mTOR inhibitors. This is valuable in dealing with ER − /EGFR + tumours. Triple negative breast cancers (TNBCs) can show enhanced EGFR expression. This synergy may benefit TNBC patients.

Selective inhibitors of mTOR are also known and indeed mTOR is often affected by inhibitors of the signalling systems it co-ordinates. Several clinical evaluations of combination of rapamycin analogues with RTK inhibitors as well as established chemotherapeutic agents are currently being carried out in many forms of early and advanced disease. The rapamycin analogues not only block mTOR signalling but also block Akt activation, possibly by attenuating the formation of the mTORC2 complex. Given the relatively moderate activity of the analogues in the clinical setting and that Akt functions upstream of mTORC1, combination of mTOR inhibitors with inhibitors of Akt have been evaluated. Studies are also being designed to look at the efficacy of combining mTOR inhibitors with trastuzumab in advanced breast cancer.

The function of these specific and transacting inhibitors have been discussed at the relevant locations in this tome. Besides this, some discussion has been directed to non-conventional agents and drugs, such as metformin, statins and bisphosphonates, used for the treatment of other pathological conditions. Resveratrol and curcumin and its analogues can target this signalling axis. Resveratrol can markedly interfere with mTOR signalling. It demonstrably suppresses NF-κB survival signalling. Curcumin induces apoptosis by the inhibition of the activations of Akt/mTOR and RAF/MEK/ERK. Both phytochemicals influence the IGF/IGFR/IRS axis. Of interest is the recognition that metformin, a conventional drug used in the treatment of type 2 diabetes, is also able to do that. The merit of metformin emanates from its ability to inhibit the relevant routes of signal transduction. It suppresses cell proliferation and cell survival signalling pathways, conspicuously PI3K/Akt/mTOR, MAPK/38-ERK and NF-κB. Working in conjunction with the tumour suppressor AMPK, metformin inhibits mTOR and possesses the potential to suppress CSC generation and propagation and can negate or mitigate resistance to mTOR inhibitors. Metformin does inhibit some angiogenic effectors, but it has not made the mark as an anti-angiogenic agent. Plumbagin suppresses NF-κB and possibly also Wnt/β-catenin signalling and inhibits invasion and angiogenesis. Combination of plumbagin with synergistically functional drugs has been explored and indeed open to further exploration. Plumbagin and metformin can collaboratively activate AMPK.

It is essential that one recognises the signalling diversity of any given response modifiers whilst devising therapeutic courses of action. It would be of interest that curcumin, resveratrol and quercetin might directly or indirectly suppress the activation of EMT and the generation and self-renewal of CSCs. This contention is amply supported by the seemingly paradoxical dual function of transforming growth factor (TGF)-β, the cybernetic interregulation of signalling outcomes and the emergence of biphasic or multiphasic and differential responses to the cytokine. The TGF-β effector proteins have offered some useful opportunities. However, TGF-β signalling by either or both canonical and non-canonical modes appears to depend upon the state of progression. One obfuscating factor is the presence of a self-regulatory mechanism involving the inhibitory Smad, which affects TGF-β action. Other inflammatory cytokines and growth factors such as EGF also come under the ambit of this self-regulatory mechanism. These issues may have limited the freedom of choosing the target. Nonetheless, the accessory receptors of the TGF-β pathway do provide discernible choices. Endoglin is a good illustration with its dual function in angiogenesis and in tumour progression. This could result from endoglin transducing its signal either by the canonical or the non-canonical route. Endoglin expression positively correlates with tumour progression and so explored for therapeutic targeting. It acts upstream of ALK5, hence inhibitors of activin-like kinases have been investigated as anti-tumour agents. The monoclonal antibodies against endoglin are a possible option.

Apoptosis is an essential element in health and disease. The deregulation of apoptosis leads to pathogenesis in several ways and importantly by the loss of the ability to delete cells in which genomic integrity is compromised. Apoptosis plays an important role in cell differentiation and embryonic development and morphogenesis. It is often quite legitimately termed as programmed cell death being strictly subject to genetic regulation together with a temporal element. The promotion or induction of apoptosis as an active means of controlling tumour growth is actively pursued. The use of cytotoxic drugs is an accepted form of treatment within the bounds of acceptable side effects. But the rapid advances in our understanding of the signalling systems have led to the exploration of new means of inducing apoptosis, besides tampering with the interacting systems.

TRAIL (TNF-related apoptosis inducing ligand) binds to and activates the so-called death receptors and induces apoptosis. This might be more than a means of inhibiting tumour growth. TNBCs displaying EMT are said to be sensitive to TRAIL-induced apoptosis. TRAIL is also an efficient suppresser of angiogenesis. Manipulation of signalling systems such as the MAPK cascade and the use of inhibitors of angiogenic pathways would enhance the effectiveness of TRAIL. This underscores the significance of the anti-tumour activity of recombinant TRAIL and agonistic death receptors antibodies and makes a valid claim for extending the present studies.

The developmental Hedgehog pathway of EMT activation and the generation of CSCs ought to be explored as a practical path to tumour initiation,

Epilogue Table 2 Angiogenic Pathways and Their Inhibitors in the Control of EMT Activation, CSC Biology and Tumour Growth

Signalling pathways
Hedgehog; SMO inhibitors LDE225, GDC-0449; cyclopamine analogue
IPI-926
Hippo; verteporfin inhibitor of YAP/TAZ
HIF-1/VEGF; thioredoxin inhibitor PX-12; pleurotin, inhibitor of thioredoxin reductase
Notch DLL γ-secretase inhibitor DAPT
HMG proteins
ID proteins
Trail death receptor agonists
Inhibitors
Allosteric inhibitors of mTOR, RTKs, dual mTOR/PI3K inhibitors
Endogenous inhibitors; TSPs; inhibitory kringles
Statins; bisphosphonates
Metformin
Suramin
Flavonoids
Selenoproteins

growth and progression (Epilogue Table 2). One can see effective approaches via both the canonical and non-canonical modes of its signalling. The SMO (smoothened, an element in Hedgehog signalling) inhibitors, LDE225 (sonidegib), GDC-0449 (vismodegib) and cyclopamine and the analogue IPI-926 (saridegib), are salient examples of successful suppressors of CSCs and EMT activation. Non-canonical pathways of activation of Gli give some additional leverage. The mTOR system also influences Hh (Hedgehog) signalling via Gli transcription. Angiopoietin-1 and angiopoietin-1-like protein have links with Hh signalling, CSCs, drug resistance and tumour progression. This wide spectrum of signalling interaction may enable synergistic inhibition of Hh.

The Hippo inhibits cell proliferation, promotes apoptosis and inhibits EMT and CSCs. The key event in the system is the suppression of the downstream effectors YAP/TAZ (Yes-associated protein/transcriptional co-activator with a PDZ-binding motif) and their ability to promote cell proliferation and survival. Hence, targeting of YAP/TAZ is an appealing prospect. The light activated drug verteporfin is an inhibitor of YAP/TAZ and has achieved some clinical success. But targeted delivery is not totally resolved. Conjugated with antibodies such as trastuzumab, verteporfin could target HER2 + tumours. Preliminary work has shown that verteporfin can be targeted to the endothelium, but directing the drug specifically to tumour-associated endothelium needs further thought. Bisphosphonate-mediated inhibition of YAP/TAZ is also an option. Some bisphononates do exhibit anti-angiogenic effects. But the perceived beneficial properties must be counterpoised with the serious side effects of the drugs (Epilogue Table 2).

Statins function within the mevalonate pathway and inhibit cholesterol synthesis. They markedly suppress cell migration and cell proliferation with induction of apoptosis. Statins and bisphosphonates, also inhibitors of cholesterol synthesis, restrain the activity of YAP/TAZ of Hippo signalling. The statins inhibit PI3K/Akt/mTOR signalling and possibly also induce apoptosis via the p38/MAPK route. They suppress NF-κB, cell adhesion and EMT activation. These findings have triggered the exploration of the clinical potential of statins. However, no unequivocal benefits have been noted. Low-grade pancreatic ductal adenocarcinoma has shown response to statins. Possibly more pre-clinical and clinical evaluations might be helpful to determine a future course of action.

The deregulation of Notch signalling leads to stem cell maintenance and propagation, cell proliferation, EMT activation and angiogenesis. The Notch ICD (the intracellular domain)/CSL transcription factor complex activates the relevant genes. The ICD is cleaved by γ-secretase. These effects are counteracted by inhibitors of γ-secretase, such as DAPT. Monoclonal antibodies against the Delta4 ligand of Notch reportedly inhibit the growth of tumours.* The thioredoxin-interacting protein (TXNIP) inhibits the NF-κB pathway. It inhibits thioredoxin and this inhibits cell proliferation and promotes apoptosis. But TXNIP is downregulated in tumours. So, attempts have been made to circumvent this by using thioredoxin inhibitors such as PX-12 or by inhibiting thioredoxin reductase, which activates thioredoxin, using pleurotin, a natural product of the mushroom *Pleurotus ostreatus*.

The generation of stem cells seems temporally to correspond with EMT activation and tumour progression. Hedgehog, Wnt, Notch, Akt/mTOR and miRNAs signalling are associated with both EMT activation and CSC development. Hence, targeting stem cells and suppressing resistance to therapy by interfering with these signalling pathways could be viable approaches. Salinomycin, a putative CSC inhibitor, targets Hedgehog signalling. Rapamycin and GDC-0449 (vismodegib) also suppress Hedgehog and mTOR pathways and synergistically inhibit CSCs. CSCs display tissue-specific tropism. This could provide a road to targeted delivery of drugs and antibodies to tumours. The benefits of combining chemotherapy with stem cell therapy have been debated but there are no reports of clear response. Some transcription factors involved with CSCs have been suggested as therapeutic targets. Of note are Sp1 and the Ets family transcription factors. The bHLH (basic helix loop helix (transcription factors)) neurogenins have also attracted much attention. Stem cell therapy is still in its infancy.

The immunomodulatory and anti-inflammatory thalidomides need to be scrutinised for their anti-cancer effects. They lower immune resistance of tumour by targeting immune checkpoint proteins, and suppress evasion of immune surveillance. They inhibit angiogenesis, cell invasion and metastasis and promote apoptosis by the conventional signalling routes. Combination with mTOR inhibition seems beneficial in multiple myeloma and other B-cell malignancies. However, more attention is needed to design drugs with reduced cytotoxicity and effective at low doses taking adequate note of the chiral stability of new analogues.

There is much discernible progress with inhibitors of checkpoint proteins. Tumours adopt certain immune checkpoint pathways especially against tumour-specific T cells. This leads to immune resistance. The CD28 family proteins PD1/CTLA4/BTLA and their ligands have held the sway in immunotherapy.

Anti-PD1 and anti-CTLA4 are antibodies being clinically evaluated. The ligand VISTA with homology to PD-L1 is in focus. Pre-clinical work has shown that its inhibition suppresses tumour growth and enhances host survival. The practical elucidation of the involved effective pathways has indicated some useful points of furthering research endeavour. Some inhibitors

Epilogue Table 3 Modes of Immunotherapy and Their Inhibitors

Immune checkpoint pathways
CD28 family PD1 CTLA4 BTLA proteins
Nivolumab; Pembrolizumab (PD1 monoclonal antibodies)
Ipilimumab (CTLA4 monoclonal antibody)
CD47/SIRP
TSP-1
Toll-like receptors
Imiquimod

function by the cereblon/lenalidomide path and the B-Raf-mediated MAPK inhibition. B-Raf inhibitors have been beneficially combined with the CTLA4 monoclonal antibody ipilimumab. CD47/SIRP-α evades immune surveillance. Blocking SIRP overcomes this. Clinical trials have emphasised the potential of combining checkpoints inhibitors with conventional chemotherapy (Epilogue Table 3).

Several extraneous inhibitors have proved their utility in the control of cancer growth in vitro and in pre-clinical models. Suramin inhibits the function of many growth factors including VEGF and bFGF and suppresses endothelial cell proliferation and angiogenesis. Suramin/bevacizumab combination has been tested in animal tumour models. Some flavonoids are gaining currency at least at the experimental level. Silymarin modulates CSC, EMT and cell proliferation pathways. It is effective at very low concentrations when combined with conventional therapeutic agents. This is positive for its safety profile. The selenoproteins inhibit cell proliferation by inhibiting ERα and PI3K/Akt signalling and induce apoptosis by activating the Bcl-apoptosis and Trail pathways. The suppression of angiogenesis seems to occur by the suppression of VEGF/FGF and the uPA/uPAI pathways. The selenium-binding protein 1 may have links with EMT suppression. Some clinical trials have investigated the effects of selenium compounds on tumour growth after resection and tumour recurrence and as potential aids for cancer prevention. There are no definitive and definable results.

Angiogenesis is a single most critical event in tumour growth and secondary spread. The concept of inhibiting angiogenesis to control tumour growth and metastasis is not new. Several signalling pathways are involved in the induction of angiogenesis, including crucial aspects relating to endothelial cell survival, migration and endothelial barrier function. Again these signalling pathways are co-ordinated by mTOR. The practical value of this is emphasised in the context of evolving new treatment strategies. As stated at the beginning of this epilogue, the signalling systems are not mutually exclusive in terms of the phenotypic effects they create or the physiological definition or distinction they deliver. Angiogenesis is a concomitant phenomenon of the activation of EMT and the generation, propagation and maintenance of CSCs. The biological effects of naturally occurring inhibitors, endogenously produced inhibitors, monoclonal antibodies raised against angiogenic agents are described together with clinical benefits of their deployment as therapeutic agents.

Rather disconcertingly some signalling systems with apparent significant link to the regulation of angiogenesis have not made the mark. Notable are Hedgehog, Hippo and TRAIL. But then the aim here is to predicate the presence of possibilities of beneficial approaches. This applies equally to other effectors of angiogenesis. For instance, thioredoxin aids cell proliferation with inhibition of apoptosis. It induces HIF-1 and VEGF and promotes angiogenesis. It is activated by thioredoxin reductase. Pleurotin, a reversible inhibitor of thioredoxin reductase, and the thioredoxin inhibitor PX-12 inhibit HIF-1 and HIF-induced VEGF production. PX-12 has not made the mark in the clinical setting. Some potential benefits of PX-12 have been identified but little progress can be noted. COX-2 has been linked with EMT activation and the generation of CSCs with implications for drug resistance. The COX-2 inhibitors celecoxib and apricoxib reputedly reverse EMT. Celecoxib together with VEGFR inhibition has had some success. Inhibitors of mTOR are said to potentiate the effects of celecoxib. Inhibition by curcumin, resveratrol and quercetin has also been attempted. The COX-2 inhibition approach has proved rather discouraging. The TRAIL, PTEN/Akt and PDCD4 pathways are seemingly involved in COX-2 function are still open to exploration. The search for small molecule inhibitors of angiogenesis has extended to inhibition of VEGFA by bevazimuab and of MMP signalling by marimastat and prinomastat, among others. Tackling of MMPs has not been particularly successful at the clinical level.

Some endogenous inhibitors of angiogenesis that have been extensively studied also suppress EMT activation and CSCs. The signalling systems they operate and their phenotypic outcome have been largely elucidated. Some of the follow-up of these studies is worthy of note. The TSPs and the mimetic drugs containing TSRs (TSP repeat elements) are being evaluated for therapeutic use as single agents or in combination with established angiogenesis inhibitors. However, the pursuit of the utility of collagen-derived inhibitors is uninspiring. Endostatin and the recombinant Endostar actively inhibit angiogenesis. So do angiostatin, a cleavage product of plasminogen, and its kringles 1–5.

The strategy to target regulators of genetic transcriptional activity apparently closely related to tumour growth and progression has not unexpectedly surfaced with some interesting findings. The HMG (high mobility group) proteins are transcriptional regulators. HMGAs bind to the AT-rich regions of the minor groove of the DNA. HMGA2 is overexpressed in some cancers. It regulates the cell cycle, activates EMT and promotes cancer invasion and metastasis. Its expression correlates with clinical stage, nodal involvement and prognosis. Some competitive inhibitors of HMGA2 such as netropsin, distamycin and berenil also inhibit tumour growth. Their anti-microbial effects have been studied. But understandably, there are concerns about possible mutagenic effects of these agents.

Although remote they might seem to the control of tumour biology, one ought to allude to the bHLH transcription factors, the IDs (inhibitors of DNA-binding proteins). Of the ID family, IDs 1–3 appear to promote angiogenesis, activate EMT and support the maintenance and expansion of CSCs, but ID4 inhibits angiogenesis. There is much experimental support for this view. But inhibition of the tumour promoter IDs or re-expression ID4 by targeted demethylation are viewed with much reservation as a possible approach.

In the context of the genetic activity associated with the tumour phenomenon, many tumour promoter and suppressor genes have been identified and their function dissected in detail in numerous works. But in the midst of this multiplicity, I have chosen to discuss two tumour promoter genes, viz. MTA and S100A4 on account of the extensive span of their signalling generating a wide spectrum of biological effects. The MTAs are metastasis-associated genes. MTA1 promotes EMT activation, tumour cell proliferation and survival, and invasion, whilst MTA3 inhibits EMT. MTA1 signalling interacts with Wnt/E-cadherin/β-catenin, Hh, notch, cell cycle regulatory and growth factor receptor and ER pathways. This signalling span emphasises the value of MTA1. In clinical samples, MTA1 expression has been debatably reported to correlate with angiogenesis, aggressive disease with risk of recurrence. Nonetheless, engaging MTA expression beneficially is also underway. Gadolinium metallofullerenol nanoparticles have been claimed to be able to suppress metastasis of pancreatic cancer, with parallel suppression of MTA1 and HIF-1α. Resveratrol inhibits MTA1 and reinstates the PI3K/Akt inhibitory action of PTEN. The LMP2A protein of Epstein–Barr virus 2 promotes EMT with mTOR intervention. Possibly mTOR inhibitors could be of use in nasopharyngeal tumours to the pathogenesis of which the virus is aetiologically linked.

The calcium-binding protein S100A4 is overexpressed due to epigenetic hypomethylation in correlation with tumour progression. S100A4 regulates cell proliferation, EMT activation, invasion and metastasis. The p53/stathmin, the apoptosis family genes and PI3K/Akt/mTOR are among the operational pathways. S100A4 modulates cytoskeletal dynamics. It activates angiogenic factors and endothelial cell proliferation. The S1004/RAGE/VEGFA is active in endothelial proliferation and angiogenesis. The inhibition of RAGE suppresses S100A4-induced angiogenesis. In vitro and xenografts studies show that niclosamide targets the Wnt/β-catenin pathway and suppresses S100A4-mediated promotion of invasion. Niclosamide also suppresses proliferative and angiogenic signalling. It inhibits EMT activation and CSCs. Among other potential agents are monoclonal S100A4 antibodies, sulindac and flavonoids. Fumagillin inhibits angiogenesis possibly by targeting methionine aminopeptidase-2 overexpressed in tumours. S100A4 binds the peptidase, postulating a potential route to inhibiting angiogenesis. These are novel approaches commended for further pre-clinical evaluation.

A few concluding words to define the structure and execution of this book might not be deemed as extravagant. It is essential to appreciate the diversity of research being pursued to identify viable molecular approaches to effectively modulate the signalling systems that influence tumour biology. This would mean recognising both the evolving and progressing areas and the overt and hidden fault lines. This is the driving force behind my motivation and execution of the book. The basic challenge I have set myself is to integrate the different aspects of tumour growth and progression and focus on the salient nodes of signalling that are amenable to beneficial manipulation. In other words, I have attempted to personally experience and hopefully provide the readership a good feel for the state of the art; hence, the brief but an intelligible and inclusive title.

The book is designed for someone with scientific background, but not for the lay person. I have provided a good background of basic information of the signalling systems involved and the molecular pathology of the growth and progression of cancer as a prelude in each section of the book before delving into practical propositions about how the aberrant aspects can be prioritised and targeted for novel therapy. To indulge in some reiteration, my effort has been to identify the foci in the signalling systems and its components that are in my view worthy of further exploration. These are what I call the growing points. I have discussed many factors that seemed interesting prima facie and were pursued by some in that perception, but had not proved their potential. In essence this has meant being selective in the discussion of works based on criteria of credibility and appropriateness for the topic. With this in mind, I have provided an overall summary of my assessment of the clinical value of each topic. Finally, in this epilogue I have attempted an integration of the concept of the molecular approach to cancer management, and the assessment, analysis and evaluation of the potential clinical benefits that could accrue from extending the boundaries of the molecular approach to some seemingly intractable problems and conundrums. Most importantly, my primary aim is to help to focus on what the readers, the graduate student, the researcher and the clinician might like to see and be interested in and find most beneficial. I do hope I have succeeded in that.

References

Abbes, M., Baati, H., Guermazi, S., Messina, C., Santulli, A., Gharsallah, N., et al., 2013. Biological properties of carotenoids extracted from Halobacterium halobium isolated from a Tunisian solar saltern. BMC Complement. Alternative Med. 13, art. no. 255.

Abu El-Asrar, A.M., Mohammad, G., Nawaz, M.I., Siddiquei, M.M., 2015. High mobility group box-1 modulates the expression of inflammatory and angiogenic signalling pathways in diabetic retina. Curr. Eye Res. 40, 1141–1152.

Adams, J.C., Lawler, J., 2011. The thrombospondins. Cold Spring Harbor Perspect Biol. . Available from: http://dx.doi.org/10.1101/cshperspect.a009712.

Adams, S., Kozhaya, L., Martiniuk, F., Meng, T.C., Chiriboga, L., Liebes, L., et al., 2012. Topical TLR7 agonist imiquimod can induce immune-mediated rejection of skin metastases in patients with breast cancer. Clin. Cancer Res. 18, 6748–6757.

Adler, J.J., Johnson, D.E., Heller, B.L., Bringman, L.R., Ranahan, W.P., Conwell, M.D., et al., 2013. Serum deprivation inhibits the transcriptional co-activator YAP and cell growth via phosphorylation of the 130-kDa isoform of Angiomotin by the LATS1/2 protein kinases. Proc. Natl Acad. Sci. USA 110, 17368–17373.

Aggarwal, B.B., Bhatt, I.D., Ichikawa, H., Ahn, K.S., Sethi, G., Sandur, S.K., et al., 2007. Curcumin: biological and medicinal properties. In: Babu, K.N., Ravindran, N., Sivarama, K. (Eds.), Turmeric; the Genus Curcuma. CRC Press, New York, 297–368.

Aikio, M., Alahuhta, I., Nurmenniemi, S., Suojanen, J., Palovuori, R., Teppo, S., et al., 2012. Arresten, a collagen-derived angiogenesis inhibitor, suppresses invasion of squamous cell carcinoma. PLoS One 7, art. no. e51044.

Algotar, A.M., Stratton, M.S., Ahmann, F.R., Ranger-Moore, J., Nagle, R.B., Thompson, P.A., et al., 2013. Phase 3 clinical trial investigating the effect of selenium supplementation in men at high-risk for prostate cancer. The Prostate 73, 328–335.

Alonso, N., Guillen, R., Chambers, J.W., Leng, F., 2015. A rapid and sensitive high-throughput screening method to identify compounds targeting protein–nucleic acids interactions. Nucleic Acids Res. 43, DOI 10.1093/nar/gkv069.

Amaoka, N., Osada, S., Kanematsu, M., Imai, H., Tomita, H., Tokuyama, Y., et al., 2007. Clinicopathological features of hepatocellular carcinoma evaluated by vascular endothelial growth factor expression. J. Gastroenterol. Hepatol. 22, 2202–2207.

Amato, R.J., Hernandez-McClain, J., Saxena, S., Khan, M., 2008. Lenalidomide therapy for metastatic renal cell carcinoma. Am. J. Clin. Oncol. Cancer Clin. Trials 31, 244–249.

Ambrosio, M.R., Di Serio, C., Danza, G., Rocca, B.J., Ginori, A., Prudovsky, I., et al., 2016. Carbonic anhydrase IX is a marker of hypoxia and correlates with higher Gleason scores and ISUP grading in prostate cancer. Diagnostic Pathol. 11, art. no. 45.

Ameis, H.M., Drenckhan, A., Freytag, M., Izbicki, J.R., Supuran, C.T., Reinshagen, K., et al., 2016. Carbonic anhydrase IX correlates with survival and is a potential therapeutic target for neuroblastoma. J. Enzyme Inhib. Med. Chem. 31, 404–409.

Andersen, K.C., 2005. Lenalidomide and thalidomide: mechanisms of action–similarities and differences. Semin. Hematol. 42, S3–8.

Ando, T., Ito, H., Arioka, Y., Ogiso, H., Seishima, M., 2015. Combination therapy with alpha-galactosylceramide and a Toll-like receptor agonist exerts an augmented suppressive effect on lung tumor metastasis in a mouse model. Oncol. Rep. 33, 826–832.

Andre, F., O'Regan, R., Ozguroglu, M., Toi, M., Xu, B.H., Jerusalem, G., et al., 2014. Everolimus for women with trastuzumab-resistant, HER2-positive, advanced breast cancer (BOLERO-3): a randomised, double-blind, placebo-controlled phase 3 trial. Lancet Oncol. 15, 580–591.

Anfossi, S., Giordano, A., Gao, H., Cohen, E.N., Tin, S., Wu, Q., et al., 2014. High serum miR-19a levels are associated with inflammatory breast cancer and are predictive of favorable clinical outcome in patients with metastatic HER2(+) inflammatory breast cancer. PLoS One 9, art. no. e83113.

Anido, J., Saez-Borderias, A., Gonzalez-Junca, A., Rodon, L., Folch, G., Carmona, M.A., et al., 2010. TGF-b receptor inhibitors target the CD44(high)/Id1(high) glioma-initiating cell population in human glioblastoma. Cancer Cell 18, 655–668.

Ansell, P.J., Zhang, H., Davidson, D.J., Harlan, J.E., Xue, J., Brodjian, S., et al., 2010. Recombinant kringle 5 from plasminogen antagonises hepatocyte growth factor-mediated signalling. Eur. J. Cancer 46, 966–973.

Apsel, B., Blair, J.A., Gonzalez, B., Nazif, T.M., Feldman, M.E., Aizenstein, B., et al., 2008. Targeted polypharmacology: discovery of dual inhibitors of tyrosine and phosphoinositide kinases. Nat. Chem. Biol. 4, 691–699.

Ardini, E., Menichincheri, M., Banfi, P., Bosotti, R., De Ponti, C., Pulci, R., et al., 2016. Entrectinib, a pan-TRK, ROS1, and ALK inhibitor with activity in multiple molecularly defined cancer indications. Mol. Cancer Ther. 15, 628–639.

Armand, P., 2015. Immune checkpoint blockade in hematologic malignancies. Blood 125, 3393–3400.

Arumugam, T., Simeone, D.M., Schmidt, A.M., Logsdon, C.D., 2004. S100P stimulates cell proliferation and survival via receptor for activated glycation end products (RAGE). J. Biol. Chem. 279, 5059–5065.

Arumugam, T., Ramachandran, V., Gomez, S.B., Schmidt, A.M., Logsdon, C.D., 2012. S100P-derived RAGE antagonistic peptide reduces tumor growth and metastasis. Clin. Cancer Res. 18, 4356–4364.

Assadian, S., El-Assaad, W., Wang, X.Q.D., Gannon, P.O., Barres, V., Latour, M., et al., 2012. p53 Inhibits angiogenesis by inducing the production of arresten. Cancer Res. 72, 1270–1279.

Atari-Hajipirloo, S., Nikanfar, S., Heydari, A., Noori, F., Kheradmand, F., 2016. The effect of celecoxib and its combination with imatinib on human HT-29 colorectal cancer cells: involvement of COX-2, Caspase-3, VEGF and NF-kappa B genes expression. Cell Mol. Biol. 62, 68–74.

Atawia, R.T., Tadros, M.G., Khalifa, A.E., Mosli, H.A., Abdel-Naim, A.B., 2013. Role of the phytoestrogenic, pro-apoptotic and anti-oxidative properties of silymarin in inhibiting experimental benign prostatic hyperplasia in rats. Toxicol. Lett. 219, 160–169.

Atkins, M.B., Gravis, G., Drosik, K., Demkow, T., Tomczak, P., Wong, S.S., et al., 2015. Trebananib (AMG 386) in combination with sunitinib in patients with metastatic renal cell cancer: an open-label, multicenter, phase II study. J. Clin. Oncol. 33, 3431–3438.

Attarha, S., Andersson, S., Mints, M., Souchelnytskyi, S., 2014. Mammalian sterile-like 1 kinase inhibits TGF beta and EGF-dependent regulation of invasiveness, migration and proliferation of HEC-1-A endometrial cancer cells. Int. J. Oncol. 45, 853–860.

Aversa, C., Rossi, V., Geuna, E., Martinello, R., Milani, A., Redana, S., et al., 2014. Metastatic breast cancer subtypes and central nervous system metastases. Breast 23, 623–628.

Aziz, M.H., Dreckschmidt, N.E., Verma, A.K., 2008. Plumbagin, a medicinal plant-derived naphthoquinone, is a novel inhibitor of the growth and invasion of hormone-refractory prostate cancer. Cancer Res. 68, 9024–9032.

Azzoni, C., Bottarelli, L., Cecchini, S., Lagrasta, C., Pizzi, S., D'Adda, T., et al., 2011. Involvement of HER2/neu and metastasis-related proteins in the development of ileal neuroendocrine tumors. Virchows Archiv 458, 525–536.

Baccelli, I., Stenzinger, A., Vogel, V., Pfitzner, B.M., Klein, C., Wallwiener, M., et al., 2014. Co-expression of MET and CD47 is a novel prognosticator for survival of luminal-type breast cancer patients. Oncotarget 5, 8147–8160.

Bachelot, T., McCool, R., Duffy, S., Glanville, J., Varley, D., Fleetwood, K., et al., 2014. Comparative efficacy of everolimus plus exemestane versus fulvestrant for hormone-receptor-positive advanced breast cancer following progression/recurrence after endocrine therapy: a network meta-analysis. Breast Cancer Res. Treat. 143, 125–133.

Bachmann, C., Grischke, E.M., Fehm, T., Staebler, A., Schittenhelm, J., Wallwiener, D., 2013. CNS metastases of breast cancer show discordant immunohistochemical phenotype compared to primary. J. Cancer Res. Clin. Oncol. 139, 551–556.

Bachran, C., Leppla, S.H., 2016. Tumor targeting and drug delivery by anthrax toxin. Toxins 8, art. no. 197.

Badura, S., Tesanovic, T., Pfeifer, H., Wystub, S., Nijmeijer, A.B., Liebermann, M., et al., 2013. Differential effects of selective inhibitors targeting the PI3K/AKT/mTOR pathway in acute lymphoblastic leukemia. PLoS One 8, e80070.

Baker, A.F., Dragovich, T., Tate, W.R., Ramanathan, R.K., Roe, D., Hsu, C.H., et al., 2006. The antitumor thioredoxin-1 inhibitor PX-12 (1-methylpropyl 2-imidazolyl disulfide) decreases thioredoxin-1 and VEGF levels in cancer patient plasma. J. Lab. Clin. Med. 147, 83–90.

Baker, A.F., Adab, K.N., Raghunand, N., Chow, H.H.S., Stratton, S.P., Squire, S.W., et al., 2013. A phase IB trial of 24-hour intravenous PX-12, a thioredoxin-1 inhibitor, in patients with advanced gastrointestinal cancers. Invest. New Drugs 31, 631–641.

Baker, L.H., Rowinsky, E.K., Mendelson, D., Humerickhouse, R.A., Knight, R.A., Qian, J., et al., 2008. Randomized, phase II study of the thrombospondin-1-mimetic angiogenesis inhibitor ABT-510 in patients with advanced soft tissue sarcoma. J. Clin. Oncol. 26, 5583–5588.

Bakker, M.F., Peeters, P.H.M., Klaasen, V.M., Bueno-de-Mesquita, H.B., Jansen, E.H.J.M., Ros, M. M., et al., 2016. Plasma carotenoids, vitamin C, tocopherols, and retinol and the risk of breast cancer in the European Prospective Investigation into Cancer and Nutrition cohort. Am. J. Clin. Nutrit. 103, 454–464.

Baksh, K., Weber, J., 2015. Immune checkpoint protein inhibition for cancer: preclinical justification for CTLA-4 and PD1 blockade and new combinations. Semin. Oncol. 42, 363–377.

Bao, Y., Peng, F., Zhou, Q.C., Yu, Z.H., Li, J.C., Cheng, Z.B., et al., 2015. Phase II trial of recombinant human endostatin in combination with concurrent chemoradiotherapy in patients with stage III non-small-cell lung cancer. Radiother. Oncol. 114, 161–166.

Barbera, M.J., Puig, I., Dominguez, D., Julien-Grille, S., Guaita-Esteruelas, S., Peiro, S., et al., 2004. Regulation of Snail transcription during epithelial to mesenchymal transition of tumor cells. Oncogene 23, 7345–7354.

Barclay, A.N., Brown, M.H., 2006. The SIRP family of receptors and immune regulation. Nat. Rev. Immunol. 6, 457–464.

Barnholz-Sloan, J.S., Sloan, A.E., Davis, F.G., Vigneau, F.D., Lai, P., Swaya, R.E., 2004. Incidence proportions of brain metastases in patients diagnosed (1973 to 2001) in the metropolitan detroit cancer surveillance system. J. Clin. Oncol. 22, 2865–2872.

Barok, M., Joensuu, H., Isola, J., 2014. Trastuzumab emtansine: mechanisms of action and drug resistance. Breast Cancer Res. 16, art. no. R22.

Batsaikhan, B.E., Yoshikawa, K., Kurita, N., Iwata, T., Takasu, C., Kashihara, H., 2014. Cyclopamine decreased the expression of sonic Hedgehog and its downstream genes in colon cancer stem cells. Anticancer Res. 34, 6339–6344.

Behr, C.A., Hesketh, A.J., Barlow, M., Glick, R.D., Symons, M., Steinberg, B.M., 2015. Celecoxib inhibits Ewing sarcoma cell migration via actin modulation. J. Surg. Res. 198, 424–433.

Belmont, L., Rabbe, N., Antoine, M., Cathelin, D., Guignabert, C., Kurie, J., et al., 2014. Expression of TLR9 in tumor-infiltrating mononuclear cells enhances angiogenesis and is associated with a worse survival in lung cancer. Int. J. Cancer. 134 (4), 765–777.

Benedito, R., Roca, C., Sorensen, I., Adams, S., Gossller, A., Fruttiger, M., et al., 2009. The Notch ligands Dll4 and Jagged1 have opposing effects on angiogenesis. Cell 137, 1124–1135.

Berghoff, A.S., Bartsch, R., Preusser, M., Ricken, G., Steger, G.G., Bago-Horvath, Z., et al., 2014. Co-overexpression of HER2/HER3 is a predictor of impaired survival in breast cancer patients. Breast 23, 637–843.

Berlingieri, M.T., Manfioletti, G., Santoro, M., Bandiera, A., ViscontiR, Giancotti, V., et al., 1995. Inhibition of HMGI-C protein synthesis suppresses retrovirally induced neoplastic transformation of rat thyroid cells. Mol. Cell. Biol. 15, 1545–1553.

Berry, D.A., Ueno, N.T., Johnson, M.M., Lei, X., Caputo, J., Smith, D.A., et al., 2011. High-dose chemotherapy with autologous hematopoietic stem-cell transplantation in metastatic breast cancer: overview of six randomized trials. J. Clin. Oncol. 29, 3224–3231.

Bhat, T.A., Nambiar, D., Tailor, D., Pal, A., Agarwal, R., Singh, R.P., 2013. Acacetin inhibits in vitro and in vivo angiogenesis and downregulates Stat signaling and VEGF expression. Cancer Prevent. Res. 6, 1128–1139.

Bi, W.Z., Li, D.A.W., Luo, S., Song, Z.G., Wang, Y., Jin, H., et al., 2015. A high risk of osteosarcoma in individuals who are homozygous for the p.D104N in endostatin. Sci. Rep. 5, art. no. 16392.

Bianco, R., Garofalo, S., Rosa, R., Damiano, V., Gelardi, T., Daniele, G., et al., 2008. Inhibition of mTOR pathway by everolimus cooperates with EGFR inhibitors in human tumours sensitive and resistant to anti-EGFR drugs. Br. J. Cancer 98, 923–930.

Bieging, K.T., Mello, S.S., Attardi, L.D., 2014. Unravelling mechanisms of p53-mediated tumour suppression. Nat. Rev. Cancer 14, 359–370.

Bielawski, K., Bielawska, A., 2008. Small-molecule based delivery systems for alkylating antineoplastic compounds. Chem. Med. Chem. 3, 536–542.

Bilandzic, M., Wang, Y., Ahmed, N., Luwor, R.B., Zhu, H.J., Findlay, J.K., et al., 2014. Betaglycan blocks metastatic behavior in human granulosa cell tumors by suppressing NFkappaB-mediated induction of MMP2. Cancer Lett. 354, 107–114.

Bin Hafeez, B., Jamal, M.S., Fischer, J.W., Mustafa, A., Verma, A.K., 2012. Plumbagin, a plant derived natural agent inhibits the growth of pancreatic cancer cells in in vitro and in vivo via targeting EGFR, Stat3 and NF-κB signaling pathways. Int. J. Cancer 131, 2175–2186.

Bin Hafeez, B., Fischer, J.W., Singh, A., Zhong, W., Mustafa, A., Meske, L., et al., 2015. Plumbagin inhibits prostate carcinogenesis in intact and castrated PTEN knockout mice via targeting PKC epsilon, Stat3, and epithelial-to-mesenchymal transition markers. Cancer Prevent. Res. 8, 375–386.

Biscetti, F., Flex, A., Pecorini, G., Angelini, F., Arena, V., Stigliano, E., et al., 2016. The role of high-mobility group box protein 1 in collagen antibody-induced arthritis is dependent on vascular endothelial growth factor. Clin. Exp. Immunol. 184, 62–72.

Biswas, D.K., Cruz, A.P., Gansberger, E., Pardee, A.B., 2000. Epidermal growth factor induced nuclear factor kappa B activation: a major pathway of cell-cycle progression in estrogen-receptor negative breast cancer cells. Proc. Natl Acad. Sci. USA 97, 8542–8547.

Blackhall, F., Cappuzzo, F., 2016. Crizotinib: from discovery to accelerated development to front-line treatment. Ann. Oncol. 27, 35–41.

Bocca, C., Bozzo, F., Cannito, S., Parola, M., Miglietta, A., 2012. Celecoxib inactivates epithelial-mesenchymal transition stimulated by hypoxia and/or epidermal growth factor in colon cancer cells. Mol. Carcinogenesis 51, 783–795.

Bono, F., De Smet, F., Herbert, C., De Bock, K., Georgiadou, M., Fons, P., et al., 2013. Inhibition of tumor angiogenesis and growth by a small-molecule multi-FGF receptor blocker with allosteric properties. Cancer Cell. 23, 477–488.

Bora-Singhal, N., Nguyen, J., Schaal, C., Perumal, D., Singh, S., Coppola, D., et al., 2015. YAP1 regulates OCT4 activity and SOX2 expression to facilitate self-renewal and vascular mimicry of stem-like cells. Stem Cells 33, 1705–1718.

Bowles, D.W., Keysar, S.B., Eagles, J.R., Wang, G.L., Glogowska, M.J., McDermott, J.D., et al., 2016. A pilot study of cetuximab and the hedgehog inhibitor IPI-926 in recurrent/metastatic head and neck squamous cell carcinoma. Oral Oncol. 53, 74–79.

Brackett, C.M., Kojouharov, B., Veith, J., Greene, K.F., Burdelya, L.G., Gollnick, S.O., et al., 2016. Toll-like receptor-5 agonist, entolimod, suppresses metastasis and induces immunity by stimulating an NK-dendritic-CD8(+) T-cell axis. Proc. Natl. Acad. Sci. U.S.A. 113, E874–E883.

Brassart-Pasco, S., Senechal, K., Thevenard, J., Ramont, L., Devy, J., Di Stefano, L., et al., 2012. Tetrastatin, the NC1 domain of the alpha 4(IV) collagen chain: a novel potent anti-tumor matrikine. PLoS One 7, art. no. e29587.

Bratt, A., Wilson, W.J., Troyanovsky, B., Aase, K., Kessler, R., Van Meir, E.G., et al., 2002. Angiomotin belongs to a novel protein family with conserved coiled-coil and PDZ binding domains. Gene 298, 69–77.

Breen, M.J., Moran, D.M., Liu, W.Z., Huang, X.K., Vary, C.P.H., Bergan, R.C., 2013. Endoglin-mediated suppression of prostate cancer invasion is regulated by activin and bone morphogenetic protein type II receptors. PLoS One 8, art. no. e72407.

Brouxhon, S.M., Kyrkanides, S., Teng, X., Athar, M., Ghazizadeh, S., Simon, M., et al., 2014. Soluble E-cadherin: a critical oncogene modulating receptor tyrosine kinases, MAPK and PI3K/Akt/mTOR signalling. Oncogene 33, 225–235.

Bryden, F., Maruani, A., Savoie, H., Chudasama, V., Smith, M.E.B., Caddick, S., et al., 2014. Regioselective and stoichiometrically controlled conjugation of photodynamic sensitizers to a HER2 targeting antibody fragment. Bioconjugate Chem. 25, 611–617.

Buchsbaum, D.J., Zhou, T., Grizzle, W.E., Oliver, P.G., Hammond, C.J., Zhang, S., et al., 2003. Antitumor efficacy of TRA-8 anti-DR5 monoclonal antibody alone or in combination with chemotherapy and/or radiation therapy in a human breast cancer model. Clin. Cancer Res. 9, 3731–3741.

Bueno, L., de Alwis, D.P., Pitou, C., Yingling, J., Lahn, M., Glatt, S., et al., 2008. Semi-mechanistic modelling of the tumour growth inhibitory effects of LY2157299, a new type I receptor TGF-β kinase antagonist in mice. Eur. J. Cancer 44, 142–1560.

Busch, A., Zeh, D., Janzen, V., Mugge, L.O., Wolf, D., Fingerhut, L., et al., 2014. Treatment with lenalidomide induces immunoactivating and counter-regulatory immunosuppressive changes in myeloma patients. Clin. Exp. Immunol. 177, 439–453.

Byun, M.R., Hwang, J.H., Kim, A.R., Kim, K.M., Hwang, E.S., Yaffe, M.B., et al., 2014. Canonical Wnt signalling activates TAZ through PP1A during osteogenic differentiation. Cell Death Diff. 21, 854–863.

Cai, G., Freeman, G.J., 2009. The CD160, BTLA, LIGHT/HVEM pathway: a bidirectional switch regulating T-cell activation. Immunol. Rev. 229, 244–258.

Cai, X.B., Hu, X., Tan, X.J., Cheng, W.J., Wang, Q.J., Chen, X.F., et al., 2015. Metformin induced AMPK activation, G0/G1 phase cell cycle arrest and the inhibition of growth of oesophageal squamous cell carcinomas in vitro and in vivo. PLoS One 10, art. no. e0133349.

Cain, R.J., Vanhaesebroeck, B., Ridley, A.J., 2010. The PI3K p110 alpha isoform regulates endothelial adherens junctions via Pyk2 and Rac1. J. Cell Biol. 188, 863–876.

Campbell, N., Greenaway, J., Henkin, J., Petrik, J., 2011. ABT-898 induces tumor regression and prolongs survival in a mouse model of epithelial ovarian cancer. Mol. Cancer Therap. 10, 1876–1885.

Cao, L., Zhou, Y., Zhai, B., Liao, J., Xu, W., Zhang, R., et al., 2011. Sphere-forming cell subpopulations with cancer stem cell properties in human hepatoma cell lines. BMC Gastroenterol. 11, art. no. 71.

Cao, Y.B., Qu, J.L., Li, C., Yang, D., Hou, K.Z., Zheng, H.C., et al., 2015. Celecoxib sensitizes gastric cancer to rapamycin via inhibition of the Cbl-b-regulated PI3K/Akt pathway. Tumor Biol. 36, 5607–5615.

Carbone, C., Piro, G., Fassan, M., Tamburrino, A., Mina, M.M., Zanotto, M., et al., 2015. An angiopoietin-like protein 2 autocrine signaling promotes EMT during pancreatic ductal carcinogenesis. Oncotarget 6, 13822–13834.

Cardillo, T.M., Trisal, P., Arrojo, R., Goldenberg, D.M., Chang, C.H., 2013. Targeting both IGF-1R and mTOR synergistically inhibits growth of renal cell carcinoma in vitro. BMC Cancer 13, art. no. 170.

Carey, D.J., 1997. Syndecans: multifunctional cell-surface co-receptors. Biochem. J. 327, 1–16.

Caronongan III, A., Venturini, B., Canuti, D., Dlay, S., Naguib, R.N.G., Sherbet, G.V., 2016. Neural analyses validate and emphasise the role of progesterone receptor in breast cancer progression and prognosis. Anticancer Res. 36, 1909–1915.

Carreira, C.M., LaVallee, T.M., Tarantini, F., Jackson, A., Lathrop, J.T., Hampton, B., et al., 2003. S100A13 is involved in the regulation of fibroblast growth factor-1 and p40 synaptotagmin-1 release in vitro. J. Biol. Chem. 273, 22224–22231.

Castellino, F.J., McCance, S.G., 1997. The kringle domains of human plasminogen. Ciba Found. Symp. 212, 46–60.

Cecchinato, V., Chiaramonte, R., Nizzardo, M., Cristofaro, B., Basile, A., Sherbet, G.V., et al., 2007. Resveratrol-induced apoptosis in human T-cell acute lymphoblastic leukaemia MOLT-4 cells. Biochem. Pharmacol. 74, 1568–1574.

Ceder, R., Haig, Y., Merne, M., Hansson, A., Zheng, X.I., Rosberg, K., et al., 2012. Differentiation-promoting culture of competent and noncompetent keratinocytes identifies biomarkers for head and neck cancer. Am. J. Pathol. 180, 457–472.

Chaiteerakij, R., Petersen, G.M., Bamlet, W.R., Chaffee, K.G., Zhen, D.B., Burch, P.A., et al., 2016. Metformin use and survival of patients with pancreatic cancer: a cautionary lesson. J. Clin. Oncol. 34, 1898–1904.

Chakravorty, A., Sugden, B., 2014. Netrospin inkhibits the growth of Burkitt's lymphoma cells by forcing the loss of Epstein-Barr virus (EBV) genomes from those cells. Eur. J. Cancer 50, S190.

Chan, S.W., Lim, C.J., Chong, Y.F., Pobbati, A.V., Huang, C., Hong, W., 2011. Hippo pathway-independent restriction of TAZ and YAP by angiomotin. J. Biol. Chem. 286, 7018–7026.

Chan, S.W., Lim, C.J., Guo, F.S., Tan, I., Leung, T., Hong, W.J., 2013. Actin-binding and cell proliferation activities of angiomotin family members are regulated by Hippo pathway-mediated phosphorylation. J. Biol. Chem. 288, 37296–37307.

Chandarlapaty, S., Sakr, R.A., Giri, D., Patil, S., Heguy, A., Morrow, M., et al., 2012. Frequent mutational activation of the PI3K-AKT pathway in Trastuzumab-resistant breast cancer. Clin. Cancer Res. 18, 6784–6791.

Chandrasekaran, S., Marshall, J.R., Messing, J.A., Hsu, J.W., King, M.R., 2014. TRAIL-mediated apoptosis in breast cancer cells cultured as 3D spheroids. PLoS One 9, art. no. e111487.

Chang, K.W., Chu, T.H., Gong, N.R., Chiang, W.F., Yang, C.C., Yang, C.-C., et al., 2013. miR-370 modulates insulin receptor substrate-1 expression and inhibits the tumor phenotypes of oral carcinoma. Oral Dis. 19, 611–619.

Chao, C.C., Kan, D., Lu, K.S., Chien, C.L., 2015. The role of microRNA-30c in the self-renewal and differentiation of C6 glioma cells. Stem Cell Res. 14, 211–223.

Chao, T.H., Tseng, S.Y., Li, Y.H., Liu, P.Y., Cho, C.L., Guey-Yueh Shi, G.Y., et al., 2012. A novel vasculo-angiogenic effect of cilostazol mediated by cross-talk between multiple signalling pathways including the ERK/p38 MAPK signalling transduction cascade. Clin. Sci. 123, 147–159.

Chaudhary, J., Sandler-Riggleman, I., Ague, J.M., Skinner, M.K., 2005. The Helix-Loop-Helix inhibitor of differentiation (ID) proteins induce post-mitotic terminally differentiated Sertoli cells to re-enter the cell cycle and proliferate. Biol. Reprod. 72, 1205–1217.

Chauhan, D., Kharbanda, S., Ogata, A., Urashima, M., Teoh, G., Robertson, et al., 1997. Interleukin-6 inhibits Fas-induced apoptosis and stress activated protein kinase activation in multiple myeloma cells. Blood 89, 227–234.

Chen, C.C., Sureshbabul, M., Chen, H.W., Lin, Y.S., Lee, J.Y., Hong, Q.S., et al., 2013. Curcumin suppresses metastasis via Sp-1, FAK19 inhibition, and E-cadherin upregulation in colorectal cancer. Evid. Based Complement Alternat Med. art. no. 541695.

Chen, H.J., Mok, T.S., Chen, Z.H., Guo, A.L., Zhang, X.C., Su, J., et al., 2009. Clinicopathologic and molecular features of epidermal growth factor receptor T790M mutation and c-MET amplification in tyrosine kinase inhibitor-resistant Chinese non-small cell lung cancer. Pathol. Oncol. Res. 15, 651–658.

Chen, M.B., Zhang, Y., Wei, M.X., Shen, W., Wu, X.Y., Yao, C., et al., 2013. Activation of AMP-activated protein kinase (AMPK) mediates plumbagin-induced apoptosis and growth inhibition in cultured human colon cancer cells. Cell Signal. 25, 1993–2002.

Chen, R., Hollborn, M., Grosche, A., Reichenbach, A., Wiedemann, P., Bringmann, A., et al., 2014. Effects of the vegetable polyphenols epigallocatechin-3-gallate, luteolin, apigenin, myricetin, quercetin, and cyanidin in primary cultures of human retinal pigment epithelial cells. Mol. Vision 20, 242–258.

Chen, T., Wong, Y.S., 2008. Selenocystine induces apoptosis of A375 human melanoma cells by activating ROS-mediated mitochondrial pathway and p53 phosphorylation. Cell. Mol. Life Sci. 65, 2763–2775.

Cheng, G.Z., Zhang, W.Z., Sun, M., Wang, Q., Coppola, D., Mansour, M., et al., 2008. Twist is transcriptionally induced by activation of STAT3 and mediates STAT3 oncogenic function. J. Biol. Chem. 283, 14665–14673.

Cheng, J.C., Klausen, C., Leung, P.C., 2013. Hypoxia-inducible factor 1 alpha mediates epidermal growth factor-induced down-regulation of E-cadherin expression and cell invasion in human ovarian cancer cells. Cancer Lett. 329, 197–206.

Chenoweth, D.M., Dervan, P.B., 2009. Allosteric modulation of DNA by small molecules. Proc. Natl Acad. Sci. 106, 13175–131279.

Chi, F., Wu, R., Jin, X.Y., Jiang, M., Zhu, X.K., 2016. HER2 induces cell proliferation and invasion of non-small-cell lung cancer by upregulating COX-2 expression via MEK/ERK signaling pathway. Oncotargets Ther. 9, 2709–2716.

Chidester, C.G., Krueger, W.C., Mizsak, S.A., Duchamp, D.J., Martin, D.G., 1981. The structure of CC-1065, a potent anti-tumor agent, and its binding to DNA. J. Am. Chem. Soc. 103, 7629–7635.

Chien, W.W., Sun, Q.Y., Lee, K.L., Ding, L.W., Wuensche, P., Torres-Fernandez, L.A., et al., 2015. Activation of protein phosphatase 2A tumor suppressor as potential treatment of pancreatic cancer. Mol. Oncol. 9, 889–905.

Chng, H.W., Camplejohns, R.S., Stone, M.G., Hart, I.R., Nicholson, L.J., 2006. A new role for the anti-apoptotic gene A20 in angiogenesis. Exp. Cell. Res. 312, 2897–2907.

Choi, C.I., Lee, Y.D., Kim, H., Kim, S.H., Suh-Kim, H., Kim, S.S., 2013. Neural induction with neurogenin 1 enhances the therapeutic potential of mesenchymal stem cells in an amyotrophic lateral sclerosis mouse model. Cell Transpl. 22, 855–870.

Choi, H.J., Kwon, Y.G., 2015. Roles of YAP in mediating endothelial cell junctional stability and vascular remodelling. BMB Rep. 48, 429–430.

Choi, J.H., Yang, Y.R., Lee, S.K., Kim, S.H., Kim, Y.H., Cha, J.Y., et al., 2008. Potential inhibition of PDK1/Akt signaling by phenothiazines suppresses cancer cell proliferation and survival. Ann. NY Acad. Sci. 1138, 393–403.

Choi, S.H., Tamura, K., Khajuria, R.K., Bhere, D., Nesterenko, I., Lawler, J., et al., 2015. Antiangiogenic variant of TSP-1 targets tumor cells in glioblastomas. Mol. Ther. 23, 235–243.

Chu, Y., Liu, H., Lou, G., Zhang, Q., Wu, C., 2014. Human placenta mesenchymal stem cells expressing exogenous kringle1-5 protein by fiber-modified adenovirus suppress angiogenesis. Cancer Gene Ther. 21, 200–208.

Chua, H.L., Bhat-Nakshatri, P., Clare, S.E., Morimiya, A., Badve, S., Nakshatri, H., 2007. NF-kappaB represses E-cadherin expression and enhances epithelial to mesenchymal transition of mammary epithelial cells: potential involvement of ZEB-1 and ZEB2. Oncogene 26, 711–724.

Chuang, M.J., Sun, K.H., Tang, S.J., Deng, M.W., Wu, Y.H., Sung, J.S., et al., 2008. Tumor-derived tumor necrosis factor-alpha promotes progression and epithelial-mesenchymal transition in renal cell carcinoma cells. Cancer Sci. 99, 905–913.

Chung, S.S., Giehl, N., Wu, Y., Vadgama, J.V., 2014. STAT3 activation in HER2-overexpressing breast cancer promotes epithelial-mesenchymal transition and cancer stem cell traits. Int. J. Oncol. 44, 403–411.

Chuong, C., Katz, J., Pauley, K.M., Bulosan, M., Cha, S., 2009. RAGE expression and NF-κB activation attenuated by extracellular domain of RAGE in human salivary gland cell line. J. Cell. Physiol. 221, 430434.

Ciccocioppo, R., Cangemi, G.C., Kruzliak, P., Gallia, A., Betti, E., Badulli, C., et al., 2015. Ex vivo immunosuppressive effects of mesenchymal stem cells on Crohn's disease mucosal T cells are largely dependent on indoleamine 2,3-dioxygenase activity and cell-cell contact. Stem Cell Res. Ther. 6, art. no. 137.

Ciocca, D.R., Gago, F.E., Fanelli, M.A., Calderwood, S.K., 2006. Co-expression of steroid receptors (estrogen receptor alpha and/or progesterone receptors) and HER2/neu: clinical implications. J. Steroid Biochem. Mol. Biol. 102, 32–40.

Cioffi, M., Trabulo, S., Hidalgo, M., Costello, E., Greenhalf, W., Erkan, M., et al., 2015. Inhibition of CD47 effectively targets pancreatic cancer stem cells via dual mechanisms. Clin. Cancer Res. 21, 2325–2337.

Clark, J.L., Dresser, K., Hsieh, C.C., Sabel, M., Kleer, C.G., Khan, A., et al., 2011. Membrane localization of insulin receptor substrate-2 (IRS-2) is associated with decreased overall survival in breast cancer. Br. Cancer Res. Treat. 130, 759–772.

Clark, L.C., Combs, G.F., Turnbull, B.W., Slate, E.H., Chalker, D.K., Chow, J., et al., 1996. Effects of selenium supplementation for cancer prevention in patients with carcinoma of the skin. A randomized controlled trial. Nutritional Prevention of Cancer Study Group. J. Am. Med. Assoc. 276, 1957–1963.

Cleynen, I., Van de Ven, W.J., 2008. The HMGA proteins: a myriad of functions (review). Int. J. Oncol. 32, 289–305.

Cobleigh, M.A., Vogel, C.L., Tripathy, D., Robert, N.J., Scholl, S., Fehrenbacher, L., et al., 1999. Multinational study of the efficacy and safety of humanized anti-HER2 monoclonal antibody in women who have HER2-overexpressing metastatic breast cancer that has progressed after chemotherapy for metastatic disease. J. Clin. Oncol. 17, 2639–2648.

Compagno, M., Lim, W.K., Grunn, A., Nandula, S.V., Brahmachary, M., Shen, Q., et al., 2009. Mutations of multiple genes cause deregulation of NFκB in diffuse large B-cell lymphoma. Nature 459, 717–721.

Coornaert, B., Carpentier, I., Beyaert, R., 2009. A20: central gatekeeper in inflammation and immunity. J. Biol. Chem. 284, 8217–8221.

Cortinovis, D., Abbate, M., Bidoli, P., Capci, S., Canova, S., 2016. Targeted therapies and immunotherapy in non-small-cell lung cancer. Ecancermed. Sci. 10, art. no. 648.

Cottalorda, A., Verscheide, C., Marcais, A., Tomkowiak, M., Musestte, P., Uemasu, S., et al., 2006. TLR2 engagement on CD8 T cells lowers the threshold for optimal antigen-induced T cell activation. Eur. J. Immunol. 36, 1684–1693.

Cottrell, G.S., Amadesi, S., Schmidlin, F., Bunnett, N., 2003. Protease-activated receptor 2: activation, signalling and function. Biochem. Soc. Trans. 31, 1191–1197.

Covington, K.R., Brusco, L., Barone, I., Tsimelzon, A., Selever, J., Corona-Rodriguez, A., et al., 2013. Metastasis tumor-associated protein 2 enhances metastatic behavior and is associated with poor outcomes in estrogen receptor-negative breast cancer. Breast Cancer Res. Treat. 141, 375–384.

Crawford, A., Wherry, E.J., 2009. Editorial: therapeutic potential of targeting BTLA. J. Leukocyte Biol. 86, 5–8.

Cui, D., Dai, J.L., Keller, J.M., Mizokami, A., Xia, S.J., Keller, E.T., 2015. Notch pathway inhibition using PF-03084014, a gamma-secretase inhibitor (GSI), enhances the antitumor effect of docetaxel in prostate cancer. Clin. Cancer Res. 21, 4619–4629.

Dai, C.X., Lv, S.Z., Shi, R.R., Ding, J., Zhong, X., Song, H.S., et al., 2015. Nuclear protein C23 on the cell surface plays an important role in activation of CXCR4 signaling in glioblastoma. Mol. Neurobiol. 52, 1521–1526.

Dahlmann, M., Okhrimenko, A., Marcinkowski, P., Osterland, M., Hermann, P., Smith, J., et al., 2014. RAGE mediates S100A4-induced cell motility via MAPK/ERK and hypoxia signaling and is a prognostic biomarker for human colorectal cancer metastasis. Oncotarget 5, 3220–3233.

D'Amato, R.J., Loughnan, M.S., Flynn, E., Folkman, J., 1994. Thalidomide is an inhibitor of angiogenesis. Proc. Natl Acad. Sci. USA 91, 4082–4085.

D'Amato, R.J., Hernandez-McClain, J., Saxena, S., Khan, M., 2008. Lenalidomide therapy for metastatic renal cell carcinoma. Am. J. Clin. Oncol. Cancer Clin. Trials 31, 244–249.

D'Alessio, A., De Luca, A., Maiello, M.R., Lamura, L., Rachiglio, A.M., Napolitano, M., et al., 2010. Effects of the combined blockade of EGFR and ErbB-2 on signal transduction and regulation of cell cycle regulatory proteins in breast cancer cells. Breast Cancer Res. Treat. 123, 387–396.

Dantas-Barbosa, C., Bergthold, G., Daudigeos-Dubus, E., Blockus, H., Boylan, J.F., Ferreira, C., et al., 2015. Inhibition of the Notch pathway using gamma-secretase inhibitor RO4929097 has limited antitumor activity in established glial tumors. Anticancer Drugs 26, 272–283.

Dave, B., Migliaccio, I., Gutierrez, M.C., Wu, M.F., Chamness, G.C., Wong, H., et al., 2011. Loss of phosphatase and tensin homolog or phosphoinositol-3 kinase activation and response to Trastuzumab or Lapatinib in human epidermal growth factor receptor 2-overexpressing locally advanced breast cancers. J. Clin. Oncol. 29, 166–173.

Davies, S., Dai, D.H., Feldman, I., Pickett, G., Leslie, K.K., 2004. Identification of a novel mechanism of NF-kappa B inactivation by progesterone through progesterone receptors in Hec50co poorly differentiated endometrial cancer cells: induction of A20 and ABIN-2. Gynec. Oncol. 94, 463–470.

Davis, M.L., LeVan, T.D., Yu, F., Sayles, H., Sololove, J., Robinson, W., et al., 2015. Associations of toll-like receptor (TLR)-4 single nucleotide polymorphisms and rheumatoid arthritis disease progression: an observational cohort study. Int. Immunopharmacol. 24, 346–352.

De, A., Dainichi, T., Rathinam, C.V., Ghosh, S., 2014. The deubiquitinase activity of A20 is dispensable for NF-kappa B signalling. EMBO Rep. 15, 775–783.

Deane, R., Singh, I., Sagare, A.P., Bell, R.D., Ross, N.T., LaRue, B., 2012. A multimodal RAGE-specific inhibitor reduces amyloid β-mediated brain disorder in a mouse model of Alzheimer disease. J. Clin. Invest. 122, 1377–1392.

De Cesare, M., Sfondrini, L., Pennati, M., De Marco, C., Motta, V., Tagliabue, E., et al., 2016. CpG-oligodeoxynucleotides exert remarkable antitumor activity against diffuse malignant peritoneal mesothelioma orthotopic xenografts. J. Transl. Med. 14, art. no. 25.

Dedes, K.J., Natrajan, R., Lambros, M.B., Geyer, F.C., Lopez-Garcia, M.A., Savage, K., et al., 2011. Down-regulation of the miRNA master regulators Drosha and Dicer is associated with specific subgroups of breast cancer. Eur. J. Cancer 47, 138–150.

De Keersmaecker, B., Fostier, K., Corthals, J., Wilgenhof, S., Heirman, C., Aerts, J.L., et al., 2014. Immunomodulatory drugs improve the immune environment for dendritic cell-based immunotherapy in multiple myeloma patients after autologous stem cell transplantation. Cancer Immunol. Immunother. 63, 1023–1036.

Della Corte, C.M., Bellevicine, C., Vicidomini, G., Vitagliano, D., Malapelle, U., Accardo, M., et al., 2015. SMO gene amplification and activation of the Hedgehog pathway as novel mechanisms of resistance to anti-epidermal growth factor receptor drugs in human lung cancer. Clin. Cancer Res. 21, 4686–4697.

De Melo, F.M., Braga, C.J.M., Pereira, F.V., Maricato, J.T., Origassa, C.S.T., Souza, M.F., et al., 2015. Anti-metastatic immunotherapy based on mucosal administration of flagellin and immunomodulatory P10. Immunol. Cell Biol. 93, 86–98.

Dempke, W.C.M., Edvardsen, K., Lu, S., Reinmuth, N., Reck, M., Inoue, A., 2015. Brain metastases in NSCLC – are TKIs changing the treatment strategy? Anticancer Res. 35, 5797–5806.

Deng, B., Gou, X.C., Chen, H., Li, L.Y., Zhong, H.X., Xu, H., et al., 2013. Targeted delivery of Neurogenin-2 protein in the treatment for cerebral ischemia-reperfusion injury. Biomaterials 34, 8786–8797.

Deng, L., Yang, H., Tang, J.W., Lin, Z., Yin, A.H., Gao, Y., et al., 2015. Inhibition of MTA1 by ER alpha contributes to protection hepatocellular carcinoma from tumor proliferation and metastasis. J. Exp. Clin. Cancer Res. 34, art. no. 128.

De Rossi, G., Whiteford, J.R., 2013. A novel role for syndecan-3 in angiogenesis. F1000 Res. 2, 270.

De Rossi, G., Evans, A.R., Kay, E., Woodfin, A., McKay, T.R., Nourshargh, S., et al., 2014. Shed syndecan-2 inhibits angiogenesis. J. Cell Sci. 127, 4788–4799.

De Souza Queiroz, K.C., Zambuzzi, W.F., De Souza, A.C.S., Da Silva, R.A., Machado, D., Justo, G.Z., et al., 2007. A possible anti-proliferative and anti-metastatic effect of irradiated riboflavin in solid tumours. Cancer Lett. 258, 126–134.

Destouches, D., Huet, E., Sader, M., Frechault, S., Carpentier, G., Ayoul, F., et al., 2012. Multivalent pseudopeptides targeting cell surface nucleoproteins inhibit cancer cell invasion through tissue inhibitor of metalloproteinases 3 (TIMP-3) release. J. Biol. Chem. 287, 43685–43693.

Destouches, D., Page, N., Hamma-Kourbali, Y., Machi, V., Chaloin, O., Frechault, S., et al., 2011. A simple approach to cancer therapy afforded by multivalent pseudopeptides that target cell-surface nucleoproteins. Cancer Res. 71, 3296–3305.

De Witte, C.J., van de Sande, A.J.M., van Beekhuizen, H.J., Koeneman, M.M., Kruse, A.J., Gerestein, C.G., 2015. Imiquimod in cervical, vaginal and vulvar intraepithelial neoplasia: a review. Gynecol. Oncol. 139, 377–384.

Dhar, S., Kumar, A., Li, K., Tzivion, G., Levenson, A.S., 2015. Resveratrol regulates PTEN/Akt pathway through inhibition of MTA1/HDAC unit of the NuRD complex in prostate cancer. Biochim. Biophys. Acta Mol. Cell Res. 1853, 265–275.

Diaby, V., Adunlin, G., Ali, A.A., Tawk, R., 2014a. Using quality-adjusted progression-free survival as an outcome measure to assess the benefits of cancer drugs in randomized-controlled trials: case of the BOLERO-2 trial. Breast Cancer Res. Treat. 146, 669–673.

Diaby, V., Adunlin, G., Zeichner, S.B., Avancha, K., Lopes, G., Gluck, S., et al., 2014b. Cost-effectiveness analysis of everolimus plus exemestane versus exemestane alone for treatment of hormone receptor positive metastatic breast cancer. Breast Cancer Res. Treat. 147, 433–441.

Di Agostino, S., Sorrentino, G., Ingallina, E., Valenti, F., Ferraiuolo, M., Silvio Bicciato, S., et al., 2016. YAP enhances the pro-proliferative transcriptional activity of mutant p53 proteins. EMBO Rep. 17, 188–201.

Díaz-Coránguez Segovia, M.J., López-Ornelas, A., Puerta-Guardo, H., Ludert, J., Chavez, B., et al., 2013. Transmigration of neural stem cells across the blood brain barrier induced by glioma cells. PLoS One 8, art. no. e60655.

Diaz-Padilla, I., Wilson, M.K., Clarke, B.A., Hirte, H.W., Welch, S.A., Mackay, H.J., et al., 2015. A phase II study of single-agent RO4929097, a gamma-secretase inhibitor of Notch signaling, in patients with recurrent platinum-resistant epithelial ovarian cancer: a study of the Princess Margaret, Chicago and California phase II consortia. Gynecol. Oncol. 137, 216–222.

Dida, F., Li, Y.F., Iwao, A., Deguchi, T., Azuma, E., Komada, Y., 2008. Resistance to TRAIL-induced apoptosis caused by constitutional phosphorylation of Akt and PTEN in acute lymphoblastic leukemia cells. Exp. Hematol. 36, 1343–1353.

Dietsch, G.N., Lu, H.L., Yang, Y., Morishima, C., Chow, L.Q., Disis, M.L., et al., 2016. Coordinated activation of toll-like receptor8 (TLR8) and NLRP3 by the TLR8 agonist, VTX-2337, ignites tumoricidal natural killer cell activity. PLoS One 11, e0148764.

Di Fazio, P., Montalbano, R., Neureiter, D., Alinger, B., Schmidt, A., Merkel, A.L., et al., 2012. Downregulation of HMGA2 by the pan-deacetylase inhibitor panobinostat is dependent on hsa-let-7b expression in liver cancer cell lines. Exp. Cell Res. 318, 1832–1843.

Di Giacomo, A.M., Margolin, K., 2015. Immune checkpoint blockade in patients with melanoma metastatic to the brain. Semin. Oncol. 42, 459–465.

Ding, Q., Keller, J.N., 2005. Evaluation of Rage isoforms, ligands, and signaling in the brain. Biochim. Biophys. Acta Mol. Cell Res. 1746, 18–27.

Dockendorff, C., Nagiec, M.M., Weiwer, M., Buhrlage, S., Ting, A., Nag, P.P., et al., 2012. Macrocyclic Hedgehog pathway inhibitors: optimization of cellular activity and mode of action studies. ACS Med. Chem. Lett. 3, 808–813.

Dong, H.L., Claffey, K.P., Brocke, S., Epstein, 2015. Inhibition of breast cancer cell migration by activation of cAMP signalling. Breast Cancer Res. Treat. 15, 17–28.

Dong, H.M., Guo, H., Xie, L.X., Wang, G., Zhong, X.Y., Khoury, T., 2013. The metastasis-associated gene MTA3, a component of the Mi-2/NuRD transcriptional repression complex, predicts prognosis of gastroesophageal junction adenocarcinoma. PLoS One 8, art. no. e62986.

Dong, Y.Q., Lu, C.W., Zhang, L., Yang, J., Hameed, W., Chen, W., 2015. Toll-like receptor 4 signaling promotes invasion of hepatocellular carcinoma cells through MKK4/JNK pathway. Mol. Immunol. 68, 671–683.

Dossing, K.B.V., Binderup, T., Kaczkowski, B., Jacobsen, A., Rossing, M., Winther, O., et al., 2015. Down-regulation of miR-129-5p and the let-7 family in neuroendocrine tumors and metastases leads to up-regulation of their targets Egr1, G3bp1, Hmga2 and Bach1. Genes 6, 1–21.

Dowling, R.J., Goodwin, P.J., Stambolic, V., 2011. Understanding the benefit of metformin use in cancer treatment. BMC Med. 9, art. no. 33.

Duan, L., Ying, G.G., Danzer, B., Perez, R.E., Shariat-Madar, Z., Levenson, V.V., et al., 2014. The prolyl peptidases PRCP/PREP regulate IRS-1 stability critical for rapamycin-induced feedback activation of PI3K and AKT. J Biol Chem 289, 21694–21705.

Duwel, A., Eleno, N., Jerkic, M., Arevalo, M., Bolanos, P., Bernabeu, C., et al., 2007. Reduced tumor growth and angiogenesis in endoglin-haploinsufficient mice. Tumor Biol. 28, 1–8.

Ebbinghaus, S., Hussain, M., Tannir, N., Gordon, M., Desai, A.A., Knight, R.A., et al., 2007. Phase 2 study of ABT-510 in patients with previously untreated advanced renal cell carcinoma. Clin. Cancer Res. 13, 6689–6695.

Echizen, K., Hirose, O., Maeda, Y., Oshima, M., 2016. Inflammation in gastric cancer: interplay of the COX-2/prostaglandin E2 and toll-like receptor/MyD88 pathways. Cancer Sci. 107, 391–397.

Efeyan, A., Sabatini, D.M., 2010. mTOR and cancer: many loops in one pathway. Curr. Opin. Cell Biol. 22, 169–176.

El-Ami, T., Moll, L., Marques, F.C., Volovik, Y., Reuveni, H., Cohen, E., 2014. A novel inhibitor of the insulin/IGF signaling pathway protects from age-onset, neurodegeneration-linked proteotoxicity. Aging Cell 13, 165–174.

Elderbroom, J.L., Huang, J.J., Gatza, C.E., Chen, J., How, T., Starr, M., et al., 2014. Ectodomain shedding of T beta RIII is required for T beta RIII-mediated suppression of TGF-beta signaling and breast cancer migration and invasion. Mol. Biol. Cell 25, 2320–2332.

El Khatib, M., Kalnytska, A., Palagani, V., Kossatz, U., Manns, M.P., Malek, N.P., et al., 2013. Inhibition of hedgehog signaling attenuates carcinogenesis in vitro and increases necrosis of cholangiocellular carcinoma. Hepatology 57, 1035–1045.

Emeagi, P.U., Van Lint, S., Goyvaerts, C., Maenhout, S., Cauwels, A., McNeish, L.A., et al., 2012. Proinflammatory characteristics of SMAC/DIABLO-induced cell death in antitumor therapy. Cancer Res. 72, 1342–1352.

Endo, H., Takenaga, K., Kanno, T., Satoh, H., Mori, S., 2002. Methionine aminopeptidase 2 is a new target for the metastasis-associated protein, S100A4. J. Biol. Chem. 77, 26396–26402.

Engelman, J.A., Chen, L., Tan, X., Crosby, K., Guimaraes, A.R., Upadhyay, R., et al., 2008. Effective use of PI3K and MEK inhibitors to treat mutant Kras G12D and PIK3CAH1047R murine lung cancers. Nat. Med. 14, 1351–1356.

Eo, H.J., Park, G.H., Jeong, J.B., 2016. Inhibition of Wnt signaling by silymarin in human colorectal cancer cells. Biomol. Ther. 24, 380–386.

ESMO (2016). Certitinib provides longer progression free survival than chemotherapy in phase II trial of ALK rearranged lung cancer treatment. Press Release, October 2016.

Estal, R.M., Suela, S.P., Jimenez, I.D., Rojas, C.E., Garcia-Casado, Z., Fita, M.J.J., et al., 2013. MicroRNA signatures in hereditary breast cancer. Breast Cancer Res. Treat. 142, 19–30.

Eto, K., Iwatsuki, M., Watanabe, M., Ida, S., Ishimoto, T., Iwagami, S., et al., 2014. The microRNA-21/PTEN pathway regulates the sensitivity of HER2-positive gastric cancer cells to Trastuzumab. Ann. Surg. Oncol. 21, 343–350.

Evangelisti, C., Florian, M.C., Massimi, I., Dominici, C., Giannini, G., Galardi, S., et al., 2009. MiR-128 up-regulation inhibits Reelin and DCX expression and reduces neuroblastoma cell motility and invasiveness. FASEB J. 23, 4276–4287.

Faes, S., Planche, A., Uldry, E., Santoro, T., Pythoud, C., Stehle, J.C., 2016. Targeting carbonic anhydrase IX improves the anti-cancer efficacy of mTOR inhibitors. Oncotarget 7, 36666–36680.

Falahi, F., Sgro, A., Blancafort, P., 2015. Epigenome engineering in cancer: fairytale or a realistic path to the clinic? Front Oncol 5, 22, art. no..

Fan, R., Kim, N.G., Gumbiner, B.M., 2013. Regulation of Hippo pathway by mitogenic growth factors via phophoinositide 5-kinase and phosphoinositide-dependent kinase-1. Proc. Natl. Acad. Sci. 110, 2569–2574.

Fan, S., Gao, M., Meng, Q., Laterra, J.J., Symons, M.H., Coniglio, S., 2005. Role of NF-kappaB signaling in hepatocyte growth factor/scatter factor-mediated cell protection. Oncogene 24, 1749–1766.

Fang, Y., Lahiri, J., Picard, L., 2003. G-protein coupled receptor microarrays for drug discovery. Drug Discov. Today 8, 755–761.

Fantozzi, A., Gruber, D.C., Pisarsky, L., Heck, C., Kunita, A., Yilmaz, M., et al., 2014. VEGF-mediated angiogenesis links EMT-induced cancer stemness to tumor initiation. Cancer Res. 74, 1566–1575.

Faronato, M., Nguyen, V.T.M., Patten, D.K., Lombardo, Y., Steel, J.H., Patel, N., 2015. DMXL2 drives epithelial to mesenchymal transition in hormonal therapy resistant breast cancer through notch hyper-activation. Oncotarget 6, 22467–22479.

Febbraio, M., Haar, D.P., Silverstein, R.L., 2001. CD36: a class B scavenger receptor involved in angiogenesis, atherosclerosis, inflammation, and lipid metabolism. J. Clin. Invest. 108, 785–791.

Fecteau, J.F., Corral, L.G., Ghia, E.M., Gaidarova, S., Futalan, D., Bharati, I.S., et al., 2014. Lenalidomide inhibits the proliferation of CLL cells via a cereblon/p21(WAF1/Cip1)-dependent mechanism independent of functional p53. Blood 124, 1637–1644.

Feldman, M.E., Apsel, B., Uotila, A., Loewith, R., Knight, Z.A., Ruggero, D., et al., 2009. Active-site inhibitors of mTOR target rapamycin-resistant outputs of mTORC1 and mTORC2. PLoS Biol. 7, art. no. e1000038.

Feng, N., Luo, J.M., Guo, X.M., 2016. Silybin suppresses cell proliferation and induces apoptosis of multiple myeloma cells via the PI3K/Akt/mTOR signaling pathway. Mol. Med. 13, 3243–3248.

Feng, W., Cai, D.W., Zhang, B., Lou, G.C., Zou, X.P., 2015. Combination of HDAC inhibitor TSA and silibinin induces cell cycle arrest and apoptosis by targeting survivin and cyclinB1/Cdk1 in pancreatic cancer cells. Biomed. Pharacother. 74, 257–264.

Ferracin, M., Bassi, C., Pedriali, M., Pagotto, S., D'Abundo, L., Zagatti, B., et al., 2013. miR-125b targets erythropoietin and its receptor and their expression correlates with metastatic potential and ERBB2/HER2 expression. Mol. Cancer 12, art. no. 130.

Fesquet, D., De Bettignies, G., Bellis, M., Espeut, J., Devault, A., 2015. Binding of Kif23-iso1/CHO1 to 14-3-3 is regulated by sequential phosphorylations at two LATS kinase consensus sites. PLoS One 10, art. no. e0117857.

Fiala, O., Pesek, M., Finek, J., Minarik, M., Benesova, L., Bortlicek, Z., et al., 2015. Statins augment efficacy of EGFR-TKIs in patients with advanced-stage non-small cell lung cancer harbouring KRAS mutation. Tumor Biol. 36, 5801–5805.

Fillmore, C.M., Kuperwasser, C., 2008. Human breast cancer cell lines contain stem-like cells that self-renew, give rise to phenotypically diverse progeny and survive chemotherapy. Br. Cancer Res. 10, R25.

Fox, C.B., Sivananthan, S.J., Duthie, M.S., Vergara, J., Guderian, J.A., Moon, E., et al., 2014. A nanoliposome delivery system to synergistically trigger TLR4 AND TLR7. J. Nanobiotechnol. 12, art. no. 17.

Fraineau, S., Monvoisin, A., Clarhaut, J., Talbot, J., Simonneau, C., Kanthou, C., et al., 2012. The vitamin K-dependent anticoagulant factor, protein S, inhibits multiple VEGF-A-induced angiogenesis events in a Mer- and SHP2-dependent manner. Blood 120, 5073–5083.

Franco, S.J., Muller, U., 2011. ECM functions during neuronal migration and lamination in the mammalian central nervous system. Dev. Neurobiol. 71, 889–900.

Frank, R.T., Edmiston, M., Kendall, S.E., Najbauer, J., Cheunr, C.W., Kassa, et al., 2009. Neural stem cells as a novel platform for tumor-specific delivery of therapeutic antibodies. PLoS One 4, art. no. e8314.

Freed-Pastor, W.A., Mizuno, H., Zhao, X., Langerod, A., Moon, S.H., Rodriguez-Barrueco, R., et al., 2012. Mutant p53 disrupts mammary tissue architecture via the mevalonate pathway. Cell 148, 244–258.

Freudlsperger, C., Bian, Y., Wise, S.C., Burnett, J., Coupar, J., Yang, X., et al., 2013. TGF-beta and NF-kappa B signal pathway cross-talk is mediated through TAK1 and SMAD7 in a subset of head and neck cancers. Oncogene 32, 1549–1559.

Frost, P., Berlanger, E., Mysore, V., Hoang, B., Yi Jiang, S., Gera, J., et al., 2013. Mammalian target of rapamycin inhibitors induce tumor cell apoptosis in vivo primarily by inhibiting VEGF expression and angiogenesis. J. Oncol. 2013, art. no. 897025.

Fujii, R., Imanishi, Y., Shibata, K., Sakai, N., Sakamoto, K., Shigetomi, S., et al., 2014. Restoration of E-cadherin expression by selective Cox-2 inhibition and the clinical relevance of the epithelial-to-mesenchymal transition in head and neck squamous cell carcinoma. J. Exp. Clin. Cancer Res. 33, art. no. 40.

Fujiwara, K., Ohuchida, K., Ohtsuka, T., Mizumoto, K., Shindo, K., Ikenaga, N., et al., 2013. Migratory activity of CD105(+) pancreatic cancer cells is strongly enhanced by pancreatic stellate cells. Pancreas 42, 1283–1290.

Fukuhara, S., Sako, K., Noda, K., Zhang, J., Minami, M., Mochizuki, N., 2010. Angiopoietin-1/Tie2 receptor signaling in vascular quiescence and angiogenesis. Histol. Hisptopathol. 25, 387–396.

Gadgeel, S.M., Gandhi, L., Riely, G., Chipport, A.A., West, H.L., Azada, M.C., et al., 2014. Safety and activity of alectinib against systemic disease and brain metastases in patients with crizotinib-resistant ALK-rearranged non-small-cell lung cancer (AF-002JG): results from the dose-finding portion of a phase 1/2 study. Lancet Oncol. 15, 1119–1128.

Gadgeel, S.M., Lew, D.L., Synold, T.W., LoRusso, P., Chung, V., Christensen, S.D., et al., 2013. Phase I study evaluating the combination of lapatinib (a Her2/Neu and EGFR inhibitor) and everolimus (an mTOR inhibitor) in patients with advanced cancers: South West Oncology Group (SWOG) Study S0528. Cancer Chemo Pharmacol. 72, 1089–1096.

Gale, N.W., Dominguez, M.G., Noguera, I., Pan, L., Hughes, V., Valenzuela, D.M., et al., 2004. Haploinsufficiency of delta-like 4 ligand results in embryonic lethality due to major defects in arterial and vascular development. Proc. Natl Acad. Sci. USA 101, 15949–15954.

Gandini, S., Puntoni, M., Heckman-Stoddard, B.M., Dunn, B.K., Ford, L., DeCensi, A., et al., 2014. Metformin and cancer risk and mortality: a systematic review and meta-analysis taking into account biases and confounders. Cancer Prevent. Res. 7, 867–885.

Ganesan, P., Piha-Paul, S., Naing, A., Falchook, G., Wheler, J., et al., 2013. Phase I clinical trial of lenalidomide in combination with temsirolimus in patients with advanced cancer. Invest. New Drugs 31, 1505–1513.

Garcia, A.G., Nedev, H., Bijian, K., Su, J., Alaoui-Jamali, M.A., Saragovi, H.U., 2013. Reduced in vivo lung metastasis of a breast cancer cell line after treatment with Herceptin mAb conjugated to chemotherapeutic drugs. Oncogene 32, 2527–2533.

Garcia-Maceira, P., Mateo, J., 2009. Silibinin inhibits hypoxia-inducible factor-1 alpha and mTOR/p70S6K/4E-BP1 signalling pathway in human cervical and hepatoma cancer cells: implications for anticancer therapy. Oncogene 28, 313–324.

Garcia-Rendueles, M.E.R., Ricarte, J.C., Untch, B.R., Landa, I., Knauf, J.A., Voza, F., et al., 2015. NF2 loss promotes oncogenic RAS-induced thyroid cancers via YAP-dependent transactivation of RAS proteins and sensitizes them to MEK inhibition. Cancer Discov. 5, 1178–1193.

Garrett, S.C., Hodgson, L., Rybin, A., Toutchkine, A., Hahn, K.M., Lawrence, D.S., et al., 2008. A biosensor of S100A4 metastasis factor activation: Inhibitor screening and cellular activation dynamics. Biochemistry 47, 986–996.

Ge, R., Rajeev, V., Ray, P., Lattime, E., Riffling, S., Medicheria, S., et al., 2006. Inhibition of growth and metastasis of mouse mammary carcinoma by selective inhibitor of transforming growth factor-beta type I receptor kinase in vivo. Clin. Cancer Res. 12, 4315–4330.

Gettinger, S.N., Horn, L., Gandhi, L., Spigel, D.R., Antonia, S.J., Rizvi, N.A., et al., 2015. Overall survival and long-term safety of nivolumab (anti-programmed death 1 antibody, BMS-936558, ONO-4538) in patients with previously treated advanced non-small-cell lung cancer. J. Clin. Oncol. 33, 2004–2012.

Giampietro, C., Disanza, A., Bravi, L., Barrios-Rodiles, M., Corada, M., Frittoli, E., et al., 2015. The actin-binding protein EPS8 binds VE-cadherin and modulates YAP localization and signalling. J. Cell Biol. 211, 1177–1192.

Giles, K.M., Brown, R.A.M., Epis, M.R., Kalinowski, F.C., Leedman, P.J., 2013. miRNA-7-5p inhibits melanoma cell migration and invasion. Biochem. Biophys. Res. Commun. 430, 706–710.

Gioia, U., Di Carlo, V., Caramanica, P., Toselli, C., Cinquino, A., Marchioni, M., et al., 2014. Mir-23a and mir-125b regulate neural stem/progenitor cell proliferation by targeting Musashi1. RNA Biol. 11, 1105–1112.

Goff, L.W., Cohen, R.B., Berlin, J.D., de Braud, F.G., Lyshchik, A., Noberasco, C., et al., 2016. A phase I study of the anti-activin receptor-like kinase 1 (ALK-1) monoclonal antibody PF-03446962 in patients with advanced solid tumors. Clin. Cancer Res. 22, 2146–2154.

Goldman, A.P., Williams, C.S., Sheng, H., Lamps, L.W., Williams, V.P., Pairet, M., et al., 1998. Meloxicam inhibits the growth of colorectal cancer cells. Carcinogenesis 19, 2195–2199.

Gonzalez-Angulo, A.M., Akcakanat, A., Liu, S., Green, M.C., Murray, J.L., Chen, H., et al., 2014. Open-label randomized clinical trial of standard neoadjuvant chemotherapy with paclitaxel followed by FEC versus the combination of paclitaxel and everolimus followed by FEC in women with triple receptor-negative breast cancer. Ann. Oncol. 25, 1122–1127.

Good, D.J., Polverini, P.J., Rastinejad, F., Le Beau, M.M., Lemons, R.S., Frazier, W.A., et al., 1990. A tumor suppressor-dependent inhibitor of angiogenesis is immunologically and functionally indistinguishable from a fragment of thrombospondin. Proc. Natl Acad. Sci. USA 87, 6624–6628.

Gorgun, G., Samur, M.K., Cowens, K.B., Paula, S., Bianchi, G., Anderson, J.E., et al., 2015. Lenalidomide enhances immune checkpoint blockade induced immune response in multiple myeloma. Clin. Cancer Res. Available from: http://dx.doi.org/10.1158/1078-0432.CCR-15-0200.

Gou, Y., Zhang, Y., Qi, J., Kong, L.L., Zhou, Z.P., Liang, S.C., et al., 2015. Binding and anticancer properties of plumbagin with human serum albumin. Chem. Biol. Drugs 86, 362–369.

Grant, M.A., Baron, R.M., Macias, A.A., Layne, M.D., Perrella, M.A., Rigby, A.C., 2009. Netropsin improves survival from endotoxaemia by disrupting HMGA1 binding to the NOS2 promoter. Biochem. J. 418, 103–112.

Gras, J., 2014. Galunistertib TGF-beta receptor type-1 (ALK5; SKR4) inhibitor Oncolytic. Drugs Future 39, 257–262.

Griffith, E.C., Su, Z., Niwayama, S., Ramsay, C.A., Chang, Y.H., Liu, J.O., 1998. Molecular recognition of angiogenesis inhibitors fumagillin and ovalicin by methionine aminopeptidase 2. Proc. Natl Acad. Sci. USA 95, 15183–15188.

Gross, N., Ranjbar, M., Evers, C., Hua, J., Martin, G., Schulze, B., et al., 2013. Choroidal neovascularization reduced by targeted drug delivery with cationic liposome-encapsulated paclitaxel or targeted photodynamic therapy with verteporfi. Mol. Vis. 19, 54–61.

Grum-Schwensen, B., Kllingelhofer, J., Beck, M., Bonefeld, C.M., Hamerlik, P., Guldberg, P., et al., 2015. S100A4-neutralizing antibody suppresses spontaneous tumor progression, pre-metastatic niche formation and alters T-cell polarization balance. BMC Cancer 15, art. no. 44.

Guan, Y., Li, A.C., Xiao, W.W., Liu, S., Chen, B.B., Lu, T.X., et al., 2015. The efficacy and safety of endostar combined with chemoradiotherapy for patients with advanced, locally recurrent nasopharyngeal carcinoma. Oncotarget 6, 33926–33934.

Guichard, S.M., Curwen, J., Bihani, T., D'Cruz, C.M., Yates, J.W.T., Grondine, M., et al., 2015. AZD2014, an inhibitor of mTORC1 and mTORC2, is highly effective in ER+ breast cancer when administered using intermittent or continuous schedules. Mol. Cancer Ther. 14, 2508–2518.

Guillerey, C., Chow, M.T., Miles, K., Olver, S., Sceneay, J., Takeda, K., et al., 2015. Toll-like receptor 3 regulates NK cell responses to cytokines and controls experimental metastasis. Oncoimmunology 4, e1027468.

Guler, M., Yilmaz, T., Ozercan, I., Elkiran, T., 2009. The inhibitory effects of trastuzumab on corneal neovascularization. Am. J. Ophthalmol. 147, 703–708.

Gunaratnam, L., Morley, M., Franovic, A., de Paulsen, N., Mekhail, K., Parolin, D.A., et al., 2003. Hypoxia inducible factor activates the transforming growth factor-alpha/epidermal growth factor receptor growth stimulatory pathway in VHL(-/-) renal cell carcinoma cells. J. Biol. Chem. 278, 44966–44974.

Guo, L.F., Chen, Y., He, T., Qi, F.F., Liu, G.H., Fu, Y., et al., 2015a. Nuclear-translocated endostatin downregulates hypoxia inducible factor-1 alpha activation through interfering with Zn(II) homeostasis. Mol. Med. Rep. 11, 3473–3480.

Guo, L.F., Song, N., He, T., Qi, F.F., Zheng, S., Xu, X.G., et al., 2015b. Endostatin inhibits the tumorigenesis of hemangioendothelioma via downregulation of CXCL1. Mol. Carcinogenesis 54, 1340–1353.

Guo, S.Z., Messmer-Blust, A.F., Wu, J.P., Song, X.X., Philbrick, M.J., Shie, J.L., et al., 2014. Role of A20 in cIAP-2 protection against tumor necrosis factor alpha (TNF-alpha)-mediated apoptosis in endothelial cells. Int. J. Mol. Sci. 15, 3816–3833.

Guo, Y., Shan, Q.Q., Gong, Y.P., Lin, J., Shi, F.F., Shi, R., et al., 2014. Curcumin induces apoptosis via simultaneously targeting AKT/mTOR and RAF/MEK/ERK survival signaling pathways in human leukemia THP-1 cells. Pharmazie 69, 229–233.

Guo, Z., Jiang, J.H., Zhang, J., Yang, H.J., Yang, F.Q., Qi, Y.P., et al., 2015. COX-2 promotes migration and invasion by the side population of cancer stem cell-like hepatocellular carcinoma cells. Medicine 94, art. no. e1806.

Gupta, P.B., Onder, T.T., Jiang, G., Tao, K., Kuperwasser, C., Weinberg, R.A., et al., 2009. Identification of selective inhibitors of cancer stem cells by high throughput screening. Cell 138, 645–659.

Gupta, V.K., Jaskowiak, N.T., Beckett, M.A., Mauceri, H.J., Grunstein, J., Johnson, R.S., et al., 2002. Vascular endothelial growth factor enhances endothelial cell survival and tumor radioresistance. Cancer J. 8, 47–54.

Gutierrez, A., Pan, L., Groen, R.W.J., Baleydier, F., Kentsis, A., Marineau, J., et al., 2014. Phenothiazines induce PP2A-mediated apoptosis in T cell acute lymphoblastic leukemia. J. Clin. Invest. 124, 644–655.

Habel, N., Vilalta, M., Bawa, O., Opolon, P., Blanco, J., Fromique, O., 2015. Cyr61 silencing reduces vascularization and dissemination of osteosarcoma tumors. Oncogene 34, 3207–3213.

Halbleib, J.M., Nelson, W.J., 2006. Cadherins in development: cell adhesion, sorting, and tissue morphogenesis. Genes Dev. 20, 3199–3214.

Han, L.H., Zhang, M.L., Wang, M.M., Jia, J.C., Zhao, M.Y., Fan, Y.M., et al., 2016. High mobility group box-1 promotes inflammation-induced lymphangiogenesis via toll-like receptor 4-dependent signalling pathway. PLoS One 11, e0154187.

Han, M.S., Moon, K.S., Lee, K.H., Cho, S.B., Lim, S.H., Jang, W.Y., et al., 2013. Brain metastasis from hepatocellular carcinoma: the role of surgery as a prognostic factor. BMC Cancer 13, 567.

Hanks, B.A., Holtzhausen, A., Evans, K.S., Jamieson, R., Gimpel, P., Campbell, O.M., 2013. Type III TGF-beta receptor downregulation generates an immunotolerant tumor microenvironment. J. Clin. Invest. 123, 3925–3940.

Haque, I., De, A., Majumber, M., Mehta, S., McGregor, D., Banerjee, S.K., et al., 2012. The matricellular protein CCN1/Cyr61 is a critical regulator of Sonic Hedgehog in pancreatic carcinogenesis. J. Biol. Chem. 287, 38569–38579.

Haque, I., Mehta, S., Majumder, M., Dhar, K., De, A., McGregor, D., et al., 2011. Cyr61/CCN1 signaling is critical for epithelial-mesenchymal transition and stemness and promotes pancreatic carcinogenesis. Mol. Cancer 10, 8.

Harris, L.G., Pannell, L.K., Singh, S., Samant, R.S., Shevde, L.A., 2012. Increased vascularity and spontaneous metastasis of breast cancer by hedgehog signaling mediated upregulation of cyr61. Oncogene 31, 3370–3380.

Hasina, R., Martin, L.E., Kasza, K., Jones, C.L., Jalil, A., Lingen, M.W., 2009. ABT-510 is an effective chemopreventive agent in the mouse 4-nitroquinoline 1-oxide model of oral carcinogenesis. Cancer Prevent. Res. 2, 385–393.

Haskins, J.W., Nguyen, D.X., Stern, D.F., 2014. Neuregulin 1-activated ERBB4 interacts with YAP to induce Hippo pathway target genes and promote cell migration. Sci. Signal. 7, art. no. ra116.

He, C., Lv, X., Hua, G., Lele, S.M., Remmenga, S., Dong, J., et al., 2015. YAP forms autocrine loops with the ERBB pathway to regulate ovarian cancer initiation and progression. Oncogene 34, 6040–6054.

He, G.F., Zhang, Y.W., Lee, J.H., Zeng, S.X., Wang, Y.Y.V., Luo, Z.J., et al., 2014. AMP-activated protein kinase induces p53 by phosphorylating MDMX and inhibiting its activity. Mol. Cell Biol. 34, 148–157.

He, J., Jing, Y., Li, W., Qian, X., Xu, Q., Li, F.S., et al., 2013. Roles and mechanism of miR-199a and miR-125b in tumor angiogenesis. PLoS One 8, e56647.

Hefferman, M.J., Murthy, N., 2005. Polyketal nanoparticles: a new pH-sensitive biodegradable drug delivery vehicle. Bioconjugate Chem. 16, 1340–1342.

Helland, A., Anglesio, M.S., George, J., Cowin, P.A., Jonstone, C.N., House, C.M., et al., 2011. Deregulation of MycN, Lin28B, and Let7 in a molecular subtype of aggressive high grade serous ovarian cancers. PLoS One 6, e18064.

Heminda, N., Lopez, B., Gonzalez, A., Dotor, J., Lasarte, J.J., Sarobe, P., 2009. A synthetic peptide from transforming growth factor-beta1 type III receptor prevents myocardial fibrosis in spontaneously hypertensive rats. Cardiovas. Res. 81, 601–609.

Herbert, C., Schieborn, U., Saxena, K., Juraszek, J., De Smet, F., Alcouffe, C., et al., 2013. Molecular mechanism of SSR128129E, an extracellularly acting, small-molecule, allosteric inhibitor of FGF receptor signaling. Cancer Cell 23, 489–501.

Hernandez, J.L., Padilla, L., Dakhjel, S., Col, T., Hervas, R., Adan, J., et al., 2013. Therapeutic targeting of tumor growth and angiogenesis with a novel anti-S100A4 monoclonal antibody. PLoS One 8, art. no. e72480.

Hicks, D.G., Short, S.M., Prescott, N.L., Tarr, S.M., Coleman, K.A., Yoder, B.J., et al., 2006. Breast cancers with brain metastases are more likely to be estrogen receptor negative, express the basal cytokeratin CK5/6, and overexpress HER2 or EGFR. Am. J. Surg. Pathol. 30, 1097–1104.

Hoang, B., Frost, P., Shi, Y., Belanger, E., Benavides, A., Pezeshkpour, G., et al., 2010. Targeting TORC2 in multiple myeloma with a new mTOR kinase inhibitor. Blood 116, 4560–4568.

Hohensee, I., Lamszus, K., Riethdorf, S., Meyer-Staeckling, S., Glatzel, M., Matschke, J., et al., 2013. Frequent genetic alterations in EGFR- and HER2-driven pathways in breast cancer brain metastases. Am. J. Pathol. 183, 83–95.

Hojjat-Farsangi, M., 2014. Small-molecule inhibitors of the receptor tyrosine kinases: promising tools for targeted cancer therapies. Int. J. Mol. Sci. 15, 13768–13801.

Hong, S.W., Shin, J.S., Moon, J.H., Kim, Y.S., Lee, J., Choi, E.K., et al., 2014. NVP-BEZ235, a dual PI3K/mTOR inhibitor, induces cell death through alternate routes in prostate cancer cells depending on the PTEN genotype. Apoptosis 19, 895–904.

Hoppmann, N., Graetz, C., Paterka, M., Poisa-Beiro, L., Larochelle, C., Hasan, M., et al., 2015. New candidates for CD4 T cell pathogenicity in experimental neuroinflammation and multiple sclerosis. Brain 138, 902–917.

Hou, L.C., Huang, F., Xu, H.B., 2016. Does celecoxib improve the efficacy of chemotherapy for advanced non-small cell lung cancer?. Br. J. Clin. Pharmacol. 81, 23–32.

Houghton, A.M., Rzymkiewicz, D.M., Ji, H.B., Gregory, A.D., Egea, E.E., Metz, H.E., et al., 2010. Neutrophil elastase-mediated degradation of IRS-1 accelerates lung tumor growth. Nat. Med. 16, 219–223.

Hsieh, A.C., Costa, M., Zollo, O., Davis, C., Feldman, M.E., Testa, J.R., et al., 2010. Genetic dissection of the oncogenic mTOR pathway reveals druggable addiction to translational control via 4EBP-eIF4E. Cancer Cell 17, 249–261.

Hsu, C.W., Huang, R.L., Khuc, T., Shou, D., Bullock, J., Grooby, S., 2016. Identification of approved and investigational drugs that inhibit hypoxia-inducible factor-1 signaling. Oncotarget 7, 8172–8183.

Hsu, Y.L., Hung, J.Y., Chou, S.H., Huang, M.S., Tsai, M.J., Lin, Y.S., et al., 2015. Angiomotin decreases lung cancer progression by sequestering oncogenic YAP/TAZ and decreasing Cyr61 expression. Oncogene 34, 4056–4068.

Hu, B., Guo, Y., Chen, C.Y., Li, Q., Niu, X., Guo, S.C., et al., 2014. Repression of SIRT1 promotes the differentiation of mouse induced pluripotent stem cells into neural stem cells. Cell Mol. Neurobiol. 34, 905–912.

Hu, Y., Hu, M.M., Shi, G.L., Han, Y., Li, B.L., 2014. Imbalance between vascular endothelial growth factor and endostatin correlates with the prognosis of operable non-small cell lung cancer. Eur. J. Surg. Oncol. 40, 1136–1142.

Hu, Z.W., Rao, B.Q., Chen, S.M., Duanmu, J., 2010. Targeting tissue factor on tumour cells and angiogenic vascular endothelial cells by factor VII-targeted verteporfin photodynamic therapy for breast cancer in vitro and in vivo in mice. BMC Cancer 10, art. no. 235.

Huang, M.C., Qiu, Q., Zeng, S., Xiao, Y.J., Shi, M.H., Zou, Y.Y., et al., 2015. Niclosamide inhibits the inflammatory and angiogenic activation of human umbilical vein endothelial cells. Inflamm. Res. 64, 1023–1032.

Huang, M.S., Wang, L., Chen, J.W., Bai, M.J., Zhou, C.R., Liu, S.J., et al., 2016. Regulation of COX-2 expression and epithelial-to-mesenchymal transition by hypoxia-inducible factor-1 alpha is associated with poor prognosis in hepatocellular carcinoma patients post TACE surgery. Int. J. Oncol. 48, 2144–2154.

Huang, S.W., Chang, S.H., Mu, S.W., Jiang, H.Y., Wang, S.T., Kao, J.K., et al., 2016. Imiquimod activates p53-dependent apoptosis in a human basal cell carcinoma cell line. J. Dermatol. Sci. 81, 182–191.

Huang, Y., Shi, H., Zhou, H., Song, X., Yuan, S., Luo, Y., 2006. The angiogenic function of nucleolin is mediated by vascular endothelial growth factor and nonmuscle myosin. Blood 107, 3564–3571.

Hung, J.J., Jeng, W.J., Chou, T.Y., Hsu, W.H., Wu, K.J., Huang, B.S., et al., 2013. Prognostic value of the new International Association for the Study of Lung Cancer/American Thoracic Society/European Respiratory Society lung adenocarcinoma classification on death and recurrence in completely resected stage I lung adenocarcinoma. Ann. Surg. 258, 1079–1086.

Hurvitz, S.A., Dalenc, F., Campone, M., O'Regan, R.M., Tjan-Heijnen, V.C., Gligorov, J., et al., 2013a. A phase 2 study of everolimus combined with trastuzumab and paclitaxel in patients with HER2-overexpressing advanced breast cancer that progressed during prior trastuzumab and taxane therapy. Breast Cancer Res. Treat. 141, 437–446.

Hurvitz, S.A., Dirix, L., Kocsis, J., Bianchi, G.V., Lu, J., Vinholes, J., et al., 2013b. Phase II randomized study of trastuzumab emtansine versus trastuzumab plus docetaxel in patients with human epidermal growth factor receptor 2-positive metastatic breast cancer. J. Clin. Oncol. 31, 1157–1163.

Hwang, G.H., Ryu, J.M., Jeon, Y.J., Choi, J., Han, H.J., Lee, Y.M., et al., 2015. The role of thioredoxin reductase and glutathione reductase in plumbagin-induced, reactive oxygen species-mediated apoptosis in cancer cell lines. Eur. J. Pharmacol. 765, 384–393.

Hwang, S., Thangapandian, S., Lee, Y., Sakkiah, S., John, S., Lee, K.W., 2011. Discovery and evaluation of potential sonic Hedgehog signalling pathway inhibitors using pharmacophore modelling and molecular dynamics simulations. J. Bioinform. Comput. Biol. 9, 15–35.

Hwang-Bo, J., Park, J.H., Chung, I.S., 2015. Tumstatin induces apoptosis mediated by Fas signaling pathway in oral squamous cell carcinoma SCC-VII cells. Oncol. Lett. 10, 1016–1022.

Hwang-Bo, J., Yoo, K.H., Park, J.H., Jeong, H.S., Chung, I.S., 2012. Recombinant canstatin inhibits angiopoietin-1-induced angiogenesis and lymphangiogenesis. Int. J. Cancer 131, 298–309.

Hyder, S.M., Liang, Y., Wu, J., 2009. Estrogen regulation of thrombospondin-1 in human breast cancer cells. Int. J. Cancer 125, 1045–1953.

Ibrahim, Y.H., Byron, S.A., Cui, X.J., Lee, A.V., Yee, D., 2008. Progesterone receptor-B regulation of insulin-like growth factor – stimulated cell migration in breast cancer cells via insulin receptor substrate-2. Mol. Cancer Res. 6, 1491–1498.

Ibuki, N., Ghaffari, M., Reuveni, H., Pandey, M., Fazli, L., Azuma, H., et al., 2014. The Tyrphostin NT157 suppresses insulin receptor substrates and augments therapeutic response of prostate cancer. Mol. Cancer Ther. 13, 2827–2839.

Iliopoulos, D., Kavousanaki, M., Ioannou, M., Boumpas, D., Verginis, P., 2011. The negative costimulatory molecule PD1 modulates the balance between immunity and tolerance via miR-21. Eur. J. Immunol. 41, 1754–1763.

Infante, J.R., Dees, E.C., Olszanski, A.J., Dhuria, S.V., Sen, S., Cameron, S., et al., 2014. Phase I dose-escalation study of LCL161, an oral inhibitor of apoptosis proteins inhibitor, in patients with advanced solid tumors. J. Clin. Oncol. 32, 3103–3110.

Ingber, D., Fujita, T., Kishimoto, S., Sudo, K., Kanamaru, T., Brem, H., et al., 1990. Synthetic analogues of fumagillin that inhibit angiogenesis and suppress tumour growth. Nature 348, 555–557.

Insinga, A., Minucci, S., Pelicci, P.G., 2005. Mechanisms of selective anticancer action of histone deacetylase inhibitors. Cell Cycle 4, 741–743.

Ishtiaq, S., Edwards, S., Sankaralingam, A., Evans, B.A.J., Elford, C., Frost, M.L., et al., 2015. The effect of nitrogen containing bisphosphonates, zoledronate and alendronate, on the production of pro-angiogenic factors by osteoblastic cells. Cytokine 71, 154–160.

Isozaki, H., Ichihara, E., Takigawa, N., Ohashi, K., Ochi, N., Yasugi, M., et al., 2016. Non-small cell lung cancer cells acquire resistance to the ALK inhibitor alectinib by activating alternative receptor tyrosine kinases. Cancer Res. 76, 1506–1516.

Ito, H., Ando, T., Arioka, Y., Saito, K., Seishima, M., 2015. Inhibition of indoleamine 2,3-dioxygenase activity enhances the anti-tumour effects of a Toll-like receptor 7 agonist in an established cancer model. Immunology 144, 621–630.

Ito, H., Ando, T., Seishima, M., 2015. Inhibition of iNOS activity enhances the anti-tumor effects of alpha-galactosylceramide in established murine cancer model. Oncotarget 6, 41863–41874.

Ito, T., Ando, H., Suzuki, T., Ogura, T., Hotta, K., Imamura, Y., 2010. Identification of a primary target of thalidomide teratogenicity. Science 327, 1345–1350.

Ivashko, I.N., Kolesar, J.M., 2016. Pembrolizumab and nivolumab: PD-1 inhibitors for advanced melanoma. Am. J. Health Syst. Pharm. 73, 193–201.

Iyer, S., Acharya, K.R., 2011. Tying the knot: the cystine signature and molecular-recognition processes of the vascular endothelial growth factor family of angiogenic cytokines. FEBS J. 278, 4304–4322.

Jackson, D., Atkinson, J., Guevara, C.I., Zhang, C.Y., Kery, V., Moon, S.J., et al., 2014. In vitro and in vivo evaluation of cysteine and site specific conjugated Herceptin antibody-drug conjugates. PLoS One 9, art. no. e83865.

Jalali, S., Huang, Y., Dumont, D.J., Hynynen, K., 2010. Focused ultrasound-mediated BBB disruption is associated with an increase in activation of AKT: experimental study in rats. BMC Neurol. 10, art. no. 114.

Janne, P.A., Ou, S.H., Kim, D.W., Oxnard, G.R., Martins, R., Kris, M.G., et al., 2014. Dacomitinib as first-line treatment in patients with clinically or molecularly selected advanced non-small-cell lung cancer: a multicentre, open-label, phase 2 trial. Lancet Oncol. 15, 1433–1441.

Janne, P.A., Shaw, A.T., Camidge, D.R., Giaccone, G., Shreeve, S.M., et al., 2016. Combined Pan-HER and ALK/ROS1/MET inhibition with dacomitinib and crizotinib in advanced non-small cell lung cancer: results of a phase I study. J. Thoracic. Oncol. 11, 737–747.

Jayachandran, A., Anaka, M., Prithviraj, P., Hudson, C., McKeown, S.J., Lo, P.H., et al., 2014. Thrombospondin 1 promotes an aggressive phenotype through epithelial-to-mesenchymal transition in human melanoma. Oncotarget 5, 5782–5797.

Jeanbart, L., Ballester, M., de Titta, A., Corthesy, P., Romero, P., Hubbell, J.A., et al., 2014. Enhancing efficacy of anticancer vaccines by targeted delivery to tumor-draining lymph nodes. Cancer Immunol. Res. 2, 436–447.

Jellbauer, S., Panthel, K., Hetrodt, J.H., Rüssmann, H., 2012. CD8 T-cell induction against vascular endothelial growth factor receptor 2 by *Salmonella* for vaccination purposes against a murine melanoma. PLoS One 7, e34214.

Jeng, K.S., Sheen, I.S., Jeng, W.J., Lin, C.C., Lin, C.K., Su, J.C., et al., 2013. High expression of patched homolog-1 messenger RNA and lioma-ssociated oncogene-1 messenger RNA of sonic hedgehog signaling pathway indicates a risk of post-resection recurrence of hepatocellular carcinoma. Ann. Surg. Oncol. 20, 464–473.

Jeon, C.Y., Pandol, S.J., Wu, B.C., Cook-Wiens, G., Gottlieb, R.A., Merz, N.B., et al., 2015. The association of statin use after cancer diagnosis with survival in pancreatic cancer patients: a SEER-medicare analysis. PLoS One 10, art. no. e012178.

Jerkic, M., Rodriguez-Barbero, A., Prieto, M., Toporsian, M., Pericacho, M., Rivas-Elena, J.V., et al., 2006. Reduced angiogenic responses in adult endoglin heterozygous mice. Cardiovasc. Res. 69, 845–854.

Jhanwar-Uniyal, M., Gillick, J.L., Neil, J., Tobias, M., Thwing, Z.E., Murali, R., 2015. Distinct signaling mechanisms of mTORC1 and mTORC2 in glioblastoma multiforme: a tale of two complexes. Adv. Biol. Regul. 57, 64–74.

Jia, H.J., Zhao, T.S., Zou, D., Jia, X.L., Gao, J., Song, X.F., 2016. Therapeutic injection of a C-type CpG ODN induced an antitumor immune response in C57/BL6 mice of orthotopically transplanted hepatocellular carcinoma. Oncol. Res. 23, 321–326.

Jiang, P., Mukthavaram, R., Chao, Y., Nomura, N., Bharati, I.S., Fogal, V., et al., 2014. In vitro and in vivo anticancer effects of mevalonate pathway modulation on human cancer cells. Br. J. Cancer 111, 1562–1571.

Jiang, S., Chen, X.P., Li, C.Y., Zhang, X.P., Zhang, T., Yue, Y.J., et al., 2012. Suramin inhibits the growth of nasopharyngeal carcinoma cells via the downregulation of osteopontin. Mol. Med. Rep. 6, 1351–1354.

Jiang, X., Guan, W., Li, M.X., Liang, W., Qing, Y., Dai, N., et al., 2015. Endostatin combined with platinum-based chemo-radiotherapy for advanced non-small cell lung cancer. Cell Biochem. Biophys. 71, 571–577.

Jimeno, A., Weiss, G.J., Miller, W.H., Gettinger, S., Eigl, B.J.C., Chang, A.L.S., et al., 2013. Phase I study of the Hedgehog pathway inhibitor IPI-926 in adult patients with solid tumors. Clin. Cancer Res. 19, 2766–2774.

Jin, R.H., Nakada, M., Teng, L., Furuta, T., Sabit, H., Hayashi, Y., et al., 2013. Combination therapy using Notch and Akt inhibitors is effective for suppressing invasion but not proliferation in glioma cells. Neurosci. Lett. 534, 316–321.

Johnson, E., Seachrist, D.D., De Leon-Rodriguez, C.M., Lozada, K.L., Miedler, J., Abdul-Karim, F. W., et al., 2010. HER2/ErbB2-induced breast cancer cell migration and invasion require p120 catenin activation of Rac1 and Cdc42. J. Biol. Chem. 285, 29491–29501.

Jonsdottir, K., Janssen, S.R., Da Rosa, F.C., Gudlaugsson, E., Skaland, I., Baak, J.P.A., et al., 2012. Validation of expression patterns for nine miRNAs in 204 lymph-node negative breast cancers. PLoS One 7, art. no. e48692.

Jung, M., Bu, S.Y., Tak, K.H., Park, J.E., Kim, E., 2013. Anticarcinogenic effect of quercetin by inhibition of insulin-like growth factor (IGF)-1 signaling in mouse skin cancer. Nutr. Res. Pract. 7, 439–445.

Kalea, A.Z., See, F., Harja, E., Arriero, M., Schmidt, A.M., Hudson, B.I., 2010. Alternatively spliced RAGEv1 inhibits tumorigenesis via suppression of JNK signalling. Cancer Res. 70, 5628–5638.

Kameyama, N., Matsuda, S., Itano, O., Ito, A., Konno, T., Arai, T., et al., 2011. Photodynamic therapy using an anti-EGF receptor antibody complexed with Verteporfin nanoparticles: a proof of concept study. Cancer Biother. Radiopharmaceut. 26, 697–704.

Kang, H.J., Lee, M.H., Kang, H.L., Kim, S.H., Ahn, J.R., Na, H., et al., 2014. Differential regulation of estrogen receptor α expression in breast cancer cells by metastasis-associated protein 1. Cancer Res. 74, 1484–1494.

Kang, S., Kim, K., Noh, J.Y., Jung, Y., Bae, O.N., Lim, K.M., et al., 2016. Simvastatin induces the apoptosis of normal vascular smooth muscle through the disruption of actin integrity via the impairment of RhoA/Rac-1 activity. Throm. Haemostasis 116, 496–505.

Kanteti, R., Riehm, J.J., Dhanasingh, I., Lennon, F.E., Mirzapoiazova, T., Mambetsariev, B., et al., 2016. PI3 kinase pathway and MET inhibition is efficacious in malignant pleural mesothelioma. Sci. Rep. 6, art. no. 32992.

Karachaliou, N., Codony-Servat, J., Teixido, C., Pilotto, S., Drozdowskyj, A., Codony-Servat, C., et al., 2015. BIM and mTOR expression levels predict outcome to erlotinib in EGFR-mutant non-small-cell lung cancer. Sci. Rep. 5, art. no. 17499.

Karagiannis, E.D., Popel, A.S., 2007. Identification of novel short peptides derived from the alpha 4, alpha 5, and alpha 6 fibrils of type IV collagen with anti-angiogenic properties. Biochem. Biophys. Rec. Commun. 354, 434–439.

Karaolis, D.K., Means, T.K., Yang, D., Takahashi, M., Yoshimura, T., Muraille, E., et al., 2007. Bacterial c-di-GMP is an immunostimulatory molecule. J. Immunol. 178, 2171–2181.

Karnevi, E., Said, K., Andersson, R., Rosendahl, A.H., 2013. Metformin-mediated growth inhibition involves suppression of the IGF-I receptor signalling pathway in human pancreatic cancer cell. BMC Cancer 13, art. no. 235.

Karp, D.D., Lee, S.J., Keller, S.M., Wright, G.S., Aisner, S., Belinsky, S.A., 2013. Randomized, double-blind, placebo-controlled, phase III chemoprevention trial of selenium supplementation in patients with resected stage I non–small-cell lung cancer: ECOG 5597. J. Clin. Oncol. 49, 2173–2185.

Katanasaka, Y., Kodera, Y., Yunokawa, M., Kitamura, Y., Tamura, T., Koizumi, F., 2014. Synergistic anti-tumor effects of a novel phosphatidyl inositol-3 kinase/mammalian target of rapamycin dual inhibitor BGT226 and gefitinib in non-small cell lung cancer cell lines. Cancer Lett. 347, 196–203.

Kattan, J., Bachour, M., Farhat, F., El Rassy, E., Assi, T., Ghosn, M., 2016. Phase II trial of weekly Docetaxel, Zoledronic acid, and Celecoxib for castration-resistant prostate cancer. Invest. New Drugs 34, 474–480.

Kaur, S., Chang, T., Singh, S.P., Lim, L., Mannan, P., Garfield, S.H., et al., 2014. CD47 signaling regulates the immunosuppressive activity of VEGF in T cells. J. Immunol. 193, 3914–3924.

Kawiak, A., Lojkowska, E., 2016. Ramentaceone, a Naphthoquinone derived from Drosera sp., induces apoptosis by suppressing PI3K/Akt signaling in breast cancer cells. PLoS One 11, art. no. e0147718.

Keane, M.M., Rubinstein, Y., Cuello, M., Ettenberg, S.A., Banerjee, P., Nau, M.M., et al., 2000. Inhibition of NF-kappaB activity enhances TRAIL mediated apoptosis in breast cancer cell lines. Br. Cancer Res. Treat. 64, 211–219.

Keifer, J.A., Guttridge, D.C., Ashburner, B.P., Baldwin Jr., A.S., 2001. Inhibition of NF-kappa B activity by thalidomide through suppression of IkappaB kinase activity. J. Biol. Chem. 276, 22382–22387.

Kele, J., Simplicio, N., Ferri, A.L., Mira, H., Guillemot, F., Arenas, E., et al., 2006. Neurogenin 2 is required for the development of ventral midbrain dopaminergic neurons. Development 133, 495–505.

Kelwick, R., Desanlis, I., Wheeler, G.N., Edwards, D.R., 2015. The ADAMTS (A Disintegrin and Metalloproteinase with Thrombospondin motifs) family. Genome Biol. 16, 113.

Kenyon, B.M., Browne, F., D'Amato, R.J., 1997. Effects of thalidomide and related metabolites in a mouse corneal model of neovascularization. Exp. Eye Res. 64, 971–978.

Keysar, S.B., Le, P.N., Anderson, R.T., Morton, J.J., Bowles, D.W., Paylor, J.J., et al., 2013. Hedgehog signaling alters reliance on EGF receptor signaling and mediates anti-EGFR therapeutic resistance in head and neck cancer. Cancer Res. 73, 3381–3392.

Khoury, M., Drake, A., Chen, Q., Dong, D., Leskov, I., Fragoso, M.F., et al., 2011. Mesenchymal stem cells secreting angiopoietin-like-5 support efficient expansion of human hematopoietic stem cells without compromising their repopulating potential. Stem Cells Dev. 20, 1371–1381.

Kim, E.J., Helfman, D.M., 2003. Characterization of the metasis-associated protein, S100A4. Role of calcium binding and dimerization in cellular localization and interaction with myosin. J. Biol. Chem. 278, 30063–30073.

Kim, H.S., Wannatung, T., Lee, S., Yang, W.K., Chung, S.H., Lim, J.S., et al., 2012. Quercetin enhances hypoxia-mediated apoptosis via direct inhibition of AMPK activity in HCT116 colon cancer. Apoptosis 17, 938–949.

Kim, H.Y., Park, S.Y., Lee, S.W., Lee, H.R., Lee, W.S., Rhim, B.Y., et al., 2014. Inhibition of HMGB1-induced angiogenesis by Cilostazol via SIRT1 activation in synovial fibroblasts from rheumatoid arthritis. PLoS One 9, art. no. e104743.

Kim, J., Lee, J., Kim, C., Choi, J., Kim, A., 2016. Anti-cancer effect of metformin by suppressing signaling pathway of HER2 and HER3 in tamoxifen-resistant breast cancer cells. Tumor Biol. 37, 5811–5819.

Kim, J.H., Gupta, S.C., Park, B., Yadav, V.R., Aggarwal, B.B., 2012. Turmeric (*Curcuma longa*) inhibits inflammatory nuclear factor (NF)-κB and NF-κB-regulated gene products and induces death receptors leading to suppressed proliferation, induced chemosensitization, and suppressed osteoclastogenesis. Mol. Nutr. Food Res. 56, 454–465.

Kim, J.H., Park, J.J., Lee, B.J., Joo, M.K., Chun, H.J., Lee, S.W., et al., 2016. Astaxanthin inhibits proliferation of human gastric cancer cell lines by interrupting cell cycle progression. Gut Liver 10, 369–374.

Kim, K.M., Lee, Y.J., 2005. Role of HER-2/neu signaling in sensitivity to tumor necrosis factor-related apoptosis-inducing ligand: enhancement of TRAIL-mediated apoptosis by amiloride. J. Cell Biochem. 96, 376–389.

Kim, M., Na, D.L., Park, S.H., Jeon, B.S., Roh, J.K., 1998. Nervous system involvement by metastatic hepatocellular carcinoma. J. Neurooncol. 36, 85–90.

Kim, R., Emi, M., Tanabe, K., 2006. Cancer immunosuppression and autoimmune disease: beyond immunosuppressive networks for tumour immunity. Immunology 119, 254–264.

Kim, S.H., Margalit, O., Katoh, H., Wang, D.Z., Wu, H., Xia, D.R., et al., 2014. CG100649, a novel COX-2 inhibitor, inhibits colorectal adenoma and carcinoma growth in mouse models. Invest. New Drugs 32, 1105–1112.

Kirane, A., Toombs, J.E., Larsen, J.E., Ostapoff, K.T., Meshaw, K.R., Zaknoen, S., et al., 2012. Epithelial-mesenchymal transition increases tumor sensitivity to COX-2 inhibition by apricoxib. Carcinogenesis 33, 1639–1646.

Kirkpatrick, L., Ramanathan, R.K., Green, S., Dragovich, T., 2005. Lowering of plasma thioredoxin by the thioredoxin inhibitor PX-12 is linked to increased patient survival in phase I clinical trial. Clin. Cancer Res. 11, 9064S.

Klickovic, U., Doberer, D., Gouva, G., Aschauer, S., Weisshaar, S., Storka, A., et al., 2014. Human pharmacokinetics of high dose oral curcumin and its effect on heme oxygenase-1 expression in healthy male subjects. Biomed. Res. Int. 2014, 458592.

Klimosch, S.N., Forsti, A., Eckert, J., Knezevic, J., Bevier, M., von Schonfels, W., et al., 2013. Functional TLR5 genetic variants affect human colorectal cancer survival. Cancer Res. 73, 7232–7242.

Klingelhofer, J., Grum-Schwensen, B., Beck, M., Nudsen, P.R.S., Grigorian, M., Lukanidin, E., et al., 2012. Anti-S100A4 antibody suppresses metastasis formation by blocking stroma cell invasion. Neoplasia 14, 1260–1268.

Knuckles, P., Vogt, M.A., Lugert, S., Milo, M., Chong, M.M.W., Hautbergue, G.M., et al., 2012. Drosha regulates neurogenesis by controlling Neurogenin 2 expression independent of microRNAs. Nat. Neurosci. 15, 962–969.

Ko, A.H., LoConte, N., Tempero, M.A., Walker, E.J., Kate Kelley, R., Lewis, S., et al., 2016. A phase I study of FOLFIRINOX plus IPI-926, a Hedgehog pathway inhibitor, for advanced pancreatic adenocarcinoma. Pancreas 45, 370–375.

Ko, Y.C., Chang, C.L., Chien, H.F., Wu, C.H., Lin, L.I., 2011. Resveratrol enhances the expression of death receptor Fas/CD95 and induces differentiation and apoptosis in anaplastic large-cell lymphoma cells. Cancer Lett. 309, 46–53.

Kodack, D.P., Chung, E., Yamashita, H., Incio, J., Duyverman, A.M.M.J., Song, Y., et al., 2012. Combined targeting of HER2 and VEGFR2 for effective treatment of HER2-amplified breast cancer brain metastases. Proc. Natl Acad. Sci. USA 109, E3119–E3127.

Koga-Yamakawa, E., Dovedi, S.J., Murata, M., Matsui, H., Leishman, A.J., Bell, J., et al., 2013. Intratracheal and oral administration of SM-276001: a selective TLR7 agonist, leads to antitumor efficacy in primary and metastatic models of cancer. Int. J. Cancer 132, 580–590.

Koike, Y., Shiratori, Y., Shiina, S., Teratani, T., Obi, S., Sato, S., et al., 2002. Randomized prospective study of prevention from tumor invasion into portal vein in 120 patients with hepatocellular carcinoma by vitamin K-II administration. Gastroenterology 416, A643.

Kolacinska, A., Cebula-Obrzut, B., Pakula, L., Chalubinska-Fendler, J., Morawiec-Sztandera, A., Pawlowska, Z., et al., 2015. Immune checkpoints: cytotoxic T-lymphocyte antigen 4 and programmed cell death protein 1 in breast cancer surgery. Oncol. Lett. 10, 1079–1086.

Komen, S.G. (2014). Breast cancer subtypes. <ww5.komen.org/BreastCancer/SubtypesofBreastCancer.html>.

Koval, A., Ahmed, K., Katanaev, V.L., 2016. Inhibition of Wnt signalling and breast tumour growth by the multi-purpose drug suramin through suppression of heterotrimeric G proteins and Wnt endocytosis. Biochem. J. 473, 371–381.

Kozak, M.M., Anderson, E.M., von Eyben, R., Pai, J.S., Poultsides, G.A., Visser, B.C., et al., 2016. Statin and metformin use prolongs survival in patients with resectable pancreatic cancer. Pancreas 45, 64–70.

Krebs, L.T., Shutter, J.R., Tanigaki, K., Honjo, T., Stark, K.L., Gridley, T., 2004. Haploinsufficient lethality and formation of arteriovenous malformations in Notch pathway mutants. Genes Dev. 18, 2469–2473.

Krop, I., Demuth, T., Guthrie, T., Wen, P.Y., Mason, W.P., Chinnaiyan, P., et al., 2012. Phase I pharmacologic and pharmacodynamic study of the gamma secretase (Notch) inhibitor MK-0752 in adult patients with advanced solid tumors. J. Clin. Oncol. 30, 2307–2313.

Krop, I., Winer, E.P., 2014. Trastuzumab Emtansine: a novel antibody-drug conjugate for HER2-positive breast cancer. Clin. Cancer Res. 20, 15–20.

Krust, B., El Khoury, D., Soundaramourty, C., Nondier, I., Hovanessian, A.G., 2011a. Suppression of tumorigenicity of rhabdoid tumor derived G401 cells by the multivalent HB-19 pseudopeptide that targets surface nucleolin. Biochimie 93, 426–433.

Krust, B., El Khoury, D., Nondier, I., Soundaramourty, C., Hovanessian, A.G., 2011b. Targeting surface nucleolin with multivalent HB-19 and related Nucant pseudopeptides results in distinct inhibitory mechanisms depending on the malignant tumor cell type. BMC Cancer 11, art. no. 333.

Kudo, N., Wolff, B., Sekimoto, T., Schreiner, E.P., Yoneda, Y., Yanagida, M., et al., 1998. Leptomycin B inhibition of signal-mediated nuclear export by direct binding to CRM1. Exp. Cell Res. 242, 540–547.

Kuimova, M.K., Bhatti, M., Deonarain, M., Yahioglu, G., Levitt, J.A., Stamati, I., 2007. Fluorescence characterisation of multiply-loaded anti-HER2 single chain Fv-photosensitizer conjugates suitable for photodynamic therapy. Photochem. Photobiol. Sci. 6, 933–939.

Kumar, R., Wang, R.A., Mazumdar, A., Talukder, A.H., Mandal, M., Yang, Z.B., et al., 2002. A naturally occurring MTA1 variant sequesters oestrogen receptor-alpha in the cytoplasm. Nature 418, 654–657.

Kumar, S., Pan, C.C., Bloodworth, J.C., Nixon, A.B., Theuer, C., Hoyt, D.G., et al., 2014. Antibody-directed coupling of endoglin and MMP-14 is a key mechanism for endoglin shedding and deregulation of TGF-beta signalling. Oncogene 33, 3970–3979.

Kumar, S., Rao, N., Ge, R., 2012. Emerging roles of ADAMTSs in angiogenesis and cancer. Cancers 4, 1252–1299.

Kuo, C.H., Chang, B.I., Lee, F.T., Chen, P.K., Lee, J.S., Shi, G.Y., et al., 2015. Development of recombinant adeno-associated virus serotype 2/8 carrying Kringle domains of human plasminogen for sustained expression and cancer therapy. Human Gene Ther. 26, 603–613.

Labropoulou, V.T., Skandalis, S.S., Ravazoula, P., Perimenis, P., Karamanos, N.K., Kalofonos, H. P., et al., 2013. Expression of syndecan-4 and correlation with metastatic potential in testicular germ cell tumours. BioMed Res. Int. 2013, 214864.

Lai, L., Liu, J.C., Zhai, D., Lin, Q.X., He, L.J., Dong, Y.M., et al., 2012. Plumbagin inhibits tumour angiogenesis and tumour growth through the Ras signalling pathway following activation of the VEGF receptor-2. Br. J. Pharmacol. 165, 1084–1096.

Lange, T., Nentwich, M.F., Luth, M., Yekebas, E., Schumacher, U., 2011. Trastuzumab has anti-metastatic and anti-angiogenic activity in a spontaneous metastasis xenograft model of esophageal adenocarcinoma. Cancer Lett. 308, 54–61.

Langer, C.J., 2015. Emerging immunotherapies in the treatment of non-small cell lung cancer (NSCLC): the role of immune checkpoint inhibitors. Am. J. Clin. Oncol. Cancer Clin. Trials 38, 422–430.

Laskowski, R.A., Gerick, F., Thronton, J.M., 2009. The structural basis of allosteric regulation in proteins. FEBS Lett. 583, 1692–1698.

Latocha, M., Zieba, A., Polaniak, R., Kusmierz, D., Nowosad, A., Jurzak, M., et al., 2015. Molecular effects of amine derivatives of phenothiazine on cancer cells C-32 and SNB-19 in vitro. Acta Poloniae Pharma 72, 909–915.

Lau, K.M., Chan, Q.K.Y., Pang, J.C.S., Ma, F.M.T., Li, K.K.W., et al., 2012. Overexpression of HMGA1 deregulates tumor growth via cdc25A and alters migration/invasion through a cdc25A-independent pathway in medulloblastoma. Acta Neuropathol. 123, 553–571.

Layden, M.J., Martindale, M.Q., 2014. Non-canonical Notch signaling represents an ancestral mechanism to regulate neural differentiation. EvoDevo 5, art. no. 30.

Le, X.F., Almeida, M.I., Mao, W.Q., Spizzo, R., Rossi, S., Nicoloso, M.S., et al., 2012. Modulation of microRNA-194 and cell migration by HER2-targeting trastuzumab in breast cancer. PLoS One 7, art. no. e41170.

Le, X.F., Mao, W.Q., Lu, C.H., Thornton, A., Heymach, J.V., Sood, A.K., et al., 2008. Specific blockade of VEGF and HER2 pathways results in greater growth inhibition of breast cancer xenografts that over express HER2. Cell Cycle 7, 3747–3758.

Leclerc, E., Fritz, G., Vetter, S.W., Heizmann, C.W., 2009. Binding of S100 proteins to RAGE: an update. Biochim. Biophys. Acta Mol. Cell Res. 1793, 993–1007.

Lee, C., Dhillon, J., Wang, M.Y.C., Gao, Y.Y., Hu, K.J., Park, E., et al., 2008. Targeting YB-1 in HER-2 overexpressing breast cancer cells induces apoptosis via the mTOR/STAT3 pathway and suppresses tumor growth in mice. Cancer Res. 68, 8661–8666.

Lee, C.J.J., Shibata, N., Wiley, M.J., Wells, P.G., 2011. Fluorothalidomide: a characterization of maternal and developmental toxicity in rabbits and mice. Toxicol Sci. 122, 157–169.

Lee, J., Hong, E.M., Jang, J.A., Park, S.W., Koh, D.H., Choi, M.H., 2016. Simvastatin induces apoptosis and suppresses insulin-like growth factor 1 receptor in bile duct cancer cells. Gut Liver 10, 310–317.

Lee, S.M., Moon, J., Redman, B.G., Chidiac, T., Flaherty, L.E., Zha, Y.Y., et al., 2015. Phase 2 study of RO4929097, a gamma-secretase inhibitor, in metastatic melanoma: SWOG 0933. Cancer 121, 432–440.

Lee, T.K.W., Cheung, V.C.H., Lu, P., Lau, Y.E.T., Ma, S., Tang, K.H., et al., 2014. Blockade of CD47-mediated cathepsin S/protease-activated receptor 2 signaling provides a therapeutic target for hepatocellular carcinoma. Hepatology 60, 179–191.

Lee, Y.S., Dutta, A., 2007. The tumor suppressor microRNA let-7 represses the HMGA2 oncogene. Genes Develop. 21, 1025–1030.

Lei, Q.Y., Zhang, H., Zhao, B., Zha, Z.Y., Bai, F., Pei, X.H., et al., 2008. AZ promotes cell proliferation and epithelial-mesenchymal transition and is inhibited by the hippo pathway. Mol. Cell Biol. 28, 2426–2436.

Leivonen, S.K., Sahlberg, K.K., Makela, R., Due, E.U., Kallioniemi, O., Borresen-Dale, A.L., et al., 2014. High-throughput screens identify microRNAs essential for HER2 positive breast cancer cell growth. Mol. Oncol. 8, 93–104.

Le Mercier, I., Chen, W.N., Lines, J.L., Day, M., Li, J.N., Sergent, P., et al., 2014. VISTA regulates the development of protective antitumor immunity. Cancer Res. 74, 1933–1944.

Leoncini, E., Edefonti, V., Hashibe, M., Parpinel, M., Cadoni, G., Ferraroni, M., et al., 2016. Carotenoid intake and head and neck cancer: a pooled analysis in the International Head and Neck Cancer Epidemiology Consortium. Eur. J. Epidemiol. 31, 369–383.

Leung, C.S., Yeung, T.L., Yip, K.P., Pradeep, S., Balasubramanian, L., Liu, J.S., et al., 2014. Calcium-dependent FAK/CREB/TNNC1 signalling mediates the effect of stromal MFAP5 on ovarian cancer metastatic potential. Nat. Commun. 5, art. no. 5092.

Lewis, K.A., Gray, P.C., Blount, A., MacConell, L.A., Wiater, E., Bilezikjian, L.M., et al., 2000. Betaglycan binds inhibin and can mediate functional antagonism of activin signalling. Nature 404, 411–414.

Li, C., Huang, S., Ma, F., Armstrong, E.A., Francis, D., Werner, L., et al., 2015. Co-inhibition of ALK and EGFR and/or c-MET on cell growth and response to radiation in ALK-positive NSCLC cells. Cancer Res. 75, Supplement.

Li, H.C., Cai, Q.Y., Shinohara, E.T., Cai, H., Cao, C., Wang, Z.F., et al., 2005. Endostatin polymorphism 4349G/A(D104N) is not associated with aggressiveness of disease in prostate [corrected] cancer. Dis. Markers 21, 37–41.

Li, J., Ye, L., Sun, P.H., Satherley, L., Hargest, R., Zhang, Z.T., et al., 2015. MTA1 is up-regulated in colorectal cancer and is inversely correlated with lymphatic metastasis. Cancer Genom. Proteom. 12, 339–345.

Li, J., Li, B., Xu, W.W., Chan, K.W., Guan, X.Y., Qin, Y.R., et al., 2016. Role of AMPK signaling in mediating the anticancer effects of silibinin in esophageal squamous cell carcinoma. Expert Opin. Ther. Targets 20, 7–18.

Li, K., Dias, S.J., Rimando, A.M., Dhar, S., Mizuno, C.S., Penman, A.D., et al., 2013. Pterostilbene acts through metastasis-associated protein 1 to inhibit tumor growth, progression and metastasis in prostate cancer. PLoS One 8, art. no. e57542.

Li, L., Ying, J., Li, H., Zhang, Y., Shu, X., Fan, Y., et al., 2012. The human cadherin 11 is a pro-apoptotic tumor suppressor modulating cell stemness through Wnt/β-catenin signaling and silenced in common carcinomas. Oncogene 31, 3901–3912.

Li, L.C., Peng, Y., Liu, Y.M., Wang, L.L., Wu, X.L., 2014. Gastric cancer cell growth and epithelial-mesenchymal transition are inhibited by gamma-secretase inhibitor DAPT. Oncol. Lett. 7, 2160–2164.

Li, T., Zhong, J.T., Dong, X.F., Xiu, P., Wang, F.H., Wei, H.L., et al., 2016. Meloxicam suppresses hepatocellular carcinoma cell proliferation and migration by targeting COX-2/PGE2-regulated activation of the beta-catenin signaling pathway. Oncol. Rep. 35, 3614–3622.

Li, W.L., Wei, W., Zhu, S.Y., Zhu, J.L., Shi, Y., Lin, T.X., et al., 2009. Generation of rat and human induced pluripotent stem cells by combining genetic reprogramming and chemical inhibitors. Cell Stem Cell 4, 16–19.

Li, X.L., Li, J., Wang, L.L., Li, A.Y., Qiu, Z.X., Qi, L.W., et al., 2016. The role of metformin and resveratrol in the prevention of hypoxia-inducible factor 1 accumulation and fibrosis in hypoxic adipose tissue. Br. J. Pharmacol. 173, 2001–2015.

Li, X.Y., Zhu, S.J., Hong, C.Q., Cai, H.Q., 2016. Angiogenesis inhibitors for patients with ovarian cancer: a meta-analysis of 12 randomized controlled trials. Curr. Med. Res. Opin. 32, 555–562.

Li, Y., He, J.M., Zhong, D.P., Li, J.J., Liang, H.J., 2015. High-mobility group box 1 protein activating nuclear factor-B to upregulate vascular endothelial growth factor C is involved in lymphangiogenesis and lymphatic node metastasis in colon cancer. J. Int. Med. Res. 43, 494–505.

Li, Y.J., Sun, L.C., He, Y., Liu, X.H., Liu, M., Wang, et al., 2009. The anti-tumor properties of two tumstatin peptide fragments in human gastric carcinoma. Acta Pharmacol. Sin. 30, 1307–1315.

Liao, H., Huang, Y., Guo, B.T., Liang, B., Liu, X.C., Ou, H.H., et al., 2015. Dramatic antitumor effects of the dual mTORC1 and mTORC2 inhibitor AZD2014 in hepatocellular carcinoma. Am. J. Cancer Res. 5, 125–139.

Lim, S.H., Kim, T.W., Hong, Y.S., Han, S.W., Lee, K.H., Kang, H.J., et al., 2015. A randomised, double-blind, placebo-controlled multi-centre phase III trial of XELIRI/FOLFIRI plus simvastatin for patients with metastatic colorectal cancer. Br. J. Cancer 113, 1421–1426.

Lin, N.U., Winer, E.P., 2007. Brain metastases: the HER2 paradigm. Clin. Cancer Res. 13, 1648–1655.

Lin, Q., Yang, X.P., Fang, D., Ren, X.R., Zhou, H.Y., Fang, J.Z., et al., 2011. High-mobility group box-1 mediates toll-like receptor 4-dependent angiogenesis. Atheroscl. Thromb. Vasc. Biol. 31, 1024–1032.

Lin, Y., Shi, R., Wang, X., Shen, H.M., 2008. Luteolin, a flavonoid with potential for cancer prevention and therapy. Curr. Cancer Drug Targets 8, 634–646.

Lin, Y.C., Chen, L.H., Varadharajan, T., Tsai, M.J., Chia, Y.C., Yuan, T.C., et al., 2014. Resveratrol inhibits glucose-induced migration of vascular smooth muscle cells mediated by focal adhesion kinase. Mol. Nutr. Food Res. 58, 1389–1401.

Lin, Z., Wan, X., Jiang, R.Q., Deng, L., Gao, Y., Tang, J.W., et al., 2014. Epstein–Barr virus-encoded latent membrane protein 2A promotes the epithelial-mesenchymal transition in nasopharyngeal carcinoma via metastatic tumor antigen 1 and mechanistic target of Rapamycin signaling induction. J. Virol. 88, 11872–11885.

Lines, J.L., Pantazi, E., Mak, J., Sempere, L.F., Wang, L., O'Connell, S., et al., 2014a. VISTA is an immune checkpoint molecule for human T cells. Cancer Res. 74, 1924–1932.

Lines, J.L., Sempere, L.F., Broughton, T., Wang, L., Noelle, R., 2014b. VISTA is a novel broad-spectrum negative checkpoint regulator for cancer immunotherapy. Cancer Immunol. Res. 2, 510–517.

Ling, Y., Yang, Y., Lu, N., You, Q.D., Wang, S., Gao, Y., et al., 2007. Endostar, a novel recombinant human endostatin, exerts antiangiogenic effect via blocking VEGF-induced tyrosine phosphorylation of KDR/Flk-1 of endothelial cells. Biochem. Biophys. Res. Commun. 361, 79–84.

Ling, Y.G., Liebes, L., Ng, B., Buckley, M., Elliott, P.J., Adams, J., et al., 2002. PS-341, a novel proteasome inhibitor, induces Bcl-2 phosphorylation and cleavage in association with G2–M phase arrest and apoptosis. Mol. Cancer Ther. 1, 841–849.

Lionello, M., Lovato, A., Staffieri, A., Blandamura, S., Turato, C., Giacomelli, L., et al., 2014. The EGFR-mTOR pathway and laryngeal cancer angiogenesis. Eur. Arch. Otorhinolaryngol. 271, 757–764.

Liou, W.S., Chen, L.J., Niu, H.S., Yang, T.T., Cheng, J.T., Lin, K.C., 2015. Herbal product silibinin-induced programmed cell death is enhanced by metformin in cervical cancer cells at the dose without influence on nonmalignant cells. J. Appl. Biomed. 13, 113–121.

Liu, C., Lou, W., Zhu, Y., Nadiminty, N., Schwartz, C.T., Evans, C.P., et al., 2014. Niclosamide inhibits androgen receptor variants expression and overcomes enzalutamide resistance in castration resistant prostate cancer. Clin. Cancer Res. 20, 3198–3210.

Liu, H., Liu, Y.Z., Zhang, F., Wang, H.S., Zhang, G., Zhou, B.H., et al., 2014. Identification of potential pathways involved in the induction of cell cycle arrest and apoptosis by a new 4-arylidene curcumin analogue T63 in lung cancer cells: a comparative proteomic analysis. Mol. Biosyst. 10, 1320–1331.

Liu, H.J., Jia, D.Y., Li, A.N., Chau, J., He, D., Ruan, X.S., et al., 2013. p53 regulates neural stem cell proliferation and differentiation via BMP-Smad1 signaling and Id1. Stem Cell Develp. 22, 913–927.

Liu, J., Yuan, Y., Chen, W.N., Putra, J., Suriawinata, A.A., Schenk, A.D., et al., 2015. Immune-checkpoint proteins VISTA and PD1 nonredundantly regulate murine T-cell responses. Proc. Natl. Acad. Sci. USA 112, 6682–6687.

Liu, J.J., Chen, X.S., Ward, T., Mao, Y., Bockhorn, J., Liu, X.F., et al., 2016. Niclosamide inhibits epithelial-mesenchymal transition and tumor growth in lapatinib-resistant human epidermal growth factor receptor 2-positive breast cancer. Int. J. Biochem. Cell Biol. 71, 12–23.

Liu, J.L., Wang, L.L., Su, Z.H., Wu, W., Cai, X.J., Li, D., et al., 2014. A reciprocal antagonism between miR-376c and TGF-beta signaling regulates neural differentiation of human pluripotent stem cells. FASEB J. 28, 4642–4656.

Liu, J.N., Wu, J.X., Zhou, L., Pan, C.C., Zhou, Y., Du, W.Y., et al., 2015. ZD6474, a new treatment strategy for human osteosarcoma, and its potential synergistic effect with celecoxib. Oncotarget 6, 21341–21351.

Liu, J.W., Dunoyer-Geindre, S., Blot-Chabaud, M., Sabatier, F., Fish, R.J., Bounameaux, H., et al., 2010. Generation of human inflammation-resistant endothelial progenitor cells by A20 gene transfer. J. Vasc. Res. 47, 157–167.

Liu, L., Eckert, M.A., Riazifar, H., Kang, D.K., Agalliu, D., Zhao, W., et al., 2013. From blood to the brain: can systemically transplanted mesenchymal stem cells cross the blood–brain barrier? Stem Cells Int. 2013, art. no. 435093.

Liu, Q.L., Yuan, W.Q., Tong, D.L., Liu, G.L., Lan, W.H., Zhang, D.Z., et al., 2016. Metformin represses bladder cancer progression by inhibiting stem cell repopulation via COX2/PGE2/STAT3 axis. Oncotarget 7, 28235–28246.

Liu, T.B., Yang, M., Yang, S.S., Ge, T.T., Gu, L.N., Lou, G., 2013. Metastasis-associated protein 1 is a novel marker predicting survival and lymph nodes metastasis in cervical cancer. Human Pathol. 44, 2275–2281.

Liu, W.M., Henry, J.Y., Meyer, B., Bartlett, J.B., Dalgleish, A.G., Galustian, C., 2009. Inhibition of metastatic potential in colorectal carcinoma in vivo and in vitro using immunomodulatory drugs (IMiDs). Br. J. Cancer 101, 803–812.

Liu, W.M., Laux, H., Henry, J.Y., Bolton, T.B., Dalgleish, A.G., Galustian, C., 2010. A microarray study of altered gene expression in colorectal cancer cells after treatment with immunomodulatory drugs: differences in action in vivo and in vitro. Mol. Biol. Rep. 37, 1801–1814.

Liu, W.M., Strauss, S.J., Chaplin, T., Shahin, S., Propper, D.J., Young, B.D., et al., 2004. s-Thalidomide has a greater effect on apoptosis than angiogenesis in a multiple myeloma cell line. Hematol. J. 5, 247–254.

Liu, W.T., Jing, Y.Y., Yu, G.F., Han, Z.P., Yu, D.D., Fan, Q.M., et al., 2015. Toll like receptor 4 facilitates invasion and migration as a cancer stem cell marker in hepatocellular carcinoma. Cancer Lett. 358, 136–143.

Liu, X., Yue, P., Zhou, Z., Khuri, F.R., Sun, S.Y., 2004. Death receptor regulation and celecoxib-induced apoptosis in human lung cancer cells. J. Natl Cancer Inst. 96, 1769–1780.

Liu, X.J., Niu, M.S., Xu, X.Y., Cai, W., Zeng, L.Y., Zhou, X.P., et al., 2014. CRM1 is a direct cellular target of the natural anti-cancer agent plumbagin. J. Pharmacol. Sci. 124, 486–493.

Liu, X.X., Li, X.B., Yin, L.H., Ding, J.X., Jin, H.Y., Feng, Y.J., 2011. Genistein inhibits placental choriocarcinoma cell line JAR invasion through ER beta/MTA3/Snail/E-cadherin pathway. Oncol. Lett. 2, 891–897.

Liu, Y., Huang, T., Zhao, X., Cheng, L., 2011. MicroRNAs modulate the Wnt signaling pathway through targeting its inhibitors. Biochem. Biophys. Res. Commun. 408, 259–264.

Liu, Y., Starr, M.D., Brady, J.C., Dellinger, A., Pang, H., Adams, B., et al., 2014. Modulation of circulating protein biomarkers following TRC105 (anti-endoglin antibody) treatment in patients with advanced cancer. Cancer Med. 3, 580–591.

Liu, Z., Kobayashi, K., van Dinther, M., van Heiningen, S.H., Valdimarsdottir, G., van Laar, T., et al., 2009. VGF and inhibitors of TGFβ type I receptor kinase synergistically promote blood vessel formation by inducing 5-integrin expression. J. Cell Sci. 122, 3294–3302.

Llopiz, D., Dotor, J., Casares, N., Bezunartea, J., Diaz-Valdes, N., Ruiz, M., et al., 2009. Peptide inhibitors of transforming growth factor-beta enhance the efficacy of antitumor immunotherapy. Int. J. Cancer 125, 2614–2623.

Lo, H.W., Hsu, S.C., Xia, W., Cao, X., Shih, J.Y., Wei, Y., et al., 2007. Epidermal growth factor receptor cooperates with signal transducer and activator of transcription 3 to induce epithelial-mesenchymal transition in cancer cells via up-regulation of TWIST gene expression. Cancer Res. 67, 9066–9076.

Lock, F.E., Underhill-Day, N., Dunwell, T., Matallanas, D., Cooper, W., Hesson, L., et al., 2010. The RASSF8 candidate tumor suppressor inhibits cell growth and regulates the Wnt and NF-kappa B signaling pathways. Oncogene 29, 4307–4316.

Longva, K.E., Pedersen, N.M., Haslekås, C., Stang, E., Madshus, I.H., 2005. Herceptin induced inhibition of ErbB2 signaling involves reduced phosphorylation of Akt but not endocytic down-regulation of ErbB2. Int. J. Cancer 116, 359–367.

Lopez, E.S., Rizzo, M.M., Croxatto, J.O., Mazzolini, G., Gallo, J.E., 2011. Suramab, a novel anti-angiogenic agent, reduces tumor growth and corneal neovascularization. Cancer Chemother. Pharmacol. 67, 723–728.

Lopez-Guerra, M., Xargay-Torrent, S., Rosich, L., Montraveta, A., Roldan, J., Matas-Cespedes, A., et al., 2015. The gamma-secretase inhibitor PF-03084014 combined with fludarabine antagonizes migration, invasion and angiogenesis in Notch1-mutated CLL cells. Leukemia 29, 96–106.

Lopez-Novoa, J.M., Bernabeu, C. (2012; updated 2016). Atlas Genet Cytogenet Oncol Haematol. <http://AtlasGeneticsOncology.org/Genes/ENGID40452ch9q34.html>.

Lotz, J.P., Cure, H., Janvier, M., Asselain, B., Morvan, F., Legros, M., et al., 2005. High-dose chemotherapy with haematopoietic stem cell transplantation for metastatic breast cancer patients: final results of the French multicentric randomised CMA/PEGASE 04 protocol. Eur. J. Cancer 41, 71–80.

Lu, L., Payvandi, F., Wu, L., Zhang, L.H., Hariri, R.J., Man, H.W., et al., 2009. The anti-cancer drug lenalidomide inhibits angiogenesis and metastasis via multiple inhibitory effects on endothelial cell function in normoxic and hypoxic conditions. Microvasc. Res. 77, 78–86.

Lu, S., Li, L., Luo, Y., Zhang, L., Wu, G., Chen, Z.W., et al., 2015. A multicenter, open-label, randomized phase II controlled study of rh-Endostatin (Endostar) in combination with chemotherapy in previously untreated extensive-stage small-cell lung cancer. J. Thoracic. Oncol. 10, 206–211.

Lu, Y., Ma, W., Mao, J., Yu, X., Hou, Z., Fan, S., et al., 2015. Salinomycin exerts anticancer effects on human breast carcinoma MCF-7 cancer stem cells via modulation of Hedgehog signaling. Chemico Biol. Int. 228, 100–107.

Lu, Y.M., Wei, C.J., Xi, Z.Q., 2014. Curcumin suppresses proliferation and invasion in non-small cell lung cancer by modulation of MTA1-mediated Wnt/beta-catenin pathway. In Vitro Cell. Develop. Biol. Anim. 50, 840–850.

Lv, M., Lv, M.L., Chen, L., Qin, T.J., Zhang, X., Liu, P.J., et al., 2015. Angiomotin promotes breast cancer cell proliferation and invasion. Oncol. Rep. 33, 1938–1946.

Lv, X.H., Jiang, H.H., Liu, Y.L., Lei, X.P., Jiao, J.W., 2014. MicroRNA-15b promotes neurogenesis and inhibits neural progenitor proliferation by directly repressing TET3 during early neocortical development. EMBO Rep. 15, 1305–1314.

Ma, Z.K., Liu, W., Zeng, J., Zhou, J.C., Guo, P., Xie, H.J., 2015. Silibinin induces apoptosis through inhibition of the mTOR-GLI1-BCL2 pathway in renal cell carcinoma. Oncol. Rep. 34, 2461–2468.

MacDonald, N.J., Murad, A.C., Fogler, W.E., Lu, Y., Sim, B.K., 1999. The tumor-suppressing activity of angiostatin protein resides within kringles 1 to 3. Biochem. Biophys. Res. Commun. 264, 469–477.

Madden, J.M., Mueller, K.L., Bollig-Fischer, A., Stemmer, P., Mattingly, R.R., Boerner, J.L., 2014. Abrogating phosphorylation of eIF4B is required for EGFR and mTOR inhibitor synergy in triple-negative breast cancer. Br. Cancer Res. Treat. 147, 283–293.

Maeshima, Y., Sudhakar, A., Lively, J.C., Ueki, K., Kharbanda, S., Kahn, C.R., et al., 2002. Tumstatin, an endothelial cell-specific inhibitor of protein synthesis. Science 295, 140–143.

Majumdar, A.P.N., Banerjee, S., Nautiyal, J., Patel, B.B., Patel, V., Du, J.H., et al., 2009. Curcumin synergizes with resveratrol to inhibit colon cancer. Nutr. Cancer Int. J. 61, 544–553.

Malashkevich, V.N., Dulyaninova, N.G., Ramagopal, U.A., Liriano, M.A., Varney, K.M., Knight, D., et al., 2010. Phenothiazines inhibit S100A4 function by inducing protein oligomerization. Proc. Natl Acad. Sci. USA 107, 8605–8610.

Man, H.W., Corral, L.G., Stirling, D.I., Muller, G.W., 2003. Alpha-fluoro-substituted thalidomide analogues. Bioorg. Med. Chem. Lett. 13, 3415–3417.

Markovic, S.N., Suman, V.J., Rao, R.A., Ingle, J.N., Kaur, J.S., Erickson, L.A., et al., 2007. A phase II study of ABT-510 (thrombospondin-1 analog) for the treatment of metastatic melanoma. Am. J. Clin. Oncol. Cancer Clin. Trials 30, 303–309.

Marlow, H., Matus, D.Q., Martindale, M.Q., 2013. Ectopic activation of the canonical wnt signaling pathway affects ectodermal patterning along the primary axis during larval development in the anthozoan Nematostella vectensis. Dev. Biol. 380, 324–334.

Marti, P., Stein, C., Blumer, T., Abraham, Y., Dill, M.T., Pikiolek, M., et al., 2015. YAP promotes proliferation, chemoresistance, and angiogenesis in human cholangiocarcinoma through TEAD transcription factors. Hepaatology 62, 1497–1510.

Martin, M.D., Hilsenbeck, S.G., Mohsin, S.K., Hopp, T.A., Clark, G.M., Osborne, C.K., et al., 2006. Breast tumors that overexpress nuclear metastasis-associated 1 (MTA1) protein have high recurrence risks but enhanced responses to systemic therapies. Breast Cancer Res. Treat. 95, 7–12.

Massarweh, S., Romond, E., Black, E.P., Van Meter, E., Shelton, B., Kadamyan-Melkumian, V., et al., 2014. A phase II study of combined fulvestrant and everolimus in patients with metastatic estrogen receptor (ER)-positive breast cancer after aromatase inhibitor (AI) failure. Breast Cancer Res. Treat. 143, 325–332.

Mata, R., Palladino, C., Nicolosi, M.L., Lo Presti, A.R., Malaguarnera, R., Ragusa, M., et al., 2016. IGF-I induces upregulation of DDR1 collagen receptor in breast cancer cells by suppressing MIR-199a-5p through the PI3K/AKT pathway. Oncotarget 7, 7683–7700.

Matsuo, M., Yamada, S., Koiz-Uyni, K., Sakurai, F., Saiki, I., 2007. Tumour-derived fibroblast growth factor-2 exerts lymphangiogenic effects through Akt/mTOR/p70S6kinase pathway in rat lymphatic endothelial cells. Eur. J. Cancer 43, 1748–1754.

Matzner, P., Sorski, L., Shaashua, L., Elbaz, E., Lavon, H., Melamed, R., et al., 2016. Perioperative treatment with the new synthetic TLR-4 agonist GLA-SE reduces cancer metastasis without adverse effects. Int. J. Cancer 138, 1754–1764.

Mazumdar, A., Wang, R.A., Mishra, S.K., Adam, L., Bagheri-Yarmand, R., Mandal, M., et al., 2001. Transcriptional repression of oestrogen receptor by metastasis-associated protein 1 corepressor. Nat. Cell Biol. 3, 30–37.

Mazumdar, T., DeVecchio, J., Agyeman, A., Shi, T., Houghton, J.A., 2011. Blocking Hedgehog survival signaling at the level of the GLI genes induces DNA damage and extensive cell death in human colon carcinoma cells. Cancer Res. 71, 5904–5914.

Mazur-Bialy, A.I., Pochec, E., 2016. HMGB1 inhibition during Zymosan-induced inflammation: the potential therapeutic action of riboflavin. Arch. Immunol. Ther. Exp. 64, 171–176.

Mazur-Bialy, A.I., Pochec, E., Plytycz, B., 2015. Immunomodulatory effect of riboflavin deficiency and enrichment. Reversible pathological response versus silencing of inflammatory activation. J. Physiol. Pharmacol. 66, 793–802.

McAllister, K.A., Grogg, K.M., Johnson, D.W., Gallione, C.J., Baldwin, M.A., Jackson, C.E., et al., 1994. Endoglin, a TGF-β binding protein of endothelial cells, is the gene for hereditary haemorrhagic telangiectasia type 1. Nat. Genet. 8, 345–351.

McCart-Reed, A.E., Song, S., Kutasovic, J.R., Reid, L.E., Valle, J.M., Vargas, A.C., et al., 2013. Thrombospondin-4 expression is activated during the stromal response to invasive breast cancer. Virchows Arch. 463, 535–545.

McCluskey, A.J., Olive, A.J., Starnbach, M.N., Collier, R.J., 2013. Targeting HER2-positive cancer cells with receptor-redirected anthrax protective antigen. Mol. Oncol. 7, 440–451.

Medinger, M., Halter, J., Heim, D., Buser, A., Gerull, S., Stern, M., et al., 2015. Angiogenic markers in plasma cell myeloma patients treated with novel agents. Anticancer Res. 35, 1085–1090.

Meiyanto, E., Putri, D.D.P., Susidarti, R.A., Murwanti, R., Sardjiman, Fitriasari, A., et al., 2014. Curcumin and its analogue (PGV-0 and PGV-1) enhance sensitivity of resistant MCF-7 cells to doxorubicin through inhibition of HER2 and NF-kB activation. Asian Pacific J. Cancer Prevent. 15, 179–184.

Mendoza, V., Vilchis-Landeros, M.M., Mendoza-Hernandez, G., Huang, T., Villarreal, M.M., Hinck, A.P., et al., 2009. Betaglycan has two independent domains required for high affinity TGF-beta binding: proteolytic cleavage separates the domains and inactivates the neutralizing activity of the soluble receptor. Biochemistry 48, 11755–11765.

Meng, F.B., Feng, W., Xin, H., Tian, Z., Zhang, Y., Zhang, L.P., 2015. 14-3-3 proteins interact with FRMD6 and regulate its subcellular localization in breast cancer cells. Chem. Res. Chin. Univ. 31, 558–563.

Meng, H., Xing, G., Bianco, E., Song, Y., Zhao, L., Sun, B., et al., 2012. Gadolinium metallofullerenol nanoparticles inhibit cancer metastasis through matrix metalloproteinase inhibition: imprisoning instead of poisoning cancer cells. Nanomedicine 8, 136–146.

Meng, Z., Gan, Y.H., 2015. Activating PTEN by COX-2 inhibitors antagonizes radiation-induced MKT activation contributing to radiosensitization. Biochem. Biophys. Res. Commun. 460, 198–204.

Menon, L.G., Shi, V.J., Carroll, R.S. (2009). Mesenchymal stromal cells as a drug delivery system. StemBook, ed. The Stem Cell Research Community, StemBook, doi/10.3824/stembook 1.35.1.

Merrell, M.A., Ilvesaro, J.M., Lehtonen, N., Sorsa, T., Gehrs, B., Rosenthal, E., et al., 2006. Toll-like receptor 9 agonists promote cellular invasion by increasing matrix metalloproteinase activity. Mol. Cancer Res. 4, 437–447.

Messersmith, W.A., Shapiro, G.I., Cleary, J.M., Jimeno, A., Dasari, A., Huang, B., et al., 2015. A phase I, dose-finding study in patients with advanced solid malignancies of the oral gamma-secretase inhibitor PF-03084014. Clin. Cancer Res. 21, 60–67.

Mhawech, P., Benz, A., Cerato, C., Greloz, V., Assaly, M., Desmond, J.C., et al., 2005. Downregulation of the 14-3-3 in ovary, prostate and endometrial carcinomas is associated with CpG island methylation. Modern Pathol. 18, 340–348.

Miao, Y., Cui, T., Leng, F., Wilson, W.D., 2008. Inhibition of high-mobility-group A2 protein binding to DNA by netropsin: a biosensor-surface plasmon resonance assay. Anal. Biochem. 374, 7–15.

Milano, S.K., Pace, H.C., Kim, Y.M., Brenner, C., Benovic, J.L., 2002. Scaffolding functions of arrestin-2 revealed by crystal structure and mutagenesis. Biochemistry 41, 3321–3328.

Miller, K.D., Weathers, T., Haney, L.G., Timmerman, R., Dickler, M., Shen, J., et al., 2003. Occult central nervous system involvement in patients with metastatic breast cancer: prevalence, predictive factors and impact on overall survival. Ann. Oncol. 14, 1072–1077.

Minisini, A.M., Moroso, S., Gerratana, L., Giangreco, M., Iacono, D., Poletto, E., et al., 2013. Risk factors and survival outcomes in patients with brain metastases from breast cancer. Clin. Exp. Metastasis 30, 951–956.

Misch, E.A., Hawn, T.R., 2008. Toll-like receptor polymorphisms and susceptibility to human disease. Clin. Sci. (Lond.) 114, 347–360.

Mishra, S.K., Mazumdar, A., Vadlamudi, R.K., Li, F., Wang, R.A., Yu, W., et al., 2003. MICoA, a novel metastasis-associated protein 1 (MTA1) interacting protein coactivator, regulates estrogen receptor-alpha transactivation functions. J. Biol. Chem. 278, 19209–19219.

Miyaaki, H., Nakashima, O., Kurogi, M., Eguchi, K., Kojiro, M., 2007. Lens culinaris agglutinin-reactive alpha-fetoprotein and protein induced by vitamin K absence II are potential indicators of a poor prognosis: a histopathological study of surgically resected hepatocellular carcinoma. J. Gastroenterol. 42, 962–968.

Moffett, J.R., Namboodiri, M.A.A., 2003. Tryptophan and the immune system. Immunol. Cell Biol. 81, 247–265.

Mohammad, G., Siddiquei, M.M., Alam, K., Nawaz, M.I., Mousa, A., Opdenakker, G., et al., 2016. High-mobility group box-1 regulates the expression of matrix metalloproteinase-9 in diabetic retina. Int. J. Clin. Exp. Pathol. 9, 828–840.

Mohammed, A., Janakiram, N.B., Madka, V., Brewer, M., Ritchie, R.L., Lightfoot, S., et al., 2015. Targeting pancreatitis blocks tumor-initiating stem cells and pancreatic cancer progression. Oncotarget 6, 15524–15539.

Mok, S.C., Bonome, T., Vathipadiekal, V., Bell, A., Johnson, M.E., Wong, K.K., et al., 2009. A gene signature predictive for outcome in advanced ovarian cancer identifies a survival factor: microfibril-associated glycoprotein 2. Cancer Cell 16, 521–532.

Moleirinho, S., Guerrant, W., Kissil, J.L., 2014. The angiomotins – from discovery to function. FEBS Lett. 588, 2693–2703.

Mollica, L., De Marchis, F., Spitalen, A., Dallacosta, C., Pennacchini, D., Zamai, et al., 2007. Glycyrrhizin binds to high mobility group box 1 protein and inhibits its cytokine activities. Chem. Biol. 14, 431–441.

Monboisse, J.C., Oudart, J.B., Ramont, L., Brassart-Pasco, S., Maquart, F.X., 2014. Matrikines from basement membrane collagens: a new anti-cancer strategy. Biochim. Biophys. Acta 1840, 2589–2598.

Mondanizadeh, M., Arefian, E., Mosayebi, G., Saidijam, M., Khansarinejad, B., Hashemi, S.M., 2015. MicroRNA-124 regulates neuronal differentiation of mesenchymal stem cells by targeting Sp1 mRNA. J. Cell Biochem. 116, 943–953.

Montgomery, A., Adeyeni, T., San, K., Heuertz, R.M., Ezekiel, U.R., 2016. Curcumin sensitizes silymarin to exert synergistic anticancer activity in colon cancer cells. J. Cancer 7, 1250–1257.

Moore, C.B., Guthrie, E.H., Huang, M.T.H., Taxman, D., 2010. Short hairpin RNA (shRNA): design, delivery, and assessment of gene knockdown. Methods Mol. Biol. 629, 141–158.

Moore, K.N., Sill, M.W., Tenney, M.E., Darus, C.J., Griffin, D., Werner, T.L., et al., 2015. A phase II trial of trebananib (AMG 386; IND#111071), a selective angiopoietin 1/2 neutralizing peptibody, in patients with persistent/recurrent carcinoma of the endometrium: an NRG/gynecologic oncology group trial. Gynecol. Oncol. 138, 513–518.

Moore, R., Chandrahas, A., Bleris, L., 2014. Transcription activator-like effectors: a toolkit for synthetic biology. ACS Synth. Biol. 3, 708–716.

Moreira, D., Zhang, Q., Hossain, D.M., Nechaev, S., Li, H., Kowalik, C.M., et al., 2015. TLR9 signaling through NF-κB/RELA and STAT3 promotes tumor-propagating potential of prostate cancer cells. Oncotarget 6, 17302-17013.

Morelli, C., Garofalo, C., Sisci, D., Del Rincon, S., Cascio, S., Tu, X., et al., 2004. Nuclear insulin receptor substrate 1 interacts with estrogen receptor alpha at ERE promoters. Oncogene 23, 7517–7526.

Moroishi, T., Hansen, C.G., Guan, K.L., 2015. The emerging roles of YAP and TAZ in cancer. Nat. Rev. Cancer 15, 73–79.

Mortensen, D.S., Fultz, K.E., Xu, S.C., Xu, W.M., Packard, G., Khambatta, G., et al., 2015. CC-223, a potent and selective inhibitor of mTOR kinase: in vitro and in vivo characterization. Mol. Cancer Ther. 14, 1295–1305.

Moser, C.V., Meissner, M., Laarmann, K., Olbrich, K., King-Himmelreich, T.S., Wolters, M.C., et al., 2016. The protein kinase IKK epsilon contributes to tumour growth and tumour pain in a melanoma model. Biochem. Pharmacol. 103, 64–73.

Moser, T.L., Enghild, J.J., Pizzo, S.V., Stac, M.S., 1993. The extracellular matrix proteins laminin and fibronectin contain binding domains for human plasminogen and tissue plasminogen activator. J. Biol. Chem. 268, 18917–18923.

Motz, G.T., Coukos, G., 2011. The parallel lives of angiogenesis and immunosuppression: cancer and other tales. Nat. Rev. Immunol. 11, 702–711.

Mu, J.S., Xu, H.N., Yang, Y., Huang, W.D., Xiao, J., Li, M.L., et al., 2014. Thioridazine, an antipsychotic drug, elicits potent antitumor effects in gastric cancer. Oncol. Rep. 31, 2107–2114.

Mundt, F., Heidari-Hamedani, G., Nilsonne, G., Metintas, M., Hjerpe, A., Dobra, K., 2014. Diagnostic and prognostic value of soluble syndecan-1 in pleural malignancies. Biomed. Res. Int. 2014, art. no. 419853.

Murata, Y., Kotani, T., Ohnishi, H., Matozaki, T., 2014. The CD47-SIRP alpha signalling system: its physiological roles and therapeutic application. J. Biochem. 155, 335–344.

Murphy, K.M., Nelson, C.A., John, R., Šedý, J.R., 2006. Balancing co-stimulation and inhibition with BTLA and HVEM. Nat. Rev. Immunol. 6, 671–681.

Na, J.H., Hwang, J.Y., Lee, K.S., Choi, Y.K., Choe, J., Kim, J.Y., et al., 2014. TRAIL negatively regulates VEGF-induced angiogenesis via caspase-8-mediated enzymatic and non-enzymatic functions. Angiogenesis 17, 179–194.

Nagao, K., Matsuytma, H., Mozawa, M., Hara, I., Nishioka, T., Komura, T., et al., 2016. Zoledronic acid combined with androgen-deprivation therapy may prolong time to castration-resistant prostate cancer in hormone-naïve metastatic prostate cancer patients – a propensity scoring approach. Asian J. Urol. 3, 33–38.

Nagaraj, S.R.M., Shilpa, P., Rachaiah, K., Salimath, B.P., 2015. Crosstalk between VEGF and MTA1 signaling pathways contribute to aggressiveness of breast carcinoma.. Mol. Carcinogenesis 54, 333–350.

Nagaria, P., Robert, C., Rasool, F.V., 2013. DNA double-strand break response in stem cells: mechanisms to maintain genomic integrity. Biochim. Biophys. Acta 1830, 2345–2353.

Nair, J.S., Sheikh, T., Ho, A.L., Schwartz, G.K., 2013. PTEN regulates sensitivity of melanoma cells to RO4929097, the gamma-secretase inhibitor. Anticancer Res. 33, 1307–1316.

Nakajima, H., Ishikawa, Y., Furuya, M., Sano, T., Ohno, Y., Horiguchi, J., et al., 2014. Protein expression, gene amplification, and mutational analysis of EGFR in triple-negative breast cancer. Breast Cancer 21, 66–74.

Nakamura, N., Hara, T., Shimizu, M., Mabuchi, R., Nagano, J., Ohno, T., et al., 2015. Effects of indoleamine 2,3-dioxygenase inhibitor in non-Hodgkin lymphoma model mice. Int. J. Hemtol. 102, 327–334.

Nakamura, S., Nagano, S., Nagao, H., Ishidou, Y., Yokouchi, M., Abematsu, M., et al., 2013. Arsenic trioxide prevents osteosarcoma growth by inhibition of GLI transcription via DNA damage accumulation. PLoS One 8, art. no. e69466.

Nakamura, T., Miyabe, H., Hyodo, M., Sato, Y., Hayakawa, Y., Harashima, H., 2015. Liposomes loaded with a STING pathway ligand, cyclic di-GMP, enhance cancer immunotherapy against metastatic melanoma. J. Control Release 216, 149–157.

Nambiar, D.K., Rajamani, P., Singh, R.P., 2015. Silibinin attenuates ionizing radiation-induced pro-angiogenic response and EMT in prostate cancer cells. Biochem. Biophys. Res. Commun. 456, 262–268.

Natale, R.B., Thongprasert, S., Greco, F.A., Thomas, M., Tsai, C.M., Sunpaweravong, P., et al., 2011. Phase III Trial of Vandetanib compared with erlotinib in patients with previously treated advanced non–small-cell lung cancer. J. Clin. Oncol. 29, 1059–1066.

Naumnik, W., Ossolinska, M., Plonska, I., Chyczewska, E., Niklinski, J., 2015. Circulating thrombospondin-2 and FGF-2 in patients with advanced non-small cell lung cancer: correlation with survival. Lung Cancer Autoimmune Dis. Adv. Exp. Med. Biol. 833, 9–14.

Nayak, L., Lee, E.Q., Wen, P.Y., 2012. Epidemiology of brain metastases. Curr. Oncol. Rep. 14, 48–54.

Necchi, A., Giannatempo, P., Mariani, L., Fare, E., Raggi, D., Pennati, M., et al., 2014. PF-03446962, a fully-human monoclonal antibody against transforming growth-factor beta (TGF beta) receptor ALK1, in pre-treated patients with urothelial cancer: an open label, single-group, phase 2 trial. Invest. New Drugs 32, 555–560.

Nguyen, L., Fifis, T., Christophi, C., 2016. Vascular disruptive agent OXi4503 and anti-angiogenic agent Sunitinib combination treatment prolong survival of mice with CRC liver metastasis. BMC Cancer 16, art. no. 533.

Nguyen, T.L., Grizzle, W.E., Zhang, K., Hameed, O., Siegal, G.P., Wei, S., 2013. Syndecan-1 overexpression is associated with nonluminal subtypes and poor prognosis in advanced breast cancer. Am. J. Clin. Pathol. 140, 468–474.

Ni, Y.H., Ding, L., Zhang, D.Y., Hou, Y.Y., Huang, X.F., Hu, Q.G., 2015. Distinct expression patterns of Toll-like receptor 7 in tumour cells and fibroblast-like cells in oral squamous cell carcinoma. Histopathology 67, 730–739.

Niculescu-Duvaz, I., 2010. Trastuzumab emtansine, an antibody-drug conjugate for the treatment of HER2 + metastatic breast cancer. Curr. Opin. Mol. Ther. 12, 350–360.

Niu, M.S., Cai, W., Liu, H.Z., Chong, Y.L., Hu, W.Q., Gao, S.F., et al., 2015. Plumbagin inhibits growth of gliomas in vivo via suppression of FOXM1 expression. J. Pharmacol. Sci. 128, 131–136.

Nocera, D.A., Roselli, E., Araya, P., Nunez, N.G., Lienenklaus, S., Jablonska, J., et al., 2016. In vivo visualizing the IFN-beta response required for tumor growth control in a therapeutic model of polyadenylic-polyuridylic acid administration. J. Immunol. 196, 2860–2869.

Noe, V., Willems, J., Vandekerchhove, Roy, F.V., Bruyneel, E., Mareel, M., 1999. Inhibition of adhesion and induction of epithelial cell invasion by HAV-containing E-cadherin-specific peptides. J. Cell Sci. 112, 127–135.

Noort, A.R., van Zoest, K.P.M., Weijers, E.M., Koolwijk, P., Maracle, C.X., Novack, D.V., et al., 2014. NF-kappa B-inducing kinase is a key regulator of inflammation-induced and tumour-associated angiogenesis. J. Pathol. 234, 375–385.

Nordstrom, T., Van Blarigan, E.L., Ngo, V., Roy, R., Weinberg, V., Song, X.L., et al., 2016. Associations between circulating carotenoids, genomic instability and the risk of high-grade prostate cancer. Prostate 76, 339–348.

Normanno, N., Campiglio, M., De, L.A., Somenzi, M., Maiello, M., Ciardiello, F., et al., 2002. Cooperative inhibitory effect of ZD1839 (Iressa) in combination with trastuzumab (Herceptin) on human breast cancer cell growth. Ann. Oncol. 13, 65–72.

Nussinov, R., Tsai, C.J., 2013. Allostery in disease and in drug discovery. Cell 153, 293–305.

Nwizu, T., Kanteti, R., Kawada, I., Rolle, C., Volkes, E., Salgia, R., 2011. Crizotinib, a potent inhibitor of EML4-ALK that is highly effective in clinical trials. In addition to its ability to inhibit ALK, it was also shown to suppress c-Met tyrosine kinase activity. Drugs Fut. 36, 91–99.

O'Brien, N.A., McDonald, K., Tong, L., von Euw, E., Kalous, O., Conklin, D., et al., 2014. Targeting PI3K/mTOR overcomes resistance to HER2-targeted therapy independent of feed-back activation of AKT. Clin. Cancer Res. 20, 3507–3520.

Ochiya, T., Takenaga, K., Asagiri, M., Nakano, K., Satoh, H., Watanabe, et al., 2015. Efficient inhibition of tumor angiogenesis and growth by a synthetic peptide blocking S100A4-methionine aminopeptidase 2 interaction. Methods Clin. Develop. 2, art. no. 15008.

O'Connell, J.T., Sugimoto, H., Cooke, V.G., MacDonald, B.A., Mehta, A.I., LeBleu, V.S., et al., 2011. VEGF-A and Tenascin-C produced by S100A4(+) stromal cells are important for metastatic colonization. Proc. Natl Acad. Sci. USA 108, 16002–16007.

Oda, H., Nakatsuru, Y., Imai, Y., Sugimura, H., Ishikawa, T., 1995. A mutational hot spot in the p53 gene is associated with hepatoblastomas. Int. J. Cancer 60, 786–790.

O'Dwyer, D.N., Armstrong, M.E., Trujillo, G., Cooke, G., Keane, M.P., Fallon, P.G., et al., 2013. The Toll-like receptor 3 L412F polymorphism and disease progression in idiopathic pulmonary fibrosis. Am. J. Respir. Crit. Care Med. 188, 1442–1450.

Oh, S.P., Kamagata, Y., Muragaki, Y., Timmons, S., Ooshima, A., Olsen, B.R., 1994. Isolation and sequencing of cDNAs for proteins with multiple domains of Gly-Xaa-Yaa repeats identify a distinct family of collagenous proteins. Proc. Natl Acad. Sci. USA 91, 4229–4233.

Oh, S.Y., Knelson, E.H., Blobe, G.C., Mythreye, K., 2013. The type III TGF beta receptor regulates filopodia formation via a Cdc42-mediated IRSp53-N-WASP interaction in epithelial cells. Biochem. J. 454, 79–89.

Okada, M., Oba, Y., Yamawaki, H., 2015. Endostatin stimulates proliferation and migration of adult rat cardiac fibroblasts through PI3K/Akt pathway. Eur. J. Pharmacol. 750, 20–26.

Okazaki, T., Honjo, T., 2007. PD1 and PD1 ligands: from discovery to clinical application. Int. Immunol. 19, 813–824.

Oliveira, M.V.M., Fraga, C.A., Barros, L.O., Pereira, C.S., Santos, S.H.S., Basile, J.R., et al., 2014. High expression of S100A4 and endoglin is associated with metastatic disease in head and neck squamous cell carcinoma. Clin. Exptl Metastasis 31, 639–649.

Olsson, E., Honeth, G., Bendahl, P.O., Saal, L.H., Gruvberger-Saul, R., Ringner, M., et al., 2011. CD44 isoforms are heterogeneously expressed in breast cancer and correlate with tumor subtypes and cancer stem cell markers. BMC Cancer 11, art. no. 418.

Orecchia, P., Conte, R., Balza, E., Petretto, A., Mauri, P., Mingari, M.C., et al., 2013. A novel human anti-syndecan-1 antibody inhibits vascular maturation and tumour growth in melanoma. Eur. J. Cancer 49, 2022–2033.

O'Reilly, M.S., 1997. Angiostatin: an endogenous inhibitor of angiogenesis and of tumor growth. Experientia Suppl. 79, 273–294.

O'Reilly, M.S., Boehm, T., Shing, Y., Chen, C., Rosenthal, R.A., Moses, M., et al., 1997. Endostatin: an endogenous inhibitor of angiogenesis and tumor growth. Cell 88, 277–285.

O'Reilly, M.S., Holmgren, L., Shing, Y., Chen, C., Rosenthal, R.A., Moses, M., et al., 1994. Angiostatin: a novel angiogenesis inhibitor that mediates the suppression of metastases by a Lewis lung carcinoma. Cell 79, 315–328.

Ortiz, A., Lee, Y.C., Yu, G.Y., Liu, H.C., Lin, S.C., Bilen, M.A., et al., 2015. Angiomotin is a novel component of cadherin-11/beta-catenin/p120 complex and is critical for cadherin-11-mediated cell migration. FASEB J. 29, 1080–1091.

Otsuka, M., Kato, N., Shao, R.X., Hoshida, Y., Ijichi, H., Koike, Y., et al., 2004. Vitamin K-2 inhibits the growth and invasiveness of hepatocellular carcinoma cells via protein kinase A activation. Hepatology 40, 243–251.

Ou, S.H., Ahn, J.S., De Petris, L., Govindan, R., Yang, J.C.H., Hughes, B., et al., 2016. Alectinib in crizotinib-refractory ALK-rearranged non-small-cell lung cancer: a phase II global study. J. Clin. Oncol. 34, 661–668.

Owen, S.C., Patel, N., Logie, J., Pan, G.H., Persson, H., Moffat, J., et al., 2013. Targeting HER2 + breast cancer cells: lysosomal accumulation of anti-HER2 antibodies is influenced by antibody binding site and conjugation to polymeric nanoparticles. J. Controlled Dis. 172, 395–404.

Palle, K., Mani, C., Tripathi, K., Athar, M., 2015. Aberrant GLI1 activation in DNA damage response, carcinogenesis and chemoresistance. Cancers 7, 2330–2351.

Pan, C.C., Bloodworth, J.C., Mythreye, K., Lee, N.Y., 2012. Endoglin inhibits ERK-induced c-Myc and cyclin D1 expression to impede endothelial cell proliferation. Biochem. Biophys. Res. Commun. 424, 620–623.

Pan, J.X., Ding, K., Wang, C.Y., 2012. Niclosamide, an old antihelminthic agent, demonstrates antitumor activity by blocking multiple signaling pathways of cancer stem cells. Chin. J. Cancer 31, 178–184.

Pan, S.T., Qin, Y.R., Zhou, Z.W., He, Z.X., Zhang, X.J., Yang, T.X., et al., 2015. Plumbagin suppresses epithelial to mesenchymal transition and stemness via inhibiting Nrf2-mediated signaling pathway in human tongue squamous cell carcinoma cells. Drug Design Develop. Ther. 9, 5511–5551.

Pan, Y.M., Wang, L.M., Kang, S.G., Lu, Y.Y., Yang, Z.X., Huynh, T., et al., 2015. Gd-Metallofullerenol nanomaterial suppresses pancreatic cancer metastasis by inhibiting the interaction of histone deacetylase 1 and metastasis-associated protein 1. ACS Nano 9, 6826–6836.

Pantuck, A.J., Zeng, G., Belldegrun, A.S., Figlin, R.A., 2003. Pathobiology, prognosis, and targeted therapy for renal cell carcinoma: exploiting the hypoxia-induced pathway. Clin. Cancer Res. 9, 4641–4652.

Paolella, B.R., Havrda, M.C., Mantani, A., Wray, C.M., Zhang, Z.H., Israel, M.A., 2011. p53 directly represses Id2 to inhibit the proliferation of neural progenitor cells. Stem Cells 29, 1090–1101.

Paramasivan, M., Sarkeshik, A., Yates III, J.R., Fernandes, M.J.G., McCollum, D., 2011. Angiomotin family proteins are novel activators of the LATS2 kinase tumor suppressor. Mol. Biol. Cell 22, 3725–3733.

Pardoll, D.M., 2012. The blockade of immune checkpoints in cancer immunotherapy. Nat. Rev. Cancer 12, 252–264.

Park, M.S., Dong, S.M., Kim, B.R., Seo, S.H., Kang, S., Lee, E.J., et al., 2014. Thioridazine inhibits angiogenesis and tumor growth by targeting the VEGFR-2/PI3K/mTOR pathway in ovarian cancer xenografts. Oncotarget 5, 4929–4934.

Park, S.Y., Lee, S.W., Kim, H.Y., Lee, W.S., Hong, K.W., Kim, C.D., 2015. HMGB1 induces angiogenesis in rheumatoid arthritis via HIF-1α activation. Eur. J. Immunol. 45, 1216–1227.

Park, Y.H., Jung, H.A., Choi, M.K., Chang, W., Choi, Y.L., Do, I.G., et al., 2014. Role of HER3 expression and PTEN loss in patients with HER2-overexpressing metastatic breast cancer (MBC) who received taxane plus trastuzumab treatment. Br. J. Cancer 110, 384–391.

Patel, D., Morton, D.J., Carey, J., Havrda, M.C., Chaudhary, J., 2015. Inhibitor of differentiation 4 (ID4): from development to cancer. Biochim. Biophys. Acta Rev. Cancer 1855, 92–103.

Patel, P.H., Kondagunta, G.V., Schwartz, L., Ishill, N., Bacik, J., DeLuca, J., et al., 2008. Phase II trial of lenalidomide in patients with metastatic renal cell carcinoma. Invest. New Drugs 26, 273–276.

Patil, A., Sherbet, G.V., 2015. Therapeutic approach to the management of HER2-positive breast cancer metastatic to the brain. Cancer Lett. 358, 93–99.

Pedrosa, A.R., Trindade, A., Carvalho, C., Graca, J., Carvalho, S., Peleteiro, et al., 2015. Endothelial Jagged1 promotes solid tumor growth through both pro-angiogenic and angiocrine functions. Oncotarget 6, 24404–24423.

Pellikainen, J.M., Ropponen, K.M., Kataja, V.V., Kelloshi, J.K., Eskelinen, M.J., Kosma, V.M., 2004. Expression of matrix metalloproteinase (MMP)-2 and MMP-9 in breast cancer with a special reference to activator protein-2, HER2, and prognosis. Clin. Cancer Res. 10, 7621–7628.

Perry, J.M., He, X.C., Sugimura, R., Grindley, J.C., Haug, J.S., Ding, S., et al., 2011. Cooperation between both Wnt/beta-catenin and PTEN/PI3K/Akt signaling promotes primitive hematopoietic stem cell self-renewal and expansion. Genes Develop. 25, 1928–1942.

Persad, S., Troussard, A.A., McPhee, T.R., Mulholland, D.J., Dedhar, S., 2001. Tumor suppressor PTEN inhibits nuclear accumulation of beta-catenin and T cell/lymphoid enhancer factor 1-mediated transcriptional activation. J. Cell Biol. 153, 1161–1174.

Peters, D.E., Hoover, B., Cloud, L.G., Liu, S.H., Molinolo, A.A., Leppla, S.H., et al., 2014. Comparative toxicity and efficacy of engineered anthrax lethal toxin variants with broad antitumor activities. Toxicol. Appl. Pharmacol. 279, 220–229.

Peterson, T.R., Laplante, M., Thorsen, C.C., Sancak, Y., Kang, S.A., Kuehl, M., et al., 2009. DEPTOR is an mTOR inhibitor whose frequent overexpression in multiple myeloma cells promotes their survival. Cell 137, 873–886.

Petz, L.N., Nadulli, A.M., 2000. Sp1 binding sites and an estrogen response element half-site are involved in regulation of the human progesterone receptor A promoter. Mol. Endocrinol. 14, 972–985.

Pianetti, S., Arsura, M., Romieu-Mourez, R., Coffey, R.J., Sonenshein, G.E., 2001. Her-2/neu overexpression induces NF-kappaB via a PI3-kinase/Akt pathway involving calpain mediated degradation of IkappaB-alpha that can be inhibited by the tumor suppressor PTEN. Oncogene 20, 1287–1299.

Piha-Paul, S.A., Munster, P.N., Hollebecque, A., Argiles, G., Dajani, O., Cheng, J.D., et al., 2015. Results of a phase 1 trial combining ridaforolimus and MK-0752 in patients with advanced solid tumours. Eur. J. Cancer 51, 1865–1873.

Porter, H.A., Perry, A., Kingsley, C., Tran, N.L., Keegan, A.D., 2013. IRS1 is highly expressed in localized breast tumors and regulates the sensitivity of breast cancer cells to chemotherapy, while IRS2 is highly expressed in invasive breast tumors. Cancer Lett. 338, 239–248.

Postow, M.A., Chesney, J., Pavlick, A.C., Robert, C., Grossmann, K., McDermott, D., et al., 2015. Nivolumab and Ipilimumab versus Ipilimumab in untreated melanoma. New Engl. J. Med. 372, 2006–2017.

Pratheeshkumar, P., Budhraja, A., Son, Y.O., Wang, X., Zhang, Z., Ding, S.Z., et al., 2012. Quercetin inhibits angiogenesis mediated human prostate tumor growth by targeting VEGFR-2 regulated AKT/mTOR/P70S6K signaling pathways. PLoS One 7, art. no. e47516.

Principi, M., Di Leo, A., Pricci, M., Scavo, M.P., Guido, R., Tanzi, S., 2013. Phytoestrogens/insoluble fibers and colonic estrogen receptor beta: randomized, double-blind, placebo-controlled study. World J. Gastroenterol. 19, 4325–4333.

Pritchard, K.I., Burris III, H.A., Ito, Y., Rugo, H.S., Dakhil, S., Hortobagyi, G.N., et al., 2013. Safety and efficacy of everolimus with exemestane vs. exemestane alone in elderly patients with HER2-negative, hormone receptor-positive breast cancer in BOLERO-2. Clin. Breast Cancer 13, 421-U113.

Pujadas, L., Gruart, A., Bosch, C., Delgado, L., Teixeira, C.M., Rossi, D., et al., 2010. Reelin regulates postnatal neurogenesis and enhances spine hypertrophy and long-term potentiation. J. Neurosci. 30, 4636–4649.

Putranto, E.W., Murata, H., Yamamoto, K.I., Kataoka, K., Yamada, H., Futami, J.I., et al., 2013. Inhibition of RAGE signaling through the intracellular delivery of inhibitor peptides by PEI cationization. Int. J. Mol. Med. 32, 938–944.

Qiao, H., Wang, T.Y., Yu, Z.F., Han, X.G., Liu, X.Q., Wang, Y.G., et al., 2016. Structural simulation of adenosine phosphate via plumbagin and zoledronic acid competitively targets JNK/Erk to synergistically attenuate osteoclastogenesis in a breast cancer model. Cell Death Dis. 7, art. no. e2094.

Qin, L., Dong, Z.Z., Zhang, J.T., 2014. Reversible epigenetic regulation of 14-3-3 sigma expression in acquired gemcitabine resistance by Uhrf1 and DNA methyltransferase 1. Mol. Pharmacol. 86, 561–569.

Qin, R., Li, K., Qi, X., Zhou, X., Wang, L., Zhang, P., et al., 2014. Beta-Arrestin1 promotes the progression of chronic myeloid leukaemia by regulating BCR/ABL H4 acetylation. Br. J. Cancer 111, 568–576.

Qiu, Z.H., Yuan, W., Chen, T., Zhou, C.Z., Liu, C., Huang, Y.K., 2016. HMGCR positively regulated the growth and migration of glioblastoma cells. Gene 576, 22–27.

Qu, W., Wang, Y., Wu, Q., Liu, J., Hao, 2015. Emodin inhibits HMGB1-induced tumor angiogenesis in human osteosarcoma by regulating SIRT1. Int. J. Clin. Exp. Med. 8, 15054–15064.

Qualtrough, D., Rees, P., Speight, B., Williams, A.C., Paraskeva, C., 2015. The Hedgehog inhibitor cyclopamine reduces beta-catenin-Tcf transcriptional activity, induces E-cadherin expression, and reduces invasion in colorectal cancer cells. Cancers 7, 1885–1899.

Quek, R.H., Morgan, J.A., Shapiro, G., Butrynski, J.E., Wang, Q., Huftalen, T., et al., 2010. Combination mTOR plus IGF-IR inhibition: phase I trial of everolimus and CP-751871 in patients (pts) with advanced sarcomas and other solid tumors. J. Clin. Oncol. 28, Suppl. Abstract 10002.

Quirk, C., Bebauer, K., De'Ambrosis, B., Slade, H.B., Meng, T.C., 2010. Sustained clearance of superficial basal cell carcinomas treated with imiquimod cream 5%: results of a prospective 5-year study. Cutis 85, 318–324.

Radhakrishnan, P., Bryant, V.C., Blowers, E.C., Rajule, R.N., Gautam, N., Anwar, M.M., et al., 2013. Targeting the NF-kappa B and mTOR pathways with a quinoxaline urea analog that inhibits IKK beta for pancreas cancer therapy. Clin. Cancer Res. 19, 2025–2035.

Radhakrishnan, V.M., Kojs, P., Young, G., Ramalingam, R., Jagadish, B., Mash, E.A., et al., 2014. pTyr421cortactin is over expressed in colon cancer and is dephosphorylated by curcumin: involvement of non-receptor type 1 protein tyrosine phosphatase (PTPN1). PLoS One 9, art no. e85796.

Radziwon-Balicka, A., Santos-Martinez, M.J., Corbalan, J., O'Sullivan, S., Treumann, A., Gilmer, J.F., et al., 2014. Mechanisms of platelet-stimulated colon cancer invasion: role of clusterin and thrombospondin 1 in regulation of the P38MAPKMMP-9 pathway. Carcinogenesis 35, 324–332.

Raghu, D., Karunagaran, D., 2014. Plumbagin downregulates Wnt signaling independent of p53 in human colorectal cancer cells. J. Nat. Prod. 77, 1130–1134.

Rago, L., Beattie, R., Taylor, V., Winter, J., 2014. miR379-410 cluster miRNAs regulate neurogenesis and neuronal migration by fine-tuning N-cadherin. EMBO J. 33, 906–920.

Rahman, M., Davis, S.R., Pumphrey, J.G., Bao, J., Nau, M.M., Meltzer, P.S., et al., 2009. TRAIL induces apoptosis in triple-negative breast cancer cells with a mesenchymal phenotype. Br. Cancer Res. Treat. 113, 217–230.

Rajeshkumar, N.V., Rasheed, Z.A., Garcia-Garcia, E., Lopenz-Rios, F., Fuiwara, K., Matsui, W.H., et al., 2010. A combination of DR5 agonistic monoclonal antibody with gemcitabine targets pancreatic cancer stem cells and results in long-term disease control in human pancreatic cancer model. Mol. Cancer Ther. 9, 2582–2592.

Ramanathan, R.K., Stephenson, J.J., Weiss, G.J., Pestano, L.A., Lowe, A., Hiscox, A., et al., 2012. A phase I trial of PX-12, a small-molecule inhibitor of thioredoxin-1, administered as a 72-hour infusion every 21 days in patients with advanced cancers refractory to standard therapy. Invest. New Drugs 30, 1591–1596.

Rani, S.G., Mohan, S.K., Yu, C., 2010. Molecular level interactions of S100A13 with Amlexanox: Inhibitor for formation of the multiprotein complex in the nonclassical pathway of acidic fibroblast growth factor. Biochemistry 49, 2585–2592.

Ravaud, A., Urva, S.R., Grosch, K., Cheung, W.K., Anak, O., Sellami, D.B., 2014. Relationship between everolimus exposure and safety and efficacy: meta-analysis of clinical trials in oncology. Eur. J. Cancer 50, 486–495.

Ravishankar, D., Watson, K.A., Boateng, S.Y., Green, R.J., Greco, F., Osborn, H.M.I., 2015. Exploring quercetin and luteolin derivatives as antiangiogenic agents. Eur. J. Med. Chem. 96, 259–274.

Reel, B., Korkmaz, C.G., Arun, Z.M., Yildirim, Y.G., Ogut, D., Kaymak, A., et al., 2015. The regulation of matrix metalloproteinase expression and role of discoidin domain receptor 1/2 signalling in zoledronate-treated PC3 cells. J. Cancer 6, 1020–1029.

Reeves, R., 2010. HMG nuclear proteins: linking chromatin structure to cellular phenotype. Biochim. Biophys. Acta 1799, 3–14.

Reginato, E., Wolf, P., Hamblin, M., 2014. Immune response after photodynamic therapy increases anti-cancer and anti-bacterial effects. World J. Immunol. 4, 1–11.

Reilly, J.E., Neighbors, J.D., Tong, H.X., Henry, M.D., Hohl, R.J., 2015. Targeting geranylgeranylation reduces adrenal gland tumor burden in a murine model of prostate cancer metastasis. Clin. Expt Metastasis 32, 555–566.

Ren, G., Hu, J., Wang, R., Han, W., Zhao, M., Zhou, G., et al., 2014. Rapamycin inhibits Toll-like receptor 4-induced pro-oncogenic function in head and neck squamous cell carcinoma. Oncol. Rep. 31, 2804–2810.

Ren, Z.H., Wang, Y.N., Jiang, W.H., Dai, W., Jiang, Y.P., 2014. Anti-tumor effect of a novel soluble recombinant human endostatin: administered as a single agent or in combination with chemotherapy agents in mouse tumor models. PLoS One 9, art. no. e107823.

Renfrow, J.J., Lesser, G.J., 2013. Molecular subtyping of brain metastases and implications for therapy. Curr. Treat. Op. Oncol. 14, 514–527.

Rengarajan, T., Rajendran, P., Nandakumar, N., Balasubramanian, M.P., Nishigaki, I., 2013. Cancer preventive efficacy of marine carotenoid fucoxanthin: cell cycle arrest and apoptosis. Nutrients 5, 4978–4989.

Reshma, R.S., Sreelatha, K.H., Somasundaram, V., Kumar, S.S., Nadhan, R., Nair, R.S., et al., 2016. Plumbagin, a naphthaquinone derivative induces apoptosis in BRCA 1/2 defective castrate resistant prostate cancer cells as well as prostate cancer stem-like cells. Pharmacol. Res. 105, 134–145.

Reuveni, H., Flashner-Abramson, E., Steiner, L., Makedonski1, K., Song, R., Shir, A., et al., 2013. Therapeutic destruction of insulin receptor substrates for cancer treatment. Cancer Res. 73, 4383–4394.

Richer, J.K., Jacobsen, B.M., Manning, N.G., Abel, M.G., Wolf, D.M., Horwitz, K.B., 2002. Differential gene regulation by the two progesterone receptor isoforms in human breast cancer cells. J. Biol. Chem. 277, 5209–5218.

Riley, J.L., 2006. PD1 signaling in primary T cells. Trends Immunol. 27, 195–201.

Rinke, A., Muller, H.H., Schade-Brittinger, C., Klose, K.J., Barth, P., Wied, M., et al., 2009. Placebo-controlled, double-blind, prospective, randomized study on the effect of octreotide LAR in the control of tumor growth in patients with metastatic neuroendocrine midgut tumors: a report from the PROMID study group. J. Clin. Oncol. 27, 4656–4663.

Ristori, E., Lopez-Ramirez, M.A., Narayanan, A., Hill-Teran, G., Moro, A., Calvo, C.F., et al., 2015. A dicer-miR-107 interaction regulates biogenesis of specific miRNAs crucial for neurogenesis. Develop. Cell 32, 546–560.

Roberts, D.D., Kaur, S., Soto-Pantoja, D.R., 2015. Therapeutic targeting of the thrombospondin-1 receptor CD47 to treat liver cancer. J. Cell Commun. Signal. 9, 101–102.

Rook, A.H., Gelfand, J.C., Wysocka, M., Troxel, A.B., Benoit, B., Surber, C., et al., 2015. Topical resiquimod can induce disease regression and enhance T-cell effector functions in cutaneous T-cell lymphoma. Blood 126, 1452–1461.

Rosen, L.S., Hurwitz, H.I., Wong, M.K., Goldman, J., Mendelson, D.S., Figg, W.D., et al., 2012. A phase I first-in-human study of TRC105 (anti-endoglin antibody) in patients with advanced cancer. Clin. Cancer Res. 18, 4820–4829.

Rousseau, M.C., Hsu, R.Y., Spicer, J.D., McDonald, B., Chan, C.H., Perera, R.M., et al., 2013. Lipopolysaccharide-induced toll-like receptor 4 signaling enhances the migratory ability of human esophageal cancer cells in a selectin-dependent manner. Surgery 154, 69–77.

Rudland, P.S., Platt-Higgins, A., El-Tanani, M., Rudland, S.D.S., Barraclough, R., Winstanley, J.H. R., et al., 2002. Prognostic significance of the metastasis-associated protein osteopontin in human breast cancer. Cancer Res. 62, 3417–3427.

Russell, P.A., Wainer, Z., Wright, G.M., Daniels, M., Conron, M., Williams, R.A., 2011. Does lung adenocarcinoma subtype predict patient survival? A clinicopathologic study based on the new International Association for the Study of Lung Cancer/American Thoracic Society/European Respiratory Society international multidisciplinary lung adenocarcinoma classification. J. Thorac. Oncol. 6, 1496–1504.

Russell, S., Duquette, M., Liu, J., Drapkin, R., Lawler, J., Petrik, J., 2015. Combined therapy with thrombospondin-1 type I repeats (3TSR) and chemotherapy advanced stage epithelial ovarian cancer. FASEB J. 29, 576–588.

Sack, U., Walther, W., Scudiero, D., Selby, M., Kobelt, D., Lemm, M., et al., 2011. Novel effect of antihelminthic Niclosamide on S100A4mediated metastatic progression of colon cancer. J. Natl Cancer Inst. 103, 1018–1036.

Saitoh, M., Nishitoh, H., Fujii, M., Takeda, K., Tobiume, K., Sawada, Y., et al., 1998. Mammalian thioredoxin is a direct inhibitor of apoptosis signal-regulating kinase (ASK) 1. EMBO J. 2596–2606.

Sakaguchi, S., Wing, K., Onishi, Y., Prieto-Martin, P., Yamaguchi, T., 2009. Regulatory T cells: how do they suppress immune responses? Int. Immunol. 21, 1105–1111.

Sallon, C., Boulay, I., Fontaine, J., Logeart-Avramoglou, D., Cayla, X., Harichaux, G., et al. (2015). A novel BMP4 binding protein synthetized by pituitary cells: thrombospondin-1 acting as BMP4 antagonist, abstract. In: Endocrine Society Annual Meeting, San Diego, CA.

Sambandam, S.A.T., Kasetti, R.B., Xue, L., Dean, D.C., Lu, Q.X., Li, Q.T., 2015. 14-3-3 Sigma regulates keratinocyte proliferation and differentiation by modulating Yap1 cellular localization. J. Invest. Dermatol. 135, 1621–1628.

Samykutty, A., Shetty, A.V., Dakshinamoorthy, G., Kalyanasundaram, R., Zheng, G.X., Chen, A.S., et al., 2013. Vitamin K2, a naturally occurring menaquinone, exerts therapeutic effects on both hormone-dependent and hormone-independent prostate cancer cells. Evid. Based Complem. Alternat. Med. 2013, art. no. 287358.

Sanchez-Capelo, A., 2005. Dual role for TGF-b1 in apoptosis. Cytokine Growth Factor Rev. 16, 15–34.

Sandur, S.K., Pandey, M.K., Sung, B., Aggarwal, B.B., 2010. 5-Hydroxy-2-methyl-1,4-naphthoquinone, a vitamin K3 analogue, suppresses STAT3 activation pathway through induction of protein tyrosine phosphatase, SHP-1: potential role in chemosensitization. Mol. Cancer Res. 8, 107–118.

Sarbassov, D.D., Ali, S.M., Kim, D.H., Guertin, D.A., Latek, R.R., Erdjument-Bromage, H., et al., 2006. Rictor, a novel binding partner of mTOR, defines a rapamycin-insensitive and raptor-independent pathway that regulates the cytoskeleton. Curr. Biol. 14, 1296–1302.

Sarbassov, D.D., Guertin, D.A., Ali, S.M., Sabatini, D.M., 2005. Phosphorylation and regulation of Akt/PKB by the rictor-mTOR complex. Science 307, 1098–1101.

Sasaki, K., Gotlib, J.R., Mesa, R.A., Newberry, K.J., Ravandi, F., Cortes, J.E., et al., 2015. Phase II evaluation of IPI-926, an oral Hedgehog inhibitor, in patients with myelofibrosis. Leukemia Lymphoma 56, 2092–2097.

Sato, T., Shimosato, T., Ueda, A., Ishigatsubo, Y., Klinman, D.M., 2015. Intrapulmonary delivery of CpG microparticles eliminates lung tumors. Mol. Cancer Ther. 14, 2198–2205.

Saura, C., Bendell, J., Jerusalem, G., Su, S., Ru, Q.H., De Buck, S., et al., 2014. Phase Ib study of Buparlisib plus Trastuzumab in patients with HER2-positive advanced or metastatic breast cancer that has progressed on Trastuzumab-based therapy. Clin. Cancer Res. 20, 1935–1945.

Savellano, M.D., Pogue, B.W., Hoopes, P.J., Vitetta, E.S., Paulsen, K.D., 2005. Multiepitope HER2 targeting enhances photoimmunotherapy of HER2-overexpressing cancer cells with pyropheophorbide-a immunoconjugates. Cancer Res. 65, 6371–6379.

Sawka-Verhelle, D., Tartare-Deckert, S., White, M.F., Van Obberghen, E., 1996. Insulin receptor substrate-2 binds to the insulin receptor through its phosphotyrosine-binding domain and through a newly identified domain comprising amino acids 591-786. J. Biol. Chem. 271, 5980–5983.

Schadler, K.L., Crosby, E.J., Zhou, A.Y., Bhang, D.H., Braunstein, L., Baek, K.H., et al., 2014. Immunosurveillance by antiangiogenesis: tumor growth arrest by T cell-derived thrombospondin-1. Cancer Res. 74, 2171–2181.

Schmidt, M., Hagner, N., Marco, A., Konig-Merediz, S.A., Schroff, M., Wittig, B., 2015. Design and structural requirements of the potent and safe TLR-9 agonistic immunomodulator MGN1703. Nucleic Acid Ther. 25, 130–140.

Schmoll, H.J., Wittig, B., Arnold, D., Riera-Knorrenschild, J., Nitsche, D., Kroening, H., et al., 2014. Maintenance treatment with the immunomodulator MGN1703, a Toll-like receptor 9 (TLR9) agonist, in patients with metastatic colorectal carcinoma and disease control after chemotherapy: a randomised, double-blind, placebo-controlled trial. J. Cancer Res. Clin. Oncol. 140, 1615–1624.

Schott, A.F., Landis, M.D., Dontu, G., Griffith, K.A., Layman, R.M., Krop, I., et al., 2013. Preclinical and clinical studies of gamma secretase inhibitors with Docetaxel on human breast tumors. Clin. Cancer Res. 19, 1512–1524.

Schultz, J., Ibrahim, S.M., Vera, J., Kunz, M., 2009. 14-3-3 Sigma gene silencing during melanoma progression and its role in cell cycle control and cellular senescence. Mol. Cancer 8, art. no. 53.

Selle, F., Gligorov, J., Richard, S., Khalil, A., Alexandre, I., Avenin, D., et al., 2015. Intensive chemotherapy as salvage treatment for solid tumors: focus on germ cell cancer. Brazil J. Med. Biol. Res. 48, 13–24.

Sethi, N., Yan, Y., Quek, D., Schupbach, T., Kang, Y., 2010. Rabconnectin-3 is a functional regulator of mammalian Notch signaling. J. Biol. Chem. 285, 34757–34764.

Sfondrini, L., Sommariva, M., Tortoreto, M., Meini, A., Piconese, S., Calvaruso, M., et al., 2013. Anti-tumor activity of CpG-ODN aerosol in mouse lung metastases. Int. J. Cancer 133, 383–393.

Shah, Y.M., Kaul, A., Dong, Y., Ip, C., Rowan, B.F., 2005. Attenuation of estrogen receptor alpha (ERalpha) signaling by selenium in breast cancer cells via downregulation of ERalpha gene expression. Br. Cancer Res. Treat. 92, 239–250.

Shakhova, O., Sommer, L. (2010). Neural crest-derived stem cells. StemBook, ed. The Stem Cell Research Community, StemBook, doi/10.3824/stembook.1.51.1.

Shakir, M., Tang, D.L., Zeh, H.J., Tang, S.W., Anderson, C.J., Bahary, N., et al., 2015. The chemokine receptors CXCR4/CXCR7 and their primary heterodimeric ligands CXCL12 and CXCL12/high mobility group box 1 in pancreatic cancer growth and development finding flow. Pancreas 44, 528–534.

Shan, S.Q., Hui, G.Y., Hou, F.G., Shi, H., Zhou, G.Q., Yan, H., et al., 2015. Expression of metastasis-associated protein 3 in human brain glioma related to tumor prognosis. Neurolog. Sci. 36, 1799–1804.

Shang, H., Braggio, D., Lee, Y.J., Al Sannaa, G.A., Creighton, C.J., Bolshakov, S., et al., 2015. Targeting the Notch pathway: a potential therapeutic approach for desmoid tumors. Cancer 121, 4088–4096.

Shao, Y.Y., Lu, L.C., Cheng, A.L., Hsu, C.H., 2011. Increasing incidence of brain metastasis in patients with advanced hepatocellular carcinoma in the era of antiangiogenic targeted therapy. The Oncologist 16, 82–86.

Shaw, A.T., Sai-Hong, I.O., Yung-Jue, B., Camidge, D.R., Solomon, B.J., Salgia, R., et al., 2014. Crizotinib in ROS1-rearranged non–small-cell lung cancer. N. Engl. J. Med. 371, 1963–1971.

Shen, J., Vil, M.D., Prewett, M., Damoci, C., Zhang, H., Li, H., et al., 2009. Development of a fully human anti-PDGFR beta antibody that suppresses growth of human tumor xenografts and enhances antitumor activity of an anti-VEGFR2 antibody. Neoplasia 11, 594–604.

Shen, Y.Y., Yuan, Y., Du, Y.Y., Pan, Y.Y., 2015. Molecular mechanism underlying the anticancer effect of simvastatin on MDA-MB-231 human breast cancer cells. Mol. Med. Rep. 12, 623–630.

Shepard, H.M., Jin, P., Slamon, D.J., Pirot, Z., Maneval, D.C., 2008. Herceptin, handbook. Exp. Pharmacol. 181, 183–219.

Sherbet, G.V., 2003. Genetic Recombination in Cancer. Academic/Elsevier, London.

Sherbet, G.V., 2008. Metastasis promoter S100A4 is a potentially valuable molecular target for cancer therapy. Cancer Lett. 280, 15–30.

Sherbet, G.V., 2011a. Growth Factors and Their Receptors in Cell Differentiation, Cancer and Cancer Therapy. Elsevier, London, ISBN: 978-0-12-387819-9.

Sherbet, G.V., 2011b. S100A4 (S100 calcium binding protein A4). Atlas Genet. Cytogenet. Oncol. Haematol. 15, 877–886 (Updated in 2013).

Sherbet, G.V., 2013. Therapeutic Strategies in Cancer Biology and Pathology. Elsevier, London, ISBN: 978-0-12-416570-0.

Sherbet, G.V., 2015a. Do thalidomides have a role in the treatment of multiple sclerosis? Br. J. Med. Practitioners 8, a828.

Sherbet, G.V., 2015b. Therapeutic potential of thalidomides and its analogues in the treatment of cancer. Anticancer Res. 35, 5767–5772.

Sherbet, G.V., Lakshmi, M.S., 1997. The Genetics of Cancer. Elsevier/Academic Press, London.

Sherbet, G.V., Lakshmi, M.S., 2006. The modus operandi of S100A4 signalling in cancer growth, progression and prognosis. In: Sherbet, G.V. (Ed.), Molecular and Cellular Pathology of Cancer Progression and Prognosis. Research Signpost, Trivandrum, pp. 359–377.

Shi, H., Huang, Y., Zhou, H., Song, X., Yuan, S., Fu, Y., et al., 2007. Nucleolin is a receptor that mediates antiangiogenic and antitumor activity of endostatin. Blood 110, 2899–2906.

Shih, K.C., Bendell, J.C., Reinert, A., Jones, S., Kelley, R.K., Infante, J.R., et al., 2012. Phase I trial of an oral TORC1/TORC2 inhibitor (CC-223) in advanced solid and hematologic cancers. J. Clin. Oncol. 30, suppl; abstr 3006.

Shimura, T., Toiyama, Y., Tanaka, K., Saigusa, S., Kitajima, T., Kondo, S., et al., 2015. Angiopoietin-like protein 2 as a predictor of early recurrence in patients after curative surgery for gastric cancer. Anticancer Res. 35, 4633–4639.

Shin, D.H., Park, J.H., Lee, J.Y., Won, H.Y., Jang, K.S., Min, K.W., et al., 2015. Overexpression of Id1 in transgenic mice promotes mammary basal stem cell activity and breast tumorigenesis. Oncotarget 6, 17276–17290.

Shindo, K., Misawa, N., 2014. New and rare carotenoids isolated from marine bacteria and their antioxidant activities. Mar. Drugs 12, 1690–1698.

Shrivastava, S., Steele, R., Sowadski, M., Crawford, S.E., Varvares, M., Ray, R.B., 2015. Identification of molecular signature of head and neck cancer stem-like cells. Sci. Rep. 5, art. no. 7819.

Simonelli, M., Zucali, P., Santoro, A., Thomas, M.B., de Braud, F.G., Broghael, H., et al., 2016. Phase I study of PF-03446962, a fully human monoclonal antibody against activin receptor-like kinase 1 in patients with hepatocellular carcinoma. Ann. Oncol. 27, 1782–1787.

Singh, B.N., Fu, J., Srivastava, R.K., Shankar, S., 2011. Hedgehog signaling antagonist GDC-0449 (Vismodegib) inhibits pancreatic cancer stem cell characteristics: molecular mechanisms. PLoS One 6, e27306.

Singh, J.C., Jhaveri, K., Esteva, F.J., 2014. HER2-positive advanced breast cancer: optimizing patient outcomes and opportunities for drug development. Br. J. Cancer 111, 1888–1898.

Singh, T., Prasad, R., Katiyar, S.K., 2016. Therapeutic intervention of silymarin on the migration of non-small cell lung cancer cells is associated with the axis of multiple molecular targets including class 1 HDACs, ZEB1 expression, and restoration of miR-203 and E-cadherin expression. Am. J. Cancer Res. 6, 1287–1301.

Singla, A.K., Bondareva, A., Jirik, F.R., 2014. Combined treatment with paclitaxel and suramin prevents the development of metastasis by inhibiting metastatic colonization of circulating tumor cells. Clin. Expt. Metastasis 31, 705–714.

Sinha, S., Pal, K., Elkhanany, A., Dutta, S., Cao, Y., Mondal, G., et al., 2013. Plumbagin inhibits tumorigenesis and angiogenesis of ovarian cancer cells in vivo. Int. J. Cancer 132, 1201–1212.

Sivendran, S., Agarwal, N., Gartrell, B., Ying, J., Boucher, K.M., Choueiri, T.K., et al., 2014. Metabolic complications with the use of mTOR inhibitors for cancer therapy. Cancer Treat. Rev. 40, 190–196.

Smolarczyk, R., Cichon, T., Matuszczak, S., Mitrus, I., Lesiak, M., Kobusinska, M., et al., 2012. The role of glycyrrhizin, an inhibitor of HMGB1 protein, in anticancer therapy. Arch. Immunol. Ther. Exp. 60, 391–399.

So, J.Y., Wahler, J., Das Gupta, S., Salerno, D.M., Maehr, H., Uskokovic, M., et al., 2015. HES1-mediated inhibition of Notch1 signaling by a Gemini vitamin D analog leads to decreased CD44(+)/CD24(−/low) tumor-initiating subpopulation in basal-like breast cancer. J. Steroid Biochem. Mol. Biol. 148, 111–121.

Sohn, K.C., Li, Z.J., Choi, D.K., Zhang, T.J., Lim, J.W., Chang, I.K., et al., 2014. Imiquimod induces apoptosis of squamous cell carcinoma (SCC) cells via regulation of A20. PLoS One 9, art. no. e95337.

Solomon, B.J., Mok, T., Kim, D.W., Wu, Y.L., Nakagawa, K., Mekhail, T., et al., 2014. First-line crizotinib versus chemotherapy in *ALK*-positive lung cancer. N. Engl. J. Med. 371, 2167–2177.

Somasundaram, V., Hemalatha, S.K., Pal, K., Sinha, S., Nair, A.S., Mukhopadhyay, D., et al., 2016. Selective mode of action of plumbagin through BRCA1 deficient breast cancer stem cells. BMC Cancer 16, art. no. 336.

Soraya, H., Farajnia, S., Khani, S., Rmeshrad, M., Khorrami, Banani, A., et al., 2012. Short-term treatment with metformin suppresses toll like receptors (TLRs) activity in isoproterenol-induced myocardial infarction in rat: are AMPK and TLRs connected?. Int. Immunopharmacol. 14, 785–791.

Sorrentino, G., Ruggieri, N., Specchia, V., Cordenonsi, M., lMano, M., Dupolnt, S., et al., 2014. Metabolic control of YAP and TAZ by the mevalonae pathway. Nat. Cell Biol. 16, 357–366.

Song, H., Kim, H., Lee, K., Lee, D.H., Kim, T.S., Song, J.Y., et al., 2012. Ablation of Rassf2 induces bone defects and subsequent haematopoietic anomalies in mice. EMBO J. 31, 1147–1159.

Soto-Pantoja, D.R., Kaur, S., Roberts, D.D., 2015. CD47 signaling pathways controlling cellular differentiation and responses to stress. Crit. Rev. Biochem. Mol. Biol. 50, 212–230.

Spagnuolo, C., Russo, G.L., Orhan, I.E., Habtemariam, S., Daglia, M., Sureda, A., et al., 2015. Genistein and cancer: current status, challenges, and future directions. Adv. Nutrit. 6, 408–419.

Spengler, G., Molnar, J., Viveiros, M., Amaral, L., 2011. Thioridazine induces apoptosis of multi-drugresistant mouse lymphoma cells transfected with the human ABCB1 and inhibits the expression of P-glycoprotein. Anticancer Res. 31, 4201–4205.

Spiekerkoetter, E., Guignabert, C., de Jesus Perez, V., Alastalo, T.P., Powers, J.M., Wang, L., et al., 2009. S100A4 and bone morphogenetic protein-2 codependently induce vascular smooth muscle cell migration via phospho-extracellular signal-regulated kinase and chloride intracellular channel 4. Circ. Res. 105, 639–647.

Spivey, K.A., Banyard, J., 2010. A prognostic gene signature in advanced ovarian cancer reveals a microfibril-associated protein (MAGP2) as a promoter of tumor cell survival and angiogenesis. Cell Adhes. Migrat. 4, 169–171.

St John, M.A., Wang, G., Luo, J., Dohadwala, M., Hu, D., Lin, Y., et al., 2012. Apricoxib upregulates 15-PGDH and PGT in tobacco-related epithelial malignancies. Br. J. Cancer 107, 707–712.

Stanton, B.Z., Peng, L.F., 2010. Small-molecule modulators of the Sonic Hedgehog signaling pathway. Mol. Biosyst. 6, 44–54.

Stein, U., Arlt, F., Smith, J., Sack, U., Herrmann, P., Walther, W., et al., 2011. Intervening in beta-catenin signaling by Sulindac inhibits S100A4-dependent colon cancer metastasis. Neoplasia 13, 131–144.

Stemmler, H.J., Schmitt, M., Willems, A., Bernhard, H., Harbeck, N., Heinemann, V., 2007. Ratio of trastuzumab levels in serum and cerebrospinal fluid is altered in HER2-positive breast cancer patients with brain metastases and impairment of blood–brain barrier. Anticancer Drugs 18, 23–28.

Sterenczak, K.A., Nolte, I., Marua Escobar, H., 2013. RAGE splicing variants in mammals. Methods Mol. Biol. 963, 265–276.

Stine, J.E., Guo, H., Sheng, X.G., Han, X.Y., Schointuch, M.N., Gilliam, T.P., et al., 2016. The HMG-CoA reductase inhibitor, simvastatin, exhibits anti-metastatic and anti-tumorigenic effects in ovarian cancer. Oncotarget 7, 946–960.

Strosberg, J.R., Yeatman, T., Weber, J., Coppola, D., Schell, M.J., Han, G., et al., 2012. A phase II study of RO4929097 in metastatic colorectal cancer. Eur. J. Cancer 48, 997–1003.

Su, M., Huang, J.J., Liu, S.Y., Xiao, Y.H., Qin, X.Y., Liu, J., et al., 2016. The anti-angiogenic effect and novel mechanisms of action of Combretastatin A-4. Sci Rep 6, art. no. 28139.

Su, Z., Zang, T., Liu, M.L., Wang, L.L., Niu, W., Zhang, C.L., 2014. Reprogramming the fate of human glioma cells to impede brain tumor development. Cell Death Dis. 5, art. no. e1463.

Sui, X.B., Ma, J.H., Han, W.D., Wang, X., Fang, Y., Li, D., et al., 2015. The anticancer immune response of anti-PD1/PD-L1 and the genetic determinants of response to anti-PD1/PD-L1 antibodies in cancer patients. Oncotarget 6, 19393–19404.

Sun, J., McKallip, R.J., 2011. Plumbagin treatment leads to apoptosis in human K562 leukemia cells through increased ROS and elevated TRAIL receptor expression. Leukemia Res. 35, 1402–1408.

Sun, M., Gomes, S., Chen, P., Frankenberger, C.A., Sankarasharma, D., Chung, C.H., et al., 2014. RKIP and HMGA2 regulate breast tumor survival and metastasis through lysyl oxidase and syndecan-2. Oncogene 33, 3528–3537.

Sun, Y., Nadal-Vicens, M., Misono, S., Lin, M.Z., Zubiaga, A., Hua, X., et al., 2001. Neurogenin promotes neurogenesis and inhibits glial differentiation by independent mechanisms. Cell 104, 365–376.

Sund, M., Hamano, Y., Sugimoto, H., Sudhakr, A., Soubasakos, M., Herramalla, U., et al., 2005. Function of endogenous inhibitors of angiogenesis as endothelium-specific tumor suppressors. Proc. Natl Acad. Sci. USA 102, 2934–2939.

Sutton, K.M., Hayat, S., Chau, N.M., Cook, S., Pouyssegur, J., Ahmed, A., et al., 2007. Selective inhibition of MEK1/2 reveals a differential requirement for ERK1/2 signalling in the regulation of HIF-1 in response to hypoxia and IGF-1. Oncogene 26, 3920–3929.

Swain, S.M., Baselga, J., Miles, D., Im, Y.H., Quah, C., Lee, L.F., et al., 2014. Incidence of central nervous system metastases in patients with HER2-positive metastatic breast cancer treated with pertuzumab, trastuzumab, and docetaxel: results from the randomized phase III study CLEOPATRA. Ann. Oncol. 25, 1116–1121.

Swanson, N., Abramovits, W., Berman, B., Kulp, J., Rigel, D.S., Levy, S., 2010. Imiquimod 2.5% and 3.75% for the treatment of actinic keratoses: results of two placebo-controlled studies of daily application to the face and balding scalp for two 2-week cycles. J. Am. Acad. Dermatol. 62, 582–590.

Szereszewski, J.M., Pampillo, M., Ahow, M.R., Offermanns, S., Bhattacharya, M., Babwah, A.V., 2010. GPR54 regulates ERK1/2 activity and hypothalamic gene expression in a G alpha(q/11) and beta-arrestin-dependent manner. PLoS One 5, e12964.

Szerszenowicz, J., Drozdowska, D., 2014. Semi-automatic synthesis, antiproliferative activity and DNA-binding properties of new Netropsin and bis-Netropsin analogues. Molecules 19, 11300–11315.

Takamatsu, M., Hirata, A., Ohtaki, H., Hoshi, M., Ando, T., Ito, H., et al., 2015. Inhibition of indoleamine 2,3-dioxygenase 1 expression alters immune response in colon tumor microenvironment in mice. Cancr Sci. 106, 1008–1015.

Talukder, A.H., Gururaj, A., Mishra, S.K., Vadlamudi, R.K., Kumar, R., 2004. Metastasis-associated protein 1 interacts with NRIF3, an estrogen-inducible nuclear receptor coregulator. Mol. Cell Biol. 24, 6581–6591.

Tan, L., Wei, X.P., Zheng, L.X., Zeng, J.C., Liu, H.B., Yang, S.J., 2016. Amplified HMGA2 promotes cell growth by regulating Akt pathway in AML. J. Cancer Res. Clin. Oncol. 142, 389–399.

Tan, Q., Li, J., Yin, H.W., Wang, L.H., Tang, W.C., Zhao, F., et al., 2010. Augmented antitumor effects of combination therapy of cisplatin with ethaselen as a novel thioredoxin reductase inhibitor on human A549 cell in vivo. Invest. New Drugs 28, 205–215.

Tan, Y.X., Bi, L.X., Zhang, P.L., Wang, F.L., Lin, F.Y., Ni, W.H., et al., 2014. Thioredoxin-1 inhibitor PX-12 induces human acute myeloid leukemia cell apoptosis and enhances the sensitivity of cells to arsenic trioxide. Int. J. Clin. Exptl Pathol. 7, 4765–4773.

Tang, K.D., Holzapfel, B.M., Liu, J., Lee, T.K.W., Ma, S., Jovanovic, L., et al., 2016. Tie-2 regulates the stemness and metastatic properties of prostate cancer cells. Oncotarget 7, 2572–2584.

Tarrado-Castellarnau, M., Cortes, R., Zanuy, M., Tarrago-Celada, J., Polat, I.H., Hill, R., 2015. Methylseleninic acid promotes antitumour effects via nuclear FOXO3a translocation through Akt inhibition. Pharmacol. Res. 102, 218–234.

Tartour, E., Pere, H., Maillere, B., Terme, M., Merillon, N., Taieb, J., et al., 2011. Angiogenesis and immunity: a bidirectional link potentially relevant for the monitoring of antiangiogenic therapy and the development of novel therapeutic combination with immunotherapy. Cancer Metastasis Rev. 30, 83–95.

Teng, Y.N., Sheu, M.J., Hsieh, Y.W., Wang, R.Y., Chiang, Y.C., Hung, C.C., 2016. Beta-carotene reverses multidrug resistant cancer cells by selectively modulating human P-glycoprotein function. Phytomedicine 23, 316–323.

Teo, W.S., Nair, R., Swarbrick, A., 2014. New insights into the role of ID proteins in breast cancer metastasis: a MET affair. Br. Cancer Res. 16, art. no. 305.

Thaker, A.I., Rao, M.S., Bishnupuri, K.S., Kerr, T.A., Foster, L., Marinshaw, J.M., et al., 2013. IDO1 metabolites activate beta catenin signaling to promote cancer cell proliferation and colon tumorigenesis in mice. Gastroenterology 145, 416–425.

Thakkar, B., Aronis, K.N., Vamvini, M.T., Shields, K., Mantzoros, C.S., 2013. Metformin and sulfonylureas in relation to cancer risk in type II diabetes patients: a meta-analysis using primary data of published studies. Metab. Clin. Exp. 62, 922–934.

Thibult, M.L., Mamessier, E., Gertner-Dardenne, J., Pastor, S., Just-Landi, S., Xern, L., et al., 2013. PD1 is a novel regulator of human B-cell activation. Int. Immunol. 25, 129–137.

Thomas, R., Butler, E., Macchi, F., Williams, M., 2015. Phytochemicals in cancer prevention and management? Br. J. Med. Practit. 8, a815.

Thuault, S., Valcourt, U., Petersen, M., Manfioletti, G., Heldin, C.H., Moustakas, A., 2006. Transforming growth factor-β employs HMGA2 to elicit epithelial–mesenchymal transition. J. Cell Biol. 174, 175–183.

Tian, Q., Xue, Y., Zheng, W., Sun, R., Ji, W., Wang, X.Y., et al., 2015. Overexpression of hypoxia-inducible factor 1 alpha induces migration and invasion through Notch signalling. Int. J. Oncol. 47, 728–738.

Tian, T.T., Li, J.S., Li, B., Wang, Y.W., Li, M.Y., Ma, D., et al., 2014. Genistein exhibits anti-cancer effects via down-regulating FoxM1 in H446 small-cell lung cancer cells. Tumor Biol. 35, 4137–4145.

Tilley, C., Deep, G., Agarwal, C., Wempe, M.F., Biedermann, D., Valentova, K., et al., 2016. Silibinin and its 2,3-dehydro-derivative inhibit basal cell carcinoma growth via suppression of mitogenic signaling and transcription factors activation. Mol. Carcinogenesis 55, 3–14.

Toh, Y., Nicolson, G.L., 2014. Identification and characterization of metastasis-associated gene/protein 1 (MTA1). Cancer Metastasis Rev. 33, 837–842.

Tojo, M., Hamashima, Y., Hanyu, A., Kajimoto, T., Saitoh, M., Miyazono, K., et al., 2005. The ALK5 inhibitor A-83-01 inhibits Smad signalling and epithelial to mesenchymal transition by tranforming growth factor β. Cancer Sci. 96, 791–800.

Tomizawa, M., Shinozaki, F., Motoyoshi, Y., Sugiyama, T., Yamamoto, S., Ishige, N., 2015. Niclosamide suppresses migration of hepatocellular carcinoma cells and downregulates matrix metalloproteinase-9 expression. Oncol. Lett. 10, 3515–3518.

Tong, D., Heinze, G., Schremmer, M., Schuster, E., Czerwenka, K., Leodolter, S., et al., 2007. Expression of the human MTA1 gene in breast cell lines and in breast cancer tissues. Oncol. Res. 16, 465–470.

Tovey, S.M., Brown, S., Doughty, J.C., Mallon, E.A., Cooke, T.G., Edwards, J., 2009. Poor survival outcomes in HER2-positive breast cancer patients with low-grade, node-negative tumours. Br. J. Cancer 100, 680–683.

Tremblay, M.R., Lescarbeau, A., Grogan, M.J., Tan, E., Lin, G., Austad, B.C., et al., 2009. Discovery of a potent and orally active Hedgehog pathway antagonist (IPI-926). J. Medicinal Chem. 52, 4400–4418.

Tricker, E.M., Xu, C.X., Uddin, S., Capelletti, M., Ercan, D., Ogino, A., et al., 2015. Combined EGFR/MEK inhibition prevents the emergence of resistance in EGFR-mutant lung cancer. Cancer Discovery 5, 960–971.

Trumbach, D., Prakash, N., 2015. The conserved miR-8/miR-200 microRNA family and their role in invertebrate and vertebrate neurogenesis. Cell Tissue Res. 161–177.

Tsai, C.C., Chuang, T.W., Chen, L.J., Niu, H.S., Chung, K.M., Cheng, J.T., et al., 2015. Increase in apoptosis by combination of metformin with silibinin in human colorectal cancer cells. World J. Gastroenterol. 21, 4169–4177.

Tseng, Y.C., Tsai, Y.H., Tseng, M.J., Hsu, K.W., Yang, M.C., Huang, K.H., et al., 2012. Notch2-induced COX-2 expression enhancing gastric cancer progression. Mol. Carcinogen 51, 939–951.

Tsubouchi, Y., Mukai, S., Kwahito, Y., Yamada, R., Kohno, M., Inoue, K., et al., 2000. Meloxicam inhibits the growth of non-small cell lung cancer. Anticancer Res. 20, 2867–2872.

Tsuchida, R., Osawa, T., Wang, F., Nishii, R., Das, B., Tsuchida, S., et al., 2014. BMP4/Thrombospondin-1 loop paracrinically inhibits tumor angiogenesis and suppresses the growth of solid tumors. Oncogene 33, 3803–3811.

Tsujimoto, A., Takemura, G., Mikami, A., Aoyama, T., Ohno, T., Maruyama, R., et al., 2006. A therapeutic dose of the lipophilic statin pitavastatin enhances oxidant-induced apoptosis in human vascular smooth muscle cells. J. Cardiovas. Pharmacol. 48, 160–165.

Turner, P.R., Denny, W.A., 1996. The mutagenic properties of DNA minor-groove binding ligands. Mutat. Res. Fundam. Mol. Mech. Mutagenesis 355, 141–169.

Uchino, K., Tateishi, R., Shiina, S., Kanda, M., Masuzaki, R., Kondo, Y., et al., 2011. Hepatocellular carcinoma with extrahepatic metastasis. Clinical features and prognostic factors. Cancer 117, 4475–4483.

Uno, M., Saitoh, Y., Mochida, K., Tsuruyama, E., Kiyono, T., Imoto, I., et al., 2014. NF-kappa B inducing kinase, a central signaling component of the non-canonical pathway of NF-kappa B contributes to ovarian cancer progression. PLoS One 9, art. no. e88347.

Uronis, H.E., Cushman, S.M., Bendell, J.C., Blobe, G.C., Morse, M.A., Nixon, A.B., et al., 2013. A phase I study of ABT-510 plus bevacizumab in advanced solid tumors. Cancer Med. 2, 316–324.

Urtasun, R., Latasa, M.U., Demartis, M.I., Balzani, S., Goni, S., Garcia-Irigoyen, O., et al., 2011. Connective tissue growth factor autocriny in human hepatocellular carcinoma: oncogenic role and regulation by epidermal growth factor receptor/Yes-associated protein-mediated activation. Hepatology 54, 2149–2158.

Vale, W., Wiater, E., Gray, P., Harrison, C., Bilezikjian, L., Choe, S., 2004. Activins and inhibits and their signalling. Ann. NY Acad. Sci. 1038, 142–147.

Valverde, A., Penarando, J., Canas, A., Lopez-Sanchez, L.M., Conde, F., Hernandez, V., 2015. Simultaneous inhibition of EGFR/VEGFR and cyclooxygenase-2 targets stemness-related pathways in colorectal cancer cells. PLoS One 10, art. no. e0131363.

Van Beijnum, J.R., Nowak-Sliwinska, P., van den Boezem, E., Hautvast, P., Buurman, W.A., Griffioen, A.W., 2013. Tumor angiogenesis is enforced by autocrine regulation of high-mobility group box 1. Oncogene 32, 363–374.

Van Meeteren, L.A., Thorikay, M., Bergqvist, S., Pardali, E., Stampino, C.G., Hu-Lowe, D., et al., 2012. Anti-human activin receptor-like kinase 1 (ALK1) antibody attenuates bone morphogenetic protein 9 (BMP9)-induced ALK1 signaling and interferes with endothelial cell sprouting. J. Biol. Chem. 287, 18551–18561.

Vassen, L., Weqrzyn, W., Kelin-Hitpass, L., 1999. Human insulin receptor substrate-2 (IRS-2) is a primary progesterone response gene. Mol. Endocrinol. 13, 485–494.

Vendrell, J.A., Ghayad, S., Ben-Larbi, S., Dumontet, C., Mechti, N., Cohen, P.A., 2007. A20/TNFAIP3, a new estrogen-regulated gene that confers tamoxifen resistance in breast cancer cells. Oncogene 26, 4656–4667.

Venturelli, S., Berger, A., Bocker, A., Busch, C., Weiland, T., Noor, S., et al., 2013. Resveratrol as a pan-HDAC inhibitor alters the acetylation status of histone [corrected] proteins in human-derived hepatoblastoma cells. PLoS One 8, art. no. e73097.

Vestermark, L.W., Larsen, S., Lindelov, B., Bastholt, L., 2008. A phase II study of thalidomide in patients with brain metastases from malignant melanoma. Acta Oncol. 47, 1526–1530.

Villarino, A.V., Laurence, A., 2015. IL-1 watches the watchman. Nat. Immunol. 16, 226–227.

Viola, K., Kopf, S., Rarova, L., Jarukamjorm, K., Kretschy, N., Teichmann, M., et al., 2013. Xanthohumol attenuates tumour cell-mediated breaching of the lymphendothelial barrier and prevents intravasation and metastasis. Arch. Toxicol. 87, 1301–1312.

Vogel, C.L., Cobleigh, M.A., Tripathy, D., Gutheil, J.C., Harris, L.N., Fehrenbacher, L., et al., 2002. Efficacy and safety of trastuzumab as a single agent in first-line treatment of HER2-overexpressing metastatic breast cancer. J. Clin. Oncol. 20, 719–726.

Vogl, D.T., Stadtmauer, E.A., 2006. High-dose chemotherapy and autologous hematopoietic stem cell transplantation for metastatic breast cancer: a therapy whose time has passed. Bone Marrow Transpl. 37, 985–987.

Voss, M.H., Bastos, D.A., Karlo, C.A., Ajeti, A., Hakimi, A.A., Feldman, D.R., et al., 2014. Treatment outcome with mTOR inhibitors for metastatic renal cell carcinoma with nonclear and sarcomatoid histologies.. Ann. Oncol. 25, 663–668.

Wachowska, M., Muchowicz, A., Firczuk, M., Gabrysiak, M., Winiarska, M., Wańczyk, M., et al., 2011. Aminolevulinic acid (ALA) as a prodrug in photodynamic therapy of cancer. Molecules 16, 4140–4164.

Wang, C., Natsume, A., Lee, H.J., Motomura, K., Nishimira, Y., et al., 2012. Neural stem cell-based dual suicide gene delivery for metastatic brain tumors. Cancer Gene Ther. 19, 796–801.

Wang, C., Zhu, X.Y., Feng, W.W., Yu, Y.H., Jeong, K.J., Guo, W., et al., 2016. Verteporfin inhibits YAP function through up-regulating 14-3-3 sigma sequestering YAP in the cytoplasm. Am. J. Cancer Res. 6, 27–37.

Wang, F., Jin, R., Zou, B.B., Li, L., Cheng, F.W., Luo, X., 2016. Activation of Toll-like receptor 7 regulates the expression of IFN-lambda 1, p53, PTEN, VEGF, TIMP-1 and MMP-9 in pancreatic cancer cells. Mol. Med. Rep. 13, 1807–1812.

Wang, F., Lin, F., Zhang, P., Ni, W., Bi, L., Wu, J., et al., 2015. Thioredoxin-1 inhibitor, 1-methylpropyl 2-imidazolyl disulfide, inhibits the growth, migration and invasion of colorectal cancer cell lines. Oncol. Rep. 33, 967–973.

Wang, H.B., Yang, Z.G., Gu, J., 2014. Therapeutic targeting of angiogenesis with a recombinant CTT peptide-endostatin Mimic-Kringle 5 protein. Mol. Cancer Ther. 13, 2674–2687.

Wang, J.C., Qin, Y., Mi, X.J., 2016. The protective effects of bone marrow-derived mesenchymal stem cell (BMSC) on LPS-induced acute lung injury via TLR3-mediated IFNs, MAPK and NF-kappa B signaling pathways. Biomed. Pharmacother. 79, 176–187.

Wang, L., Le Mercier, I., Putra, J., Chen, W., Liu, J., Schenk, A.D., et al., 2014. Disruption of the immune-checkpoint *VISTA* gene imparts a proinflammatory phenotype with predisposition to the development of autoimmunity. Proc. Natl Acad. Sci. USA 111, 14846–14851.

Wang, P., Bai, Y.J., Song, B.R., Wang, Y.D., Liu, D., Lai, Y.Q., et al., 2011. PP1A-mediated dephosphorylation positively regulates YAP2 activity. PLoS One 6, e24288.

Wang, Q., Ding, H., Liu, B., Li, S.H., Li, P., Ge, H., et al., 2014. Addition of the Akt inhibitor triciribine overcomes antibody resistance in cells from ErbB2/Neu-positive/PTEN-deficient mammary tumors. Int. J. Oncol. 44, 1277–1283.

Wang, T.T., Seah, S., Loh, X., Chan, C.W., Hartman, M., Goh, B.C., et al., 2016. Simvastatin-induced breast cancer cell death and deactivation of PI3K/Akt and MAPK/ERK signalling are reversed by metabolic products of the mevalonate pathway. Oncotarget 7, 2532–2544.

Wang, W., Chen, P., Tang, M., Li, J.L., Pei, Y.F., Cai, S., et al., 2015. Tumstatin 185-191 increases the sensitivity of non-small cell lung carcinoma cells to cisplatin by blocking proliferation, promoting apoptosis and inhibiting Akt activation. Am. J. Transl. Res. 7, 1332–1344.

Wang, Y., Ding, Q., Yen, C.J., Xia, W., Izzo, J.G., Lang, J.Y., et al., 2012. The crosstalk of mTOR/S6K1 and Hedgehog pathways. Cancer Cell 21, 374–387.

Wang, Y., Gapstur, S.M., Gaudet, M.M., Furtado, J.D., Campos, H., McCullough, M.L., 2015. Plasma carotenoids and breast cancer risk in the Cancer Prevention Study II Nutrition Cohort. Cancer Causes Control 26, 1233–1244.

Wang, Y.C., Chao, T.K., Chang, C.C., Yo, Y.T., Yu, M.H., Lai, H.C., 2013. Drug screening identifies niclosamide as an inhibitor of breast cancer stem-like cells. PLoS One 8, art. no. e74538.

Wang, Y.G., Xu, L., Jia, R.R., Wu, Q., Wang, T., Wei, J., et al., 2016. DDR2 induces gastric cancer cell activities via activating mTORC2 signaling and is associated with clinicopathological characteristics of gastric cancer. Digest. Dis. Sci. 61, 2272–2283.

Wang, Y.H., Xu, Z.H., Guo, S.T., Zhang, L., Sharma, A., Robertson, G.P., et al., 2013. Intravenous delivery of siRNA targeting CD47 effectively inhibits melanoma tumor growth and lung metastasis. Mol. Ther. 21, 1919–1929.

Wang, Z.W., Qi, H., Shen, Q.R., Lu, G.D., Li, M.Y., Bao, K., et al., 2016. 4,5-Diaryl-3H-1,2-dithiole-3-thiones and related compounds as combretastatin A-4/oltipraz hybrids: synthesis, molecular modelling and evaluation as antiproliferative agents and inhibitors of tubulin. Eur. J. Med. Chem. 122, 520–529.

Warita, K., Warita, T., Beckwitt, C.H., Schurdak, M.E., Vazquez, A., Wells, A., et al., 2014. Statin-induced mevalonate pathway inhibition attenuates the growth of mesenchymal-like cancer cells that lack functional E-cadherin mediated cell cohesion. Sci. Rep. 4, art. no. 7593.

Watanabe, S., Ueda, Y., Akaboshi, S., Hino, Y., Sekita, Y., Nakao, M., 2009. HMGA2 maintains oncogenic RAS-induced epithelial-mesenchymal transition in human pancreatic cancer cells. Am. J. Pathol. 174, 854–868.

Weber, J.S., Kähler, K.C., Hauschild, A., 2012. Management of immune-related adverse events and kinetics of response with ipilimumab. J. Clin. Oncol. 30, 2691–2697.

Wegner, M., Grummt, F., 1990. Netropsin, distamycin and berenil interact differentially with a high-affinity binding site for the high mobility group protein HMG-I. Biochem. Biophys. Res. Commun. 166, 1110–1117.

Wei, C.H., Wei, L.X., Lai, M.Y., Chen, J.Z., Mo, X.J., 2013. Effect of silencing of high mobility group A2 gene on gastric cancer MKN-45 cells. World J. Gastroenterol. 19, 1239–1246.

Weihrauch, M.R., Richly, H., von Bergwelt-Baildon, M.S., Becker, H.J., Schmidt, M., Hacker, U.T., et al., 2015. Phase I clinical study of the toll-like receptor 9 agonist MGN1703 in patients with metastatic solid tumours. Eur. J. Cancer 51, 146–156.

Wein, A.N., Liu, S.H., Zhang, Y., McKenzie, A.T., Leppla, S.H., 2013. Tumor therapy with a urokinase plasminogen activator-activated anthrax lethal toxin alone and in combination with paclitaxel. Invest. New Drugs 31, 206–212.

Welsh, S.J., Williams, R.R., Birmingham, A., Newman, D.J., Kirkpatrick, D.L., Powis, G., 2003. The thioredoxin redox inhibitors 1-methylpropyl 2-imidazolyl disulfide and pleurotin inhibit hypoxia-induced factor 1alpha and vascular endothelial growth factor formation. Mol. Cancer Ther. 2, 235–243.

Wickstrom, M., Dyberg, C., Shimokawa, T., Milosevic, J., Baryawno, N., Fuskevag, O.M., et al., 2013. Targeting the hedgehog signal transduction pathway at the level of GLI inhibits neuroblastoma cell growth in vitro and in vivo. Int. J. Cancer 132, 1516–1524.

Wienkers, L.C., Padbury, G.E., 2012. Stereochemical elements associated with drug metabolism and toxicity. Part VII. Role of Metabolism in Toxicology and Pharmacology. Wiley On Line Library, Encyclopaedia Drug Interactions. DOI: 10.1002/9780470921920.edm081.

Wilson, K.E., Yang, N., Mussel, A.L., Zhang, J., 2016. The regulatory role of KIBRA and PTPN14 in Hippo signaling and beyond. Gene 7, art. no. 23.

Wolchok JD. (2015). Nivolumab, ipilimumab combination effective in advanced melanoma; cost questions raised. ASCO Annual Meeting. <https://am.asco.org/asco-plenary-nivolumab-ipilimumab-combination-effective-advanced-melanoma>.

Wolfe, A.R., Debeb, B.G., Lacerda, L., Larson, R., Bambhroliya, A., Huang, X.L., et al., 2015. Simvastatin prevents triple-negative breast cancer metastasis in pre-clinical models through regulation of FOXO3a. Br. Cancer Res. Treat. 154, 495–508.

Won, M., Park, K.A., Byun, H.S., Sohn, K.C., Kim, Y.R., Jeon, J., et al., 2010. Novel anti-apoptotic mechanism of A20 through targeting ASK1 to suppress TNF-induced JNK activation. Cell Death Differentiat. 17, 1830–1841.

Wong, S.H., Hamel, L., Chevalier, S., Phillip, A., 2000. Endoglin expression on human microvascular endothelial cells association with betaglycan and formation of higher order complexes with TGF-beta signalling receptors. Eur. J. Biochem. 267, 5550–5560.

Woo, J.K., Kang, J.H., Jang, Y.S., Ro, S., Cho, J.M., Kim, H.M., et al., 2015. Evaluation of preventive and therapeutic activity of novel non-steroidal anti-inflammatory drug, CG100649, in colon cancer: increased expression of TNF-related apoptosis-inducing ligand receptors enhance the apoptotic response to combination treatment with TRAIL. Oncol. Rep. 33, 1947–1955.

Wood, L.J., Mukherjee, M., Dolde, C.E., Xu, Y., Maher, J.F., Bunton, T.E., et al., 2000. HMG-I/Y, a new c-Myc target gene and potential oncogene. Mol. Cell Biol. 20, 5490–5502.

Workman, P., 2005. New cancer drugs on the horizon. Fut. Oncol. 1, 315–318.

Wu, J., Savooji, J., Liu, D., 2016. Second- and third-generation ALK inhibitors for non-small cell lung cancer. J. Hematol. Oncol. 9, art. no. 19.

Wu, J.M., LoRusso, P.M., Matherly, L.H., Li, J., 2012. Implications of plasma protein binding for pharmacokinetics and pharmacodynamics of the gamma-secretase inhibitor 04929097. Clin. Cancer Res. 18, 2066–2079.

Wu, L., Zhu, J.J., Prokop, L.J., Murad, M.H., 2015. Pharmacologic therapy of diabetes and overall cancer risk and mortality: a meta-analysis of 265 studies. Sci. Rep. 5, art. no. 10147.

Wu, S.F., Zhou, B., Xu, L., Sun, H.Z., 2010. Interaction between nuclear insulin receptor substrate-2 and NF-kappa B in IGF-1 induces response in breast cancer cells. Oncol. Rep. 24, 1541–1550.

Xiang, R., Luo, Y., Niethammer, A.G., Reisfeld, R.A., 2008. Oral DNA vaccines target the tumor vasculature and microenvironment and suppress tumor growth and metastasis. Immunol. Rev. 222, 117–128.

Xiao, W., Chen, X.Y., Liu, X.L., Luo, L.X., Ye, S.B., Liu, Y.Z., 2014. Trichostatin A, a histone deacetylase inhibitor, suppresses proliferation and epithelial- mesenchymal transition in retinal pigment epithelium cells. J. Cell Mol. Med. 18, 646–655.

Xiao, X., Liu, Z.G., Wang, R., Wang, J.Y., Zhang, S., Cai, X.Q., et al., 2015. Genistein suppresses FLT4 and inhibits human colorectal cancer metastasis. Oncotarget 6, 3225–3239.

Xiao, Z.Y., Chung, H.I., Banan, B., Manning, P.T., Ott, K.C., Lin, S., et al., 2015. Antibody mediated therapy targeting CD47 inhibits tumor progression of hepatocellular carcinoma. Cancer Lett. 360, 302–309.

Xing, X.F., Zhang, L.H., Wen, X.Z., Wang, X.H., Cheng, X.J., Du, H., et al., 2014. PP242 suppresses cell proliferation, metastasis, and angiogenesis of gastric cancer through inhibition of the PI3K/AKT/mTOR pathway. Anticancer Drugs 25, 1129–1140.

Xing, Y.N., Deng, P., Xu, H.M., 2014. Canstatin induces apoptosis in gastric cancer xenograft growth in mice through the mitochondrial apoptotic pathway. Biosci. Rep. 34, 189–194.

Xu, C., Wang, W., Wang, Y., Zhang, X., Yan, J., Yu, L., 2016. Serum angiopoietin-2 as a clinical marker for lung cancer in patients with solitary pulmonary nodules. Ann. Clin. Lab. Sci. 46, 60–64.

Xu, G.M., Zhang, H.N., Tian, X.F., Sun, M., Fang, X.D., 2012. Effect of HMGA2 shRNA on the cell proliferation and invasion of human colorectal cancer SW480 cells In vitro. Chem. Res. Chin. Univ. 28, 264–268.

Xu, J., Acharya, S., Sahin, O., Zhang, Q.L., Saito, Y., Yao, J., et al., 2015. 14-3-3 Zeta turns TGF-beta's function from tumor suppressor to metastasis promoter in breast cancer by contextual changes of Smad partners from p53 to Gli2. Cancer Cell 27, 177–192.

Xu, J.F., Pan, X.H., Zhang, S.J., Zhao, C., Qiu, B.S., Gu, H.F., et al., 2015. CD47 blockade inhibits tumor progression human osteosarcoma in xenograft models. Oncotarget 6, 23662–23670.

Xu, T., Wu, S.H., Yuan, Y., Yan, G.X., Xiao, D.J., 2014. Knockdown of phosphodiesterase 4D inhibits nasopharyngeal carcinoma proliferation via the epidermal growth factor receptor signaling pathway. Oncol. Lett. 8, 2110–2116.

Xu, X., Mao, W., Chen, Q., Zhuang, Q., Wang, L., Dai, J., et al., 2014. Endostar, a modified recombinant human endostatin, suppresses angiogenesis through inhibition of Wnt/β-catenin signaling pathway. PLoS One 9 (9), e107463.

Xu, Z.B., Wang, Z.G., Jia, X.L., Wang, L.X., Chen, Z.G., Wang, et al., 2016. MMGZ01, an anti-DLL4 monoclonal antibody, promotes nonfunctional vessels and inhibits breast tumor growth. Cancer Lett. 372, 118–127.

Yabuuchi, S., Pai, S.G., Campbell, N.R., de Wilde, R.F., De Oliveira, E., Korangath, P., et al., 2013. Notch signaling pathway targeted therapy suppresses tumor progression and metastatic spread in pancreatic cancer. Cancer Lett. 335, 41–51.

Yamasaki, K., Chuang, V.T., Maruyama, T., Otagiri, M., 2013. Albumin-drug interaction and its clinical implication. Biochim. Biophys. Acta 1830, 5435–5443.

Yamashita, S., Miyagi, C., Carmany-Rampey, A., Shimizu, T., Fujii, R., Schier, A.F., et al., 2002. Stat3 controls cell movements during zebrafish gastrulation. Dev. Cell 2, 363–375.

Yamashita, S., Miyagi, C., Fukada, T., Kagara, N., Che, Y.S., Hirano, T., et al., 2004. Zinc transporter LIVI controls epithelial-mesenchymal transition in zebrafish gastrula organizer. Nature 429, 298–302.

Yamazaki, M., Yamashita, Y., Kubo, N., Yashiro, M., Ohira, M., Ako, E., et al., 2012. Concurrent biological targeting therapy of squamous cell carcinoma of the esophagus with cetuximab and Trastuzumab. Oncol. Rep. 28, 49–54.

Yan, B., Lu, M.S., Wang, L., Mo, X.F., Luo, W.P., Du, Y.F., et al., 2016. Specific serum carotenoids are inversely associated with breast cancer risk among Chinese women: a case-control study. Br. J. Nutrit. 115, 129–137.

Yan, H., Chen, W., 2010. 3',5'-Cyclic diguanylic acid: a small nucleotide that makes big impacts. Chem. Soc. Rev. 39, 2914–2924.

Yan, L., DeMars, L.C., 2012. Dietary supplementation with methylseleninic acid, but not selenomethionine, reduces spontaneous metastasis of Lewis lung carcinoma in mice. Int. J. Cancer 131, 1260–1266.

Yan, W., Sun, T.Y., Yang, C.M., Jia, M., Li, J., Tang, H.L., et al., 2015. CpG ODN 1826 enhances radiosensitivity of the human lung cancer cell line A549 in a rat model. Genet. Mol. Res. 14, 9804–9812.

Yan, W., Tu, B., Liu, Y.Y., Wang, T.Y., Qiao, H., Zhai, Z.J., et al., 2013. Suppressive effects of plumbagin on invasion and migration of breast cancer cells via the inhibition of STAT3 signaling and downregulation of inflammatory cytokine expressions. Bone Res. 1, 362–370.

Yang, H., Antoine, D.J., Andersson, U., Tracey, K.J., 2013. The many faces of HMGB1: molecular structure-functional activity in inflammation, apoptosis, and chemotaxis. J. Leukoc. Biol. 93, 865–873.

Yang, H., Yamazaki, T., Pietrocola, F., Zhou, H., Zitvogel, L., Ma, Y., et al., 2015. STAT3 inhibition enhances the therapeutic efficacy of immunogenic chemotherapy by stimulating type 1 interferon production by cancer cells. Cancer Res. 75, 3812–3822.

Yang, L., Carbone, D.P., 2004. Tumor host immune interactions and dendritic cell dysfunction. Adv. Cancer Res. 82, 13–27.

Yang, M.Y., Lee, H.T., Chen, C.M., Shen, C.C., Ma, H.I., 2014. Celecoxib suppresses the phosphorylation of STAT3 protein and can enhance the radiosensitivity of medulloblastoma-derived cancer stem-like cells. Int. J. Mol. Sci. 15, 11013–11029.

Yang, S.H., Lin, H.Y., Changou, C.A., Chen, C.H., Liu, Y.R., Wang, J.H., et al., 2016. Integrin beta 3 and LKB1 are independently involved in the inhibition of proliferation by lovastatin in human intrahepatic cholangiocarcinoma. Oncotarget 7, 362–373.

Yao, E., Zhou, W., Lee-Hoeflich, S.T., Truong, T., Haverty, P.M., Eastham-Anderson, J., et al., 2009. Suppression of HER2/HER3-,ediated growth of breast cancer cells with combinations of GDC-0941 PI3K inhibitor, trastuzumab, and pertuzumab. Clin. Cancer Res. 15, 4147–4156.

Yao, H.J., Zhang, Y.G., Sun, L., Liu, Y., 2014. The effect of hyaluronic acid functionalized carbon nanotubes loaded with salinomycin on gastric cancer stem cells. Biomaterials 35, 9208–9223.

Yao, M.H., Wang, Y.D., Zhang, P., Chen, H., Xu, Z.H., Jiao, J.W., et al., 2014. BMP2-SMAD signaling represses the proliferation of embryonic neural stem cells through YAP. J. Neurosci. 34, 12039–12048.

Yao, Y., Feng, S.T., Xiao, M.M., Li, Y., Yang, L., Gong, J., et al., 2015. MTA1 promotes proliferation and invasion in human gastric cancer cells. Oncotargets Ther. 8, 1785–1794.

Yap, Y.S., Cornelio, G.H., Devi, B.C.R., Khorprasert, C., Kim, S.B., Kim, T.Y., et al., 2012. Brain metastases in Asian HER2-positive breast cancer patients: anti-HER2 treatments and their impact on survival. Br. J. Cancer 107, 1075–1082.

Yardley, D.A., Noguchi, S., Pritchard, K.I., Burris, H.A., Baselga, J., Gnant, M., et al., 2013. Everolimus plus exemestane in postmenopausal patients with HR+ breast cancer: BOLERO-2 final progression-free survival analysis. Adv. Ther. 30, 870–884.

Yee, A.J., Hari, P., Marcheselli, R., Mahindra, A.K., Cirstea, D.D., Scullen, T.A., et al., 2014. Outcomes in patients with relapsed or refractory multiple myeloma in a phase I study of everolimus in combination with lenalidomide. Br. J. Heamatol. 166, 401–409.

Yee, D., Temiz, N.A., Levitzki, A., Yang, Y., 2016. Insulin receptor substrate (IRS) targeting by the tyrophostin NT157 inhibits breast cancer cell growth [abstract]. Cancer Res. 76, Suppl Abstract No. PD2-07.

Ying, Q., Ansong, E., Diamond, A.M., Lu, Z.X., Yang, W.C., Bie, X.M., 2015. Quantitative proteomic analysis reveals that anti-cancer effects of selenium-binding protein 1 in vivo are associated with metabolic pathways. PLoS One 10, art. no. e0126285.

Yoshida, K., Tsujimoto, H., Matsumura, K., Kinoshita, M., Takahata, R., Matsumoto, Y., et al., 2015. CD47 is an adverse prognostic factor and a therapeutic target in gastric cancer. Cancer Med. 4, 1322–1333.

Yoshimura, Y., Kurasawa, M., Yorozu, K., Puig, O., Bordogna, W., Harada, N., 2016. Antitumor activity of alectinib, a selective ALK inhibitor, in an ALK-positive NSCLC cell line harboring G1269A mutation. Cancer Chemother. Pharmacol. 77, 623–628.

You, B.R., Shin, H.R., Park, W.H., 2014. PX-12 inhibits the growth of A549 lung cancer cells via G2/M phase arrest and ROS-dependent apoptosis. Int. J. Oncol. 44, 301–308.

You, H.J., How, T., Blobe, G.C., 2009. The type III transforming growth factor-beta receptor negatively regulates nuclear factor kappa B signaling through its interaction with beta-arrestin2. Carcinogenesis 30, 1281–1287.

Young, K., Tweedie, E., Conley, B., Ames, J., FitzSimons, M., Brooks, P., et al., 2015. BMP9 crosstalk with the Hippo pathway regulates endothelial cell matricellular and chemokine responses. PLoS One 10, art. no. e0122892.

Youreva, V., Kapakos, G., Srivastava, A.K., 2013. Insulin-like growth-factor-1-induced PKB signaling and Egr-1 expression is inhibited by curcumin in A-10 vascular smooth muscle cells. Can. J. Physiol. Pharmacol. 91, 241–247.

Yousefi, M., Ghaffari, S.H., Zekri, A., Hassani, S., Alimoghaddam, K., Ghavamzadeh, A., 2014. Silibinin induces apoptosis and inhibits proliferation of estrogen receptor (ER)-negative breast carcinoma cells through suppression of nuclear factor kappa B activation. Arch. Iran Med. 17, 366–371.

Yu, K.R., Park, S.B., Jung, J.W., Seo, M.S., Hong, I.S., Kim, H.S., et al., 2013. HMGA2 regulates the in vitro aging and proliferation of human umbilical cord blood-derived stromal cells through the mTOR/p70S6K signaling pathway. Stem Cell Res. 10, 156–165.

Yuan, T.Z., Zhang, H.H., Liu, B.Q., Zhang, Q., Liang, Y., Zheng, R.H., et al., 2014. Expression of MTA1 in nasopharyngeal carcinoma and its correlation with prognosis. Med. Oncol. 31, art. no. 330.

Zaiman, A.L., Pdowski, M., Medicheria, S., Gordy, K., Xu, F., Zhen, L., et al., 2008. Role of the TGF-β/Alk5 signaling pathway in monocrotaline-induced pulmonary hypertension. Am. J. Resp. Crit. Care Med. 177, 896–905.

Zan, J.H., He, X., Long, W., Liu, P.X., 2012. Insights into binding modes of tumstatin peptide T7 with the active site of alpha(v)beta(3) integrin. Mol. Simulat. 38, 498–508.

Zarranz-Ventura, J., Fernández-Robredo, P., Recalde, S., Salinas-Alamán, A., Borrás-Cuesta, F., Dotor, J., et al., 2013. Transforming growth factor-beta inhibition reduces progression of early choroidal neovascularization lesions in rats: P17 and P144 peptides. PLoS One 8, art. no. e65434.

Zeng, Z., Shi, Y.X., Tsao, T., Qiu1, Y.H., Kornblau, S.M., Baggerly, K.A., et al., 2012. Targeting of mTORC1/2 by the mTOR kinase inhibitor PP242 induces apoptosis in AML cells under conditions mimicking the bone marrow microenvironment. Blood 120, 2679–2689.

Zhang, C.C., Kaba, M., Iizuka, S., Huynh, H., Lodish, H.F., 2008. Angiopoietin-like 5 and IGFBP2 stimulate ex vivo expansion of human cord blood hematopoietic stem cells as assayed by NOD/SCID transplantation. Blood 111, 3415–3423.

Zhang, C.C., Yan, Z.M., Giddabasappa, A., Lappin, P.B., Painter, C.L., Zhang, Q., et al., 2014. Comparison of dynamic contrast-enhanced MR, ultrasound and optical imaging modalities to evaluate the antiangiogenic effect of PF-03084014 and sunitinib. Cancer Med. 3, 462–471.

Zhang, H., Cheng, S., Zhang, M., Ma, X., Zhang, L., Wang, Y., et al., 2014. Prostaglandin E2 promotes hepatocellular carcinoma cell invasion through upregulation of YB-1 protein expression. Int. J. Oncol. 44, 769–780.

Zhang, H.R., Chen, J.M., Zeng, Z.Y., Que, W.Z., 2013. Knockdown of DEPTOR inhibits cell proliferation and increases chemosensitivity to melphalan in human multiple myeloma RPMI-8226 cells via inhibiting PI3K/AKT activity. J. Int. Med. Res. 41, 584–595.

Zhang, J., Yang, W., Zhao, D.Y., Han, Y., Liu, B., Zhao, H., et al., 2014. Correlation between TSP-1, TGF-beta and PPAR-gamma expression levels and glioma microvascular density. Oncol. Lett. 7, 95–100.

Zhang, J.M., Ji, J.Y., Yu, M., Overholtzer, M., Smolen, G.A., Wang, R., et al., 2009. YAP-dependent induction of amphiregulin identifies a non-cell-autonomous component of the Hippo pathway. Nat. Cell Biol. 11, 1444–1450.

Zhang, K.Q., Gao, H.L., Wu, X.W., Wang, J.H., Zhou, W.D., Sun, G.H., et al., 2014. Frequent overexpression of HMGA2 in human atypical teratoid/rhabdoid tumor and its correlation with let-7a3/let-7b miRNA. Clin. Cancer Res. 20, 1179–1189.

Zhang, M.J., Liu, Y.H., Gao, Y., Li, S.Y., 2015. Silibinin-induced glioma cell apoptosis by PI3K-mediated but Akt-independent downregulation of FoxM1 expression. Eur. J. Pharmacol. 765, 346–354.

Zhang, P., Bai, H.Y., Liu, G.T., Wang, H.Y., Chen, F., Zhang, B.S., et al., 2015. MicroRNA-33b, upregulated by EF24, a curcumin analog, suppresses the epithelial-to-mesenchymal transition (EMT) and migratory potential of melanoma cells by targeting HMGA2. Toxicol. Lett. 234, 151–161.

Zhang, R.R., Zhang, P., Wang, H., Hou, D.M., Li, W.T., Xiao, G.S., et al., 2015. Inhibitory effects of metformin at low concentration on epithelial-mesenchymal transition of CD44(+)CD117 (+) ovarian cancer stem cells. Stem Cell Res. Ther. 6, art. no. 262.

Zhang, S., Chung, W.C., Miele, L., Xu, K., 2014. Targeting Met and Notch in the Lfng-deficient, Met-amplified triple-negative breast cancer. Can. Biol. Ther. 15, 633–642.

Zhang, S., Wang, G., Liu, D., Baao, Z., Fernig, D.G., Rudland, P.S., et al., 2005. The C-terminal region of S100A4 is important for its metastasis-inducing properties. Oncogene 24, 4401–4411.

Zhang, X.Q., Yang, C.Y., Rao, X.F., Xiong, J.P., 2016. Plumbagin shows anti-cancer activity in human breast cancer cells by the upregulation of p53 and p21 and suppression of G1 cell cycle regulators.. Eur. J. Gynaelcol. Oncol. 37, 30–35.

Zhang, Y., Wang, Y., Bao, C., Xu, Y., Shen, H., Chen, J., et al., 2012. Metformin interacts with AMPK through binding to gamma subunit. Mol. Cell Biochem. 368, 69–76.

Zhang, Y.L., Keng, Y.F., Zhao, Y., Wu, L., Zhang, Z.Y., 1998. Suramin is an active site-directed, reversible, and tight-binding inhibitor of protein-tyrosine phosphatases. J. Biol. Chem. 273, 12281–12287.

Zhao, B., Li, L., Lu, Q., Wang, L.H., Liu, C.Y., Lei, Q., et al., 2011. Angiomotin is a novel Hippo pathway component that inhibits YAP oncoprotein. Genes Dev. 25, 51–63.

Zhao, B.M., Hoffmann, F.M., 2006. Inhibition of transforming growth factor-beta1-induced signaling and epithelial-to-mesenchymal transition by the Smad-binding peptide aptamer Trx-SARA. Mol. Biol. Cell 17, 3819–3831.

Zhao, D., Pan, C., Skun, J., Gilbert, C., Drews-elger, K., Azzam, D.J., et al., 2015. VEGF drives cancer-initiating stem cells through VEGFR-2/Stat3 signaling to upregulate Myc and Sox2. Oncogene 34, 3107–3119.

Zhao, H., Tang, J.Y., Xu, J.Y., Cao, L., Jia, G., Long, D.B., et al., 2015. Selenoprotein genes exhibit differential expression patterns between hepatoma HepG2 and normal hepatocytes LO2 cell lines. Biol. Trace Element Res. 167, 236–241.

Zhao, W.E., Shi, G.Q., Gu, H.H., Ngoc, N.B., 2016. Role of PPAR gamma in the nutritional and pharmacological actions of carotenoids. Res. Rep. Biochem. 6, 13–24.

Zhao, X.P., Zhang, H., Jiao, J.Y., Tang, D.X., Wu, Y.L., Pan, C.B., 2016. Overexpression of HMGA2 promotes tongue cancer metastasis through EMT pathway. J. Transl. Med. 14, art. no. 26.

Zheng, N., Liu, L., Liu, W.W., Zhang, P., Huang, H., Zang, L.H., et al., 2016. ER beta up-regulation was involved in silibinin-induced growth inhibition of human breast cancer MCF-7 cells. Arch. Biochem. Biophys. 591, 141–149.

Zheng, Y.H., Zou, F.Y., Wang, J.J., Yin, G.F., Le, V., Fei, Z.W., et al., 2015. Photodynamic therapy-mediated cancer vaccination enhances stem-like phenotype and immune escape, which can be blocked by thrombospondin-1 signaling through CD47 receptor protein. J. Biol. Chem. 290, 8975–8986.

Zhou, N., Wang, H.J., Liu, H.X., Xue, H.S., Lin, F., Meng, X.T., et al., 2015. MTA1-upregulated EpCAM is associated with metastatic behaviors and poor prognosis in lung cancer. J. Exp. Clin. Cancer Res. 34, art. no. 157.

Zhou, X., Shi, X., Ren, K., Fan, G.T., Wu, S.J., et al., 2015. Celecoxib inhibits cell growth and modulates the expression of matrix metalloproteinases in human osteosarcoma MG-63 cell line. Eur. Rev. Med. Pharmacol. Sci. 19, 4087–4094.

Zhou, Y., Feng, X., Liu, Y.L., Ye, S.C., Wang, H., Tan, W.K., et al., 2013. Down-regulation of miR-126 is associated with colorectal cancer cells proliferation, migration and invasion by targeting IRS-1 via the AKT and ERK1/2 signaling pathways. PLoS One 8, art. no. e81203.

Zhou, Y.X., Mokhtari, R.B., Pan, J., Cutz, E., Yeger, H., 2015. Carbonic anhydrase II mediates malignant behavior of pulmonary neuroendocrine tumors. Am. J. Resp. Cell Mol. Biol. 52, 183–192.

Zhou, Y.Y., Hu, Z.G., Zeng, F.J., Han, J., 2016. Clinical profile of cyclooxygenase-2 inhibitors in treating non-small cell lung cancer: a meta-analysis of nine randomized clinical trials. PLoS One 11, art. no. e0151939.

Zhou, Z.W., Li, X.X., He, Z.X., Pan, S.T., Yang, Y.X., Zhang, X.J., et al., 2015. Induction of apoptosis and autophagy via sirtuin1- and PI3K/Akt/mTOR-mediated pathways by plumbagin in human prostate cancer cells. Drug Design Develop. Ther. 9, 1511–1554.

Zhu, L.Y., Ren, L., Chen, Y.X., Fang, J.Y., Ge, Z.Z., Li, X.B., et al., 2015. Redox status of high-mobility group box 1 performs a dual role in angiogenesis of colorectal carcinoma. J. Cell Mol. Med. 19, 2128–2135.

Zhu, P., Davis, M., Blackwelder, A.J., Bachman, N., Liu, B.L., Edgerton, S., et al., 2014. Metformin selectively targets tumor-initiating cells in ErbB2-overexpressing breast cancer models. Cancer Prevent Res. 7, 199–210.

Zhu, S.J., Moore, T.W., Morii, N., Howard, R.B., Culver, D., Arrendale, R.F., et al., 2014. Synthetic curcumin analog UBS109 inhibits the growth of head and neck squamous cell carcinoma xenografts. Curr. Cancer Drug Targets 14, 380–393.

Zhu, Y., Shah, K., 2014. Multiple lesions in receptor tyrosine kinase pathway determine glioblastoma response to pan-ERBB inhibitor PF-00299804 and PI3K/mTOR dual inhibitor PF-05212384. Cancer Biol. Ther. 15, 815–822.

Zhuo, W.L., Tao, G.L., Zhang, L., Chen, Z.T., 2013. Vector-mediated selective expression of lethal factor, a toxic element of Bacillus Anthracis, damages A549 cells via inhibition of MAPK and AKT pathways. Int. J. Med. Sci. 10, 292–298.

Zidi, S., Sghaier, I., Gazouani, E., Mezlini, A., Yacoubi-Loueslati, B., 2016. Evaluation of toll-like receptors 2/3/4/9 gene polymorphisms in cervical cancer evolution. Pathol. Oncol. Res. 22, 323–330.

Zipori, D., 2009. Biology of Stem Cells and the Molecular Basis of the Stem State. Springer Verlag, New York.

Zubeldia, I.G., Bleau, A.M., Redrado, M., Serrano, D., Agliano, A., Gil-Puig, C., et al., 2013. Epithelial to mesenchymal transition and cancer stem cell phenotypes leading to liver metastasis are abrogated by the novel TGF beta 1-targeting peptides P17 and P144. Exp. Cell Res. 319, 12–22.

Zuo, C.H., Qiu, X.X., Liu, N.L., Yang, D.R., Xia, M., Liu, J.S., et al., 2015. Interferon-alpha and cyclooxygenase-2 inhibitor cooperatively mediates TRAIL-induced apoptosis in hepatocellular carcinoma. Exp. Cell Res. 333, 316–326.

Zuo, M., Rashid, A., Churi, C., Vauthey, J.N., Chang, P., Li, Y., et al., 2015. Novel therapeutic strategy targeting the Hedgehog signalling and mTOR pathways in biliary tract cancer. Br. J. Cancer 112, 1042–1051.

Index

Note: Page numbers followed by "*f*" and "*t*" refer to figures and tables, respectively.

B

N

Q

R

S

U

V

W

FSC
www.fsc.org
MIX
Papier | Fördert
gute Waldnutzung
FSC® C083411

Kolibri 360 GmbH
Ferdinand-Jühlke-Straße 7
99095 Erfurt, Deutschland
produktsicherheit@kolibri360.de